Physicians as Leaders

Who, How, and Why Now?

Mindi K. McKenna, PhD, MBA
Perry A. Pugno, MD, MPH, CPE

with

William H. Frist, MD

Foreword by

André L. Delbecq, DBA, MBA, FACPE

Jason,
Live well and
lead well !
Cheers,
Mindi McKenna

Radcliffe Publishing
Oxford • Seattle

Radcliffe Publishing Ltd
18 Marcham Road
Abingdon
Oxon OX14 1AA
United Kingdom

www.radcliffe-oxford.com
Electronic catalogue and worldwide online ordering facility.

British Library Cataloguing in Publication Data

A catalogue record for this book is available from the British Library.

ISBN: 1 85775 788 2

Typeset by Action Publishing Technology Ltd, Gloucester, UK
Printed and bound by TJ International Ltd, Padstow, Cornwall, UK

Contents

Foreword

Mature physician leaders considering whether to bother opening another book on leadership may experience hesitations similar to my own. In all honesty, the thoughts immediately flashing across my already overloaded mental "I should read" screen were:

- Not another leadership book!
- I'm bored with the topic.
- What can be sufficiently new to warrant my time?

Such negative thoughts reflect realities mature professionals share. At the stage in life when they engage in important leadership roles they have already been inundated for years with leadership books and training programs. The first and second book/program/symposium are very helpful. After that, additional experiences are subject to diminishing value. The "next" book seldom adequately connects with our "lived-in" leadership space. Given all the other forms of professional development required by our fields, we are appropriately skeptical.

Yet, there are rare moments when leadership comes alive even for the combat-weary professional. For me it has often been when exiting a particularly stimulating presentation in the company of gifted friends who join together to break bread. In a small circle of trust, we wrestle with the realities of our shared leadership, avoiding illusions of romantic perfection, admitting to hardships, and plumbing the richness of each individual's life lessons. In such dialog hope is sustained and new efforts inspired.

In *Physicians as Leaders*, McKenna, Pugno and Frist extend just such an invitation to a shared conversation. Indeed, not just one conversation, but several interrelated conversations bridging diverse leadership themes. Following provocative, conceptually clear but terse reminders of important leadership concepts, we then can enjoy as companions some of our nation's most capable physician leaders who open both mind and heart. This makes for an "enjoyable read," but never a superficial treatment.

Would you refuse such an invitation? All that is needed is to for you to provide your own hors d'oeuvres, a favorite beverage, and a little quiet time for self-reflection. (I can assure you self-reflection is very much stimulated by these conversations!)

Or for those who are extroverts, consider inviting a couple colleagues to share their reactions to one of the conversations at your regular "get together." I promise the exchange will be more fun and stimulating than small talk.

To summarize, I came to think of this book as "dinner conversations" that were memorable, provocative, and informative. Physicians concerned with transformational leadership requirements for creating a new future for healthcare will likewise savor the dialog.

André L. Delbecq, DBA, FACPE DBA, MBA, FACPE
Emeritus Dean
School of Business
Santa Clara University
July 2005

Why Read This Book?

Perhaps you're wondering whether to read this book, considering that your time is limited and your work requires you to read too much already. We'd like to help you decide. We believe you'll find time invested in this book well spent if...

- You secretly wish you'd chosen another profession.
- You'd like to know how to get patients (or staff) to trust and follow your direction.
- You keep experiencing a nagging sense of discontent – a gut feeling that your work ought to bring more joy than it does.
- You're doing work you love, but want to be better at it.
- You're extraordinarily gifted and wonder why you aren't achieving extraordinary results.
- You're tired of racing through each day exhausted and frazzled.
- You're uncomfortable with expectations being thrust upon you and aren't sure what to do.
- You believe you're a fairly good leader, but would like to be more effective or fulfilled.
- You're a skilled physician, but a weak leader.
- You believe you have what it takes – but you lack training and proper guidance.
- You have big hopes and dreams, but don't know how to bring them about.
- You have great ideas, but can't get others to listen.
- You're convinced healthcare needs to change – but can't imagine the gridlock ever breaking.
- You're stuck working with someone who makes your life miserable.
- You want to leave a legacy worthy of your calling and your profession.

This book is packed with advice from many contemporary physician leaders. Their stories are inspiring, thought-provoking, and, frankly, perhaps a bit intimidating. Perhaps you may already count yourself among the ranks of leading physicians; or perhaps you are not yet anywhere near that point – having just recently begun your journey toward becoming an effective and fulfilled physician leader. Either way, you'll likely identify with their depictions of exhausting yet rewarding work.

The physician leaders who are profiled or quoted in our book were chosen in part because they set forth such high standards. They inspire us to be and do far more than we might have imagined. And yet, these physicians are accessible – the type of colleagues you might run into at a conference, or chat with while waiting in line at the movies. Diverse in their specialties, work styles, and aspirations – these leading physicians share at least one thing in common. They're all passionate about making a positive difference in medicine. We're talking about genuine, heartfelt, live-it-out-each-and-every-day passion for truly great healthcare. The kind of excellent healthcare we all want for our own children and grandchildren, our parents and grandparents. So while you'll find a great deal of variety in these physicians' accomplishments, you'll also notice that the truths they illuminate are really universal. Learn from them.

About the Authors

Mindi K. McKenna, PhD, MBA holds a faculty appointment in the MBA in Health Care Leadership Program in the Helzberg School of Management at Rockhurst University. She is also the Executive Director of the Healthcare Leadership Group, through which she helps physicians become effective and fulfilled leaders. Dr. McKenna is an internationally recognized expert on leadership, ethics, individual and organizational effectiveness. She frequently delivers general session keynote presentations at medical conferences and continuing professional development/CME training seminars for medical societies, professional associations, hospitals medical staffs and medical group practices. Author of the book *High Tech Medicine: Building Your Medical Practice Using Computers and the Internet*, Dr. McKenna's articles have been published in the *Journal of Health Administration Education*, the *Journal of Invasive Cardiology, Family Practice Medicine*, the *Leadership and Organizational Development Journal*, the *Journal of Business and Strategy*, and many other medical/management journals, including those published by the American College of Physician Executives and the American Hospital Association.

Dr. McKenna has over 24 years' executive leadership experience in healthcare, having been Vice President of Marketing at Cerner Corporation, and Director of Organizational Development, National Accounts and Federal Sales at Marion Laboratories (now Sanofi-Aventis). She earned a PhD in Pharmaceutical Science Administration with an emphasis in health care marketing from UMKC School of Pharmacy, an MBA from Webster University, and a BA in Industrial Psychology and Personnel Administration from the University of Kansas. Dr. McKenna is certified through the Physician Leadership Coaching Institute. She is a member of the prestigious National Speakers Association – an "organization for experts who speak professionally" – and serves on the Board of the Institute for Spirituality in Health. Dr. McKenna is active in the Alliance for Continuing Medical Education, the American College of Healthcare Executives, the Association for University Programs in Health Administration, the Health Care Management division of the Academy of Management and the Medical Group Management Association.

Perry A. Pugno, MD, MPH, CPE is Director of the Division of Medical Education for the American Academy of Family Physicians, the professional association representing the nation's family doctors. He is also the Director of the Residency Assistance Program, a peer-based, criterion-referenced nationwide consulting group for graduate medical education that establishes the "excellence criteria" for the discipline of family medicine. Dr. Pugno is an internationally recognized expert in physician education and assessment. He has written and spoken extensively on such diverse topics as leadership development, graduate medical education, medical ethics, time management, financial management, domestic violence and physician performance assessment. Dr. Pugno's writings have been published in the nation's leading medical journals including the *Journal of the American Medical Association, Academic Medicine*, the *Journal of Clinical Ethics*, the *Western Journal of Medicine, Family Medicine,* the *Journal of the American Board of Family Practice, Family Practice Management,* and the electronic publications of the American College of Physician Executives.

Dr. Pugno has over 27 years' experience in educational administration and leadership, and is the founding chair of the Academic Council of the National Institute for Program Director Development. His diverse experience as a physician leader includes public, private, managed care, and academic settings. He has worked as a postgraduate training director in multiple settings, as the director of an urban trauma center, and as a corporate vice president for Catholic Healthcare West, one of the largest integrated healthcare systems in the western United States. He earned his MD from the University of California, an MPH from Loma Linda University, and is board certified in Family Medicine, Emergency Medicine and Medical Management.

William H. Frist, MD graduated in 1974 from Princeton University where he specialized in healthcare policy at the Woodrow Wilson School of Public and International Affairs and in 1978 from Harvard Medical School; spending the next seven years in surgical training at Massachusetts General Hospital; Southampton General Hospital, Southampton, England; and Stanford University Medical Center. He is board certified in both general surgery and heart surgery.

In 1985, Dr. Frist joined the faculty at Vanderbilt University Medical Center where he founded and directed the multi-disciplinary Vanderbilt Transplant Center, which under his leadership became a nationally renowned center of multi-organ transplantation. He has performed over 150 heart and lung transplant procedures, including the first successful combined heart-lung transplant in the Southeast. Dr. Frist has written five books and more than 100 articles, chapters, and abstracts on medical research.

First elected to the U.S. Senate on November 8, 1994, and re-elected on November 7, 2000, Dr. Frist was the first practicing physician elected to the Senate since 1928. In 2000, Dr. Frist was unanimously elected chairman of the National Republican Senatorial Committee (NRSC) for the 107th Congress and in 2002, was unanimously elected Majority Leader of the U.S. Senate. Dr. Frist is particularly passionate about confronting the global AIDS pandemic. He frequently takes medical mission trips to Africa to perform surgery and care for those in need. As Senate Majority Leader, he continues to raise awareness about the HIV/AIDS crisis throughout the world.

Senator Frist and his wife, Karyn, have three sons: Harrison, Jonathan, and Bryan. He enjoys flying, writing, running marathons, and medical mission trips to Africa.

The Foreword writer, **André L. Delbecq,** DBA, MBA, FACPE is currently the Emeritus Dean, Santa Clara University, School of Business. Dr. Delbecq earned a Bachelor's degree in Business Administration from the University of Toledo, an MBA and a Doctorate in Business Administration from Indiana University with emphasis in Sociology and Applied Economic Analysis.

Dr. Delbecq began his academic career as a faculty lecturer at the University of Toledo in 1959. After teaching at Indiana University and the University of Toledo, he accepted an appointment as Associate Professor of Management at the University of Wisconsin, Graduate School of Business in 1968, where he served also as Chair of the Department of Management, Professor of

Administration, School of Social Work. Dr. Delbecq's academic pursuits involved Fellowships at the Western Australian Institute of Technology and the American Counsel of Learned Societies Contemplative Practice, and a Distinguished Lecturer at the University of South Africa. He became Dean of the Leavey School of Business and Administration at Santa Clara University in 1979, later serving as the Thomas J. and Kathleen L. McCarthy Professor of Management. Dr. Delbecq has been Director of the Institute for Spirituality of Organization Leadership at Santa Clara University since 1998.

Dr. Delbecq has been named by the American College of Physician Executives as faculty member providing the single most valuable course and has been named an Honorary Member of the American Academy of Medical Directors in recognition of contributions to the education of Physician Managers. He is a recipient of the Leavey School of Business Dean's Award for Exceptional Teaching, Research and Service, and of the Western Academy of Management's Presidential Award for Exceptional Contributions to Teaching, Scholarship and Service.

Dr. Delbecq currently serves on the Board of Scholars of the Chief Executive Leadership Institute, the Board of Directors of the Colleagues in Jesuit Business Education, and the Board of Trustees of Ascension Health in St. Louis. Dr. Delbecq has served as a member of the Editorial Boards of the *Academy of Management Journal, Health Services Research*, the *Journal of Management Education*, and as Executive Editor of the *Academy of Management Review Journal*.

Dr. Delbecq has researched organizational leadership, governance, administration, and innovation, having been awarded educational grants from the Department of Health, Education and Welfare, the Department of Labor, the American Academy of Medical Group Practices, the American College of Physician Executives, the American Group Practice Foundation, the Estes Park Institute, and the National Health Service in London.

Dr. Delbecq's works have been published in many prestigious journals including *Administrative Science Quarterly*, the *Academy of Management Review*, the *American Journal of Public Health, Health Care Management Review, Health Services Management, Health Services Research, Hospital and Health Services Administration*, the *Journal of Applied Behavioral Science*, the *Journal of Management Education*, the *Journal of Management Inquiry*, the *Medical Director*, the *Physician Executive*, the *Training and Development Journal*, and in many books and conference proceedings.

Dr. Delbecq has been a frequent lecturer and guest speaker at various academic and practitioner-oriented conferences, congresses, forums, retreats, seminars and symposium, including, for example, the American Academy of Medical Directors, the American Association of Medical Directors, the American College of Physician Executives, the American Osteopathic Hospital Association, the Institute for Health Care Improvement, the National Academy of Sciences, and the Society for Teachers of Family Medicine, where he has spoken on a variety of topics including medical management, organizational governance, strategic alliances, innovation, change, and, perhaps most significantly, the importance of spirituality in healthcare leadership.

Dr. Delbecq's service to academic and practitioner-oriented organizations has been remarkable. He has served as a consultant to the American Nursing Association, the Deans of the American Medical Schools, the Department of

Health and Social Services, the National Science Foundation, and to many hospitals and medical centers. He is a Fellow and past Governor, Board Director, Committee Chair and President of the National Academy of Management and many of its subsidiary divisions, past President of the Association of Deans of Jesuit Schools and Colleges of Business, past Board Director for the American Journal of Nursing Company, and past Chair of the National Advisory Committee of the American College of Physician Executives.

List of Contributors

Monte L. Anderson, MD
Gastroenterologist
Consultant in Gastroenterology, Hepatology, and Transplantation
Mayo Clinic Scottsdale
Scottsdale, Arizona 85259

Bruce Bagley, MD
Family Physician
Medical Director for Quality Improvement
The American Academy of Family Physicians
Leawood, Kansas 66211

Nancy J. Baker, MD
Family Physician
University of Minnesota
Minneapolis, MN 55455

Mark H. Belfer, DO, FAAFP
Family Physician
Residency Director
Akron General Medical Center/NEOUCOM
Akron, Ohio 44307

Richard B. Birrer, MD, MPH, MMM, CPE
Family, Emergency, Sports, and Geriatric Medicine Physician
Locust Whey, New York 11560

Edward T. Bope, MD
Family Physician
Program Director
Riverside Family Practice Residency Program
697 Thomas Lane
Columbus, Ohio 43214

John R. Bucholtz, DO
Family Physician
Director of Medical Education
Program Director, Family Practice Residency Program
1900 10th Avenue, Suite 100
Columbus, Georgia 31902

Daniel S. Durrie, MD
Ophthalmologist
President, Durrie Vision Center
Overland Park, Kansas 66211

David G. Fairchild, MD, MPH
Internist
Chief of General Medicine
Tufts – New England Medical Center
Boston, Massachusetts 02115

Kevin S. Ferentz, MD
Family Physician
Past President, Maryland Academy of Family Physicians
Residency Director, Department of Family Medicine, and
Associate Professor, University of Maryland School of Medicine
Baltimore, MD 21201

Michael O. Fleming, MD
Family Physician
Past President, American Academy of Family Physicians
Shreveport, Louisiana 71103

Senator William H. Frist, MD
Thoracic Surgeon
Senate Majority Leader, U.S. Congress
Washington, D.C. 20008

Francine R. Gaillour, MD, MBA, FACPE
Internist
Founder and Director of Creative Strategies in Physician Leadership
Bellevue, Washington 98008

J. Peter Geerlofs, MD
Family Physician
Chief Medical Officer
Allscripts Healthcare Solutions Inc.
Libertyville, Illinois 60048

Roland A. Goertz, MD, MBA
Family Physician
President, McClennan County Medical Education and Research Foundation
Waco, Texas 76707

Larry A. Green, MD
Family Physician
Director, The Robert Graham Center for Policy Studies in Family Medicine and
Primary Care
Washington, D.C. 20101

Reverend Pamela S. Harris, MD
Physical Medicine and Rehabilitation Physician
Clinic Chief, Kansas City Veteran's Administration Hospital
Minister of Health, United Methodist Church of the Resurrection
Roeland Park, KS 66205

Douglas E. Henley, MD, FAAFP
Family Physician
Executive Vice President
American Academy of Family Physicians
Leawood, KS 66211

Steven G. Hull, MD, FCCP, FAASM
Director of Sleep Disorders, Pain Management and Vaccine Research
Vince and Associates Clinical Research
Medical Director, somniTech, Inc.
Overland Park, Kansas 66211

Charles Jaffe, MD, PhD
Vice President Life Sciences
SAIC
West Chester, Pennsylvania 19382

William F. Jessee, MD, FACMPE
Former Pediatrician, Emergency Medicine and Preventive Medicine Physician
President, Medical Group Management Association
Englewood, Colorado 80112

Norman B. Kahn, Jr., MD
Family Physician
Vice President, Science and Education
American Academy of Family Physicians
Leawood, Kansas 66211

Kieren P. Knapp, DO, FACOFP
Family Physician
Past President, American College of Osteopathic Family Physicians
Jacobus, Pennsylvania 17407

Melanie Susan Kraft, MD, MRO, AMEt
Family Physician
Faculty Physician – Baptist Lutheran Medical Center
Family Medicine Residency Program
Kansas City, MO 64131

Jeffrey B. Kramer, MD
Cardiothoracic Surgeon
Kansas University Medical Center
3901 Rainbow Boulevard
Kansas City, Kansas 66160

Alma B. Littles, MD
Family Physician
Associate Dean of Academic Affairs
Florida State University
Tallahassee, Florida 32352

Erich H. Loewy, MD
Internist and Bioethicist
Professor of Medicine (emeritus)
Founding Alumni Association Chair of Bioethics
Associate, Department of Philosophy
University of California, Davis 95817

Donald R. Lurye, MD, MMM
Family Physician
Chief Medical Officer
Welborn Clinic
Evansville, Indiana 47713

Bridgett M. McCandless, MD
Internist
Medical Director
Jackson County Free Health Clinic
Independence, MO 64050

Deborah S. McPherson, MD, FAAFP
Family Physician
Associate Director, Family Medicine Residency Program
Kansas University Medical Center
Kansas City, Kansas 66160

Gary B. Morsch, MD, MPH
Family and Emergency Medicine Physician
U.S. Army Reserves
Founder of Heart to Heart International, Physicians Who Care, and Priority
Physician Placement
Bucyrus, Kansas 66013

Tim A. Munzing, MD
Family Physician
Director, Medical Education
Kaiser Permanente – Orange County
Santa Ana, California 92705

John R. Musich, MD, MBA
Obstetrician and Gynecologist
Past Chair, Council for Resident Education in Obstetrics and Gynecology
Troy, Michigan 48098

Randall Oates, MD
Family Physician
President and CEO, Docs, Inc.
Springdale, Arkansas 72764

Elissa J. Palmer, MD, FAAFP
Family Physician
Director, Altoona Family Physicians Residency, Pregnancy Care Center and
Women's Health and Wellness of Altoona Regional Health System
Altoona, Pennsylvania 16601

John M. Pascoe, MD, MPH
Pediatrician
Professor of Pediatrics and Chief, General and Community Pediatrics
Wright State University School of Medicine (WSUSOM)
Dayton, Ohio 45404

Ronald N. Riner, MD
Cardiologist
President, The Riner Group
St. Louis, Missouri 63117

Burton N. Routman, DO, FACOFP
Family Physician
Professor of Family Medicine
Western University of Health Sciences College of Osteopathic Medicine of the
Pacific
RCH Cucamonga, California 91730

Daniel Z. Sands, MD, MPH
General Internist, Beth Israel Deaconess Medical Center
Assistant Professor of Medicine, Harvard Medical School
Chief Medical Officer and Vice President of Clinical Strategies, Zix Corporation
Boston, Massachusetts 02215

Andrew M. Schwartz, MS, MD
Cardiothoracic Surgeon and Vice President, Medical Staff Services
Shawnee Mission Medical Center
Shawnee Mission, Kansas 66204

Michael J. Scotti, Jr., MD
Family Physician
Retired Vice President for Medical Education and Senior Vice President for
Professional Issues, American Medical Association
2540 North Randolph Street
Arlington, VA 22207

Kevin J. Soden, MD, MPH, MPA
Emergency Medicine Physician
Medical Correspondent, NBC News
Soden Consulting Services
2510 Danbury Street
Charlotte, North Carolina 28211

Jeannette E. South-Paul, MD
Family Physician
Chair, Department of Family Medicine
University of Pittsburgh School of Medicine
Pittsburgh, Pennsylvania 15213

Penny Tenzer, MD
Family Physician
Vice Chair, Department of Family Medicine and Community Health
Director, Family Medicine Residency Program
University of Miami School of Medicine 33101

Nikitas J. Zervanos, MD
Family Physician
Semi-Retired Director Emeritus, Family Practice Residency Program
Lancaster General Hospital
Lancaster, Pennsylvania 17603

About the Illustrator

Benjamin James Pugno, MA has been recognized for his artistic gifts since childhood. He is the recipient of numerous awards for artistic design, and has received recognition from the Boy Scouts of America for his creation of activity patches for that organization over a period of several years. He was involved in updating the National Historical Landmarks survey, and helped created the Internet Brochures for the National Park Service's National Register for Historic Places in 2000.

Ben's art is characterized by whimsical humor and the capacity to use familiar metaphors to communicate complex concepts. The creation of illustrations for inclusion in this book is his first commercial venture. Ben holds a "day job" as an instructor and doctoral candidate in history at the University of Houston in Houston, Texas. His areas of expertise include the Anglo-Saxon period and the transition of healthcare expertise from the clergy to the laity in the British Isles.

Acknowledgements

We want to acknowledge our heartfelt gratitude to
the many contributors to this book –
in particular, the physician leaders whose insights are incorporated
throughout,
and their staff who so capably assisted with the process.

We appreciate the critiques and suggestions from the physicians, medical residents, medical students, and nurse executives who reviewed early drafts of this manuscript while studying leadership with Dr. McKenna in the Health Care Leadership Program at Rockhurst University. Those individuals include Brandon Brevig; Christie Brock; Jimmy Dang; Eddie Eldred; Dan Hancock, MD; Shannon Hopen; Melanie Susan Kraft, MD, MRO, AMEt; Tinh Le; Josh Linebaugh; Andy Maes; Bridget M. McCandless, MD; Michele L. McDonnell; Ankur D. Mehta; Elizabeth Morris, RN; and Eric Terpstra. We also wish to thank Crystal Goodman and Lynn Ross for their support in copy-editing and reference verification.

We are particularly grateful to Myles P. Gartland, PhD, MBA, for sharing his analytical expertise and his deep knowledge of the healthcare industry, both of which have significantly enhanced the depth of our research reported in this and other publications. And we appreciate the supportiveness of James Daley, PhD, Dean of the Helzberg School of Management at Rockhurst University, for educational endeavours that equip healthcare professionals to enhance their effectiveness as leaders.

We also want to thank the staff and leadership of the American Academy of Family Physicians, the Association of Family Medicine Residency Directors and the Society of Teachers of Family Medicine for their support, encouragement and suggestions on content for the book.

We especially wish to acknowledge the enthusiasm and expertise of our colleagues at Radcliffe Publishing, whose collaboration has been essential to the successful completion of this book. We are particularly grateful to Gillian Nineham, Jamie Etherington, Paula Moran, and Lisa Abbott for their valuable editorial insights and support. We appreciate the marketing support provided by Martin Hill, Gregory Moxon, Susan Rabson, Iti Singh and Angela Francis in order to ensure this book is visible and accessible to all those who may wish to read it or adopt it for inclusion in undergraduate medical education, graduate residency program, or continuing medical education curricula.

*   *   *

Diligent effort has been made to identify the source of all material used in this book.
However, many of the materials have been gathered over quite literally the past several decades, including unidentified clippings and excerpts forwarded to us from all over the world.
If you know the correct source for any items now labeled "Source unknown," please contact us so that proper credit can be given in future printings.

Dedication

This book is dedicated to **Joe McKenna** and **Terry Pugno**, our loving partners in life, without whose encouragement and support this book would
never have been written
and to
physician leaders around the world – from years past and years to come –
whose passion and purpose, talents and time,
are contributing to ever-greater progress in the provision of healthcare
services.
A portion of the proceeds from this book
will be donated to not-for-profit educational organizations
that are dedicated to
enhancing the effectiveness and fulfillment of physician leaders around the
world.

Prologue

"Renewed physician leadership in the U.S. at this juncture may depend fundamentally on restoring in the mind of the public that physicians actually place and will continue to place highest priority on the interest of patients. Without public trust, physician leadership may be an oxymoron."

Larry A. Green, MD
Family Physician
Past-Director, The Robert Graham Center: Policy Studies in Family
Medicine and Primary Care

Nearly everyone agrees that healthcare should be "better" – in fact many would say healthcare needs an "extreme makeover." Yet few expect significant improvements anytime soon. We are doing what we can to prevent the tragic cases of those who die too young, or those who live too long. We keep on striving to help and to heal, even while the practice of medicine becomes ever more challenging.

The issues are complex; answers are elusive. Some have succumbed to engaging in blame games; contributing to the problems rather than collaborating toward new solutions. With increasing frequency and urgency, people are pleading for physician leaders to guide the way through the complexities of contemporary healthcare. Some call upon physicians to help out of belief that the solutions will require perspectives only practitioners can provide. Others believe that without physician involvement, efforts to change will be met with resistance.

Regardless of the motivation behind this growing demand for physician leadership, two things are certain. First, physicians are being called upon to help lead significant transformational improvements in healthcare, and are being called to do so more urgently than at any previous point in history. Second, until physicians are able to lead others, they will be unable to bring about significant improvements in healthcare. Yet, despite widespread agreement on these notions, few of us can identify physician leaders, articulate what they do, or explain how they lead. Now more than ever before we need a clear and compelling picture of physician leadership. Someone must help the healers heed the call.

This book is a practical guide for all physician leaders who want to be more effective and fulfilled in their work, and who want to make a positive difference by helping others be more effective and fulfilled in their work. Whether you have sought leadership roles or had leadership responsibilities thrust upon you, this book will help you become a more compelling leader.

Many of the notions included in this book are evidence-based and grounded in rigorous research – our own and that of other experts. Also included are opinions and insights from many leading physicians who were interviewed for this book and whose success stories we've profiled for your benefit. We trust their words of wisdom will inspire and enlighten you.

Throughout this book you will encounter many thought-provoking questions and suggestions for action. You will find guidance for making decisions, taking action, and building relationships that equip you to set and achieve meaningful goals. By using the tips and tools provided in this book, you will be able to more clearly conceive what *physician leadership* means to you and to determine the types of leadership you are willing and able to provide in light of your unique work style, interests, abilities, and circumstances. Perhaps most importantly, you will experience the satisfaction that comes from becoming who you want to be and achieving what you aspire to achieve.

This book is written for physicians in several situations. First, it is written as a "leader launch pad" for those who are fairly new to the profession and are just beginning to think about physician leadership – those who have not yet identified how to make a unique contribution to the profession. Second, this book is written for experienced leaders who want resources and insights for increased job satisfaction and effectiveness. Whether you are, for example, a hospital department head, chief medical officer, medical group executive, or volunteer leader within your professional society or community, we intend to help you increase your effectiveness and fulfillment as a physician leader.

This book is also written for those whose current professional responsibilities neither optimize their abilities nor satisfy their yearnings. Are you vaguely – or desperately – sensing a need to redirect your passions, but not yet clear about how to take the next step? This book is for you. It will help you find ways of leading that are optimally suited to your unique interests, values, and aspirations.

You will probably find this book an easy read, but don't expect its insights to be easily applied. Anyone who plans to skim this book quickly, file it away and be miraculously transformed will surely be disappointed. You will gain far more value from this book by using it as a handy reference guide on your lifelong journey toward ever-increasing effectiveness and fulfillment.

Section I begins by offering great news! Physicians *can* be well-suited to lead. Chapter One explains why, pointing out that clinical and administrative leadership are synergistic. In fact, only by leveraging the potential synergies of clinical leadership and administrative leadership can anyone hope to maximize patients' outcomes *and* professional incomes. (Yes, we are capitalists. We believe that well-educated, highly dedicated professionals – including physicians – ought to be compensated fairly for doing important work.) Section I also describes special challenges often faced by physician leaders, with tips for overcoming those challenges. In this first section, we will build the foundational claim that leading is everyone's responsibility. Leading, that is, not managing. You see, the art of leading is in fact quite distinct from – though complementary to – the science of managing. We lead people. We manage projects, facilities, and budgets. Managing involves the oversight of tasks to ensure predictable results. Leading involves the forging of strong relationships to guide transformational change.

By reading this book, you will glimpse a high level overview of leadership principles from experts in the field. You will read candid acknowledgment of ways in which traditional management education can sometimes go wrong and find tips for recognizing common misconceptions about leadership.

Are you familiar with the six "core competencies" now being required of physicians? If not, you will definitely want to read this part of the book to discover what these six competencies entail, and why competencies have become a widely-used framework for assessing and developing professional proficiency. If you are already aware of the physician competency outcome project, we believe you will appreciate reading how it compares with other competency initiatives currently underway – in medicine and in general. This first foundational section of the book also reports results from research we have conducted regarding the work styles, motivational values, and beliefs held about the work of leading physicians by many leading physicians. And physician educators. And physicians in training.

Section II contains a framework for considering various pathways that physician leaders may pursue and various types of contributions that physician leaders make. The ideas we offer are not drawn solely from our own experience and research. This book contains advice and "lessons learned" from over four dozen leading physicians who have graciously invested time and energy to share their insights with you. We are confident you will be inspired, perhaps intrigued, by what they have to say about leading physicians. For example, you will discover how *clinical experts* serve as standard bearers to "raise the bar" of clinical excellence in their specialties. You will learn how *physician executives* govern healthcare organizations to enhance the quality and efficiency of healthcare delivery. You will glimpse ways in which *pioneers* are guiding the invention and discovery of new drugs, devices, procedures, and practices; then accelerating the diffusion of those innovations into mainstream healthcare delivery – by promoting evidence-based medicine and evidence-based management.

You will also read insights from *activists* – courageous and often selfless advocates who are challenging the status quo and championing change, serving as catalysts for reform in healthcare policy, funding, laws and regulations. In fact, this book includes a true insider's perspective on the impact that elected officials can have on the advancement of healthcare quality, access, and affordability. Senate Majority Leader, Dr. William Frist – widely respected for his clinical skills as a heart/lung transplant surgeon *and* for his leadership skills in building coalitions of support – has written our chapter on physician leadership in government. We believe you will find the chapter written by Dr. Frist to be both enlightening and thought-provoking. Section II concludes with insights about leading in the context of several unique settings including the public domain and the military, academia and rural areas, in policy setting bodies, public health clinics, and in your community at large.

In Section III you will find a mental model we call "Stepping Stones for Successful Leadership." Despite the fact that leadership is a broad and sometimes difficult-to-define notion, most people do believe that we "know it when we see it." Why? People recognize leadership when we see (or experience) it because certain insights, skills, and attitudes are universally applied by those who lead well. The five "stepping stones" model described in this book is certainly not the only way to conceptualize successful leadership. Rather, it is a practical framework for use as a reference by physicians who aspire to greater levels of excellence in the art of leading. The five stepping stones for successful leadership we describe in this book include *credibility* (through competence and character), *clarity* (of vision and communication), *collaboration* (through commitment and teamwork), *coordination* (of decisions and actions) and *change* (including resilience and renewal). We believe these stepping stones are essential for leading people to achieve remarkable results – inside and outside of healthcare.

Physicians as a group are accustomed to *"learning by doing."* Thus we trust you will appreciate the way Section IV helps you learn *about* leading physicians *by actually leading* physicians. This section offers practical tips for assessing your present realities and future possibilities; for determining appropriate goals, roles, ground rules, and resources; for engaging the commitment and collaboration you will need from others in order to attain those goals; and ultimately, for making decisions and taking action so that you and those you lead are able to achieve truly remarkable results. This section will help you become a more compelling physician leader by helping you apply the book's insights toward your own continuing professional development.

Be forewarned. It will require effort on your part! For the concept of leadership seems simple enough when described, but is exceedingly difficult to practice on a day in, day out basis. (Not unlike parenting, competitive sports, or any other *easy-to-do-marginally but difficult-to-master* endeavors.) We encourage you to invest time in reflection after reading this book. Through reflection, you will gain awareness of yourself and others, and gain clarity about your focus and goals. To assist you in this endeavor, we offer words of wisdom from many successful physician leaders.

Perhaps you – by preference or necessity – will learn to lead by "practicing" leadership on the job. Think of it as re-engineering an airplane mid-flight. The fact is, learning on the job – whether your "real job" or a volunteer role in your professional medical society, an organizational committee, or a community-wide initiative – can be a great way of enhancing your leadership effectiveness *if* you approach it consciously and thoughtfully, rather than by random trial and error. Do you have a mentor? Do you mentor others? This section reveals what many leading physicians have to say about the importance of finding mentors – of learning all you can from all the relationships that you can in all the situations that you can.

But the book doesn't stop there! For the mark of a true leader is the development of other leaders. That's right. Gardeners grow gardens; leaders develop leaders – purposefully and enthusiastically. So you will find a section containing many tips to *help you help others* enhance their effectiveness. How? By investing time and attention in your relationships with colleagues. By creating and nurturing a culture that respects individual diversity even while encouraging fiercely loyal teamwork. Are you ready to extend your leadership influence beyond the scope of those with whom you interact regularly? Then find out how compelling physician leaders "make a difference" in healthcare by teaching and training, research and publishing, speaking and consulting, by advocating on behalf of educational and reimbursement reforms that are necessary to support physician leadership development.

Section V is your own personal *Leader Launcher Tool Kit™*, with an extensive array of instruments and activities for use in assessing and enhancing your leadership effectiveness. You see, we would not have fulfilled our commitment to you, our readers, simply by sharing stories about other physicians. You deserve straightforward assistance for applying the guidance provided in this book. We want to help you enhance your effectiveness and find more fulfillment in your work by helping you gain insights, skills, relationships, and experiences you will need for becoming the physician leader you are capable of being.

The final part of the book includes brief biographical descriptions of the physician leaders who have so generously shared their stories and their words of wisdom. These remarkable individuals have invested time to share their tips and tales in order to illuminate stepping stones for your journey toward greater success and fulfillment as a physician leader.

We wish each of those leading physicians, and each of you, our very best.
May you lead well and live well.

Section 1

Exploring Physician Leadership

"Physicians who are effective leaders must help us envision better approaches and influence their peers to adopt those better approaches. This is true for all of the changes that are needed in healthcare – changes in medical education and also in health policy, in the financing and the delivery of care."

William F. Jessee, MD, FAAP, FACPM
Pediatric, Preventive and Emergency Medicine Physician
President
Medical Group Management Association

Now, more than ever before in the history of civilization, we urgently need physicians to lead. Why? *Because our current healthcare delivery system is simply not good enough.* Healthcare can and should be better. How, specifically should it be *"better?"* We know that more consistency is possible in the quality of care that's delivered. We know that increased access to care is possible for those who need it. We know that more cost-effectively delivered care is possible for the benefit of patients and

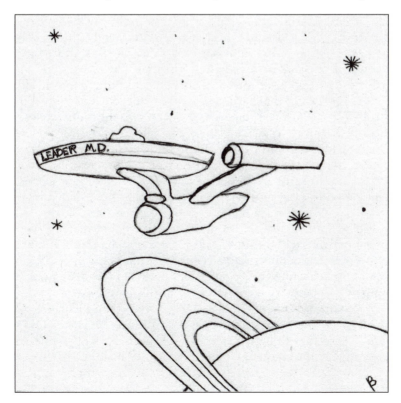

providers alike. We also know that progress toward these universally accepted goals is complex and elusive for many reasons. Some would conclude, in fact, that significant improvement to the healthcare system is nearly impossible.

> "Physicians must be in leadership roles if we are to address the demanding issues of cost and quality in our American health model. A physician can, if desire is present, learn the equivalent business knowledge a formally trained business manager learns. However, it is unlikely that formally trained business managers will go to medical school to learn the medical knowledge. If the market model is used to answer questions without physicians in leadership roles who have learned both the medical and business aspects of the process, you may end up with an economist deciding which medications patients should be receiving or what surgery your loved ones may have."
>
> Roland A. Goertz, MD, MBA
> Family Physician
> President, McLennan County Medical Education and Research Foundation

Responses to the Issues in Healthcare

The options, it seems, are three-fold. First, we could choose to accept the status quo. We could decide to "live with" (or "die with," as the case may be) our current healthcare delivery system, despite our awareness of all its hassles, headaches, and heartbreaks. No thanks! Why not? Too many of our loved ones will die too young and linger too long; too much money will be wasted on inefficient and ineffective procedures and practices; too many gifted clinicians will leave the profession in search of more lucrative, less risky endeavors. Patients deserve better. Taxpayers deserve better. Clinicians deserve better.

Second, we could abdicate the responsibility for "improving healthcare" to others. We could leave the hard work that's needed up to the non-clinical administrators and business managers. After all, they are well-trained to manage projects and processes, facilities and budgets. They are *not*, however, well-trained to understand or deal with health and disease, life and death, or the myriad of clinical, scientific, ethical and human complexities that cannot be separated from our clinical obligations and professional responsibilities. Haven't we all had enough of the more-harmful-than-helpful misguided interventions (i.e., meddling) by well-meaning – let's presume at least some of them are, anyway – albeit unenlightened administrators who mistakenly believe that "medicine is just another business." And yet, leaving the responsibility to "lead" up to the non-clinical administrators is exactly what many of us have done – by default if not by deliberate choice. (This has occurred for many understandable reasons, many of which we'll explore later in this book.)

Third, we could do something! That's right, we could recognize the importance of physician involvement in leading improvements to our healthcare system and take action to help physicians regain their rightful role. Physicians could agree to lead the changes we need in today's healthcare delivery system. Simply by reading this page in this book, you are, perhaps unconsciously, considering the validity of this third option.

Points to Ponder

1 Do you believe healthcare delivery could and should be significantly better?
2 Have you resigned yourself to accept (or tolerate) the status quo?
3 Are you hoping others will take the lead in bringing about needed improvements?
4 Are you willing and able to help lead the needed changes? If so, where and how would you like to become involved?
5 If not, what is preventing you from being willing or able to help?

"How to have a 'positive influence' and how to 'be effective' are key issues for docs who want to raise the bar. Phrases like those are challenging, though, because the expressions themselves have become tainted with other connotations and are now a turnoff. Still, those physicians who want to be good leaders want to learn how to be more effective, how to have a positive impact, and how to promote excellence."

Randall Oates, MD
Family Physician
Founder and President, Docs, Inc.

The Need for Physician Leaders

Perhaps you, like many of your colleagues, believe that any significant improvements in the delivery of healthcare must include the perspectives of physicians. A rapidly growing number of physicians have become convinced that successful change and improvement will be possible only if physicians embrace the "need to lead." Why? Because only actively practicing "in-the-trenches-physicians" can truly understand the role of medicine in the overall delivery of healthcare; only physicians can inspire collaboration and commitment to make the difficult changes in attitudes, skills, behaviors, and habits that those active in the practice of medicine must make in order for significant improvement to occur in our healthcare system.

Let's face it. Physicians are the primary decision makers regarding patients' diagnosis and care, and as such have a major influence on healthcare quality and, to some extent, the costs or at least quantity of medical procedures performed. Thus physicians *must* be integrally involved in leading the way to improve the healthcare system. Period. Physicians must contribute to the solutions (not the problems) in healthcare today.

"Hey wait," you may be thinking to yourself. "Easy for others to place the burden on us. Hasn't anyone noticed physicians today are at or beyond our capacity to absorb more expectations, more time commitments, more pressures, more obligations – especially those involving complex challenges we were never prepared to tackle! I'm exhausted, discouraged – how could I possibly tackle the monumental task of improving the practice of medicine overall? I'm frankly more interested in improving the practice of yours truly! That's plenty enough challenge for me, thank you very much!"

We understand. We empathize. We acknowledge the perturbing paradox facing physicians today. Society is asking, even demanding, that physicians lead the way toward improved healthcare delivery, and yet our current approach to medical education and training does little to equip physicians to lead or even participate in improving our healthcare system. We've educated physicians to work in the system, yet now we expect them to work on the system. To do so effectively, physicians need a multitude of insights, skills, and attitudes that are vastly different than those developed through typical medical education, experiences, roles, and relationships. Until now.

It should not surprise us that there has recently been explosive growth in an emerging field often referred to as "physician leadership." All over the United States, and in some instances around the world, medical schools and business schools are partnering together to offer "dual degree programs" in medicine and management. In fact, as of mid-2004, the AAMC listed 41 schools that offer MD/MBA combined degree programs, 61 MD/MPH programs and 1 MD/MHA program. There is a rise in the number of osteopathic medical schools that offer dual degrees as well – some in partnership with the business schools of other universities, such as the DO/MBA program launched by the Kansas City University of Medicine and Biosciences (formerly known as the University of Health Sciences – College of Osteopathic Medicine) and Rockhurst University's Helzberg School of Management.

Practicing physicians who have already completed their medical education are returning to school in record numbers to earn graduate degrees in management or business administration. Though many enroll in general MBA or executive EMBA programs, nearly 2000 have opted for the physician-specific Masters in Medical Management (MMM) degree through one of three ACPE-affiliated programs at Carnegie Mellon University, Tulane University, or the University of Southern California. The ACPE also collaborates with the University of Massachusetts, Amherst in a completely online MBA program.

Other organizations are also involved in this explosively growing trend. Commercial, publicly held firms are collaborating with private, not-for-profit foundations, professional associations, and medical societies in unprecedented and uniquely innovative ways to offer programs targeted specifically toward the development of clinical leaders. In fact, similar trends are occurring in the field of nursing and other healthcare professions, though that topic is beyond the scope and focus of this book.

Many Types of Physician Leadership

The fact is, there is an increasingly urgent call for physician leaders. And let's be clear. We're not just talking about "physician executives" – clinically trained administrators who govern the human and financial resources within healthcare organizations – though certainly there is a growing need for people with those skills in those roles. Nor are we simply referring to "clinical experts" – individual contributors who "raise the bar" by exemplifying excellence and serving as "thought leaders" to influence, directly and indirectly, the practice of medicine within a given specialty. They, too, are needed in their roles. Both physician executives and clinical experts make important contributions to the advancement of medicine by working *in* the healthcare system. Their primary impact is targeted toward the health status of those patients directly served by their organizations.

Experts and *executives*, while certainly necessary, are not sufficient for the type and degree of discontinuous, remarkable improvements so fervently sought after in the field of healthcare. The world also has a need for leading physicians to work *on* the healthcare system itself. We need "activists" who refuse to accept the status quo, who champion change – often by building coalitions of support to reform the laws and regulations, policies and infrastructures that constrain and enable the delivery of care. We need "pioneers" whose innovations guide the discovery and invention of new drugs and devices, new practices and procedures; those who have the training and experience to prevent beneficial new ideas from becoming additional financial burdens. The world also needs physicians whose focus extends beyond their own individual creativity, those who are willing and able to accelerate the diffusion of innovations across medicine, who are actively promoting mainstream adoption of better practices among all physicians, so better outcomes are enjoyed by all patients.

What healthcare needs today is not just one "superhero" archetype to single-handedly lead the charge and save the system. We need many leading physicians, and we need many approaches to leadership. The world will always need physicians who are traditionally-oriented professionals, individual professionals who choose to follow their calling by treating patients one encounter at a time. Theirs is a noble and worthy calling. The world also needs physicians who are trailblazers; leaders who are willing and able to lead the way in shaping a new approach to practicing the profession of medicine. We need physicians working *in* and *on* the healthcare system in the executive office and in the exam room or on the hospital ward. Working in the system and working on the system are both essential for making a difference – in the lives of individual patients and for the benefit of patients overall. Dr. Geerlofs explains:

> "Lyall Watson and Ken Kesey have both written about the Hundredth Monkey Phenomenon (Watson, 1992) to illustrate the concept of 'an idea whose time has come.' The story describes several monkeys on a remote Japanese island who learn to wash the gritty dirt off sweet potatoes. Slowly, other monkeys adopt the behavior. After about 100 monkeys have learned it, the behavior spreads like wild fire among the remaining monkeys on the island. Remarkably, at roughly the same time, monkeys on distant islands with no possible communication began showing the same behavior.
>
> I believe the Hundredth Monkey Phenomenon will soon happen in healthcare delivery. The notion of a new kind of 'physician leader' transforming the way care is delivered is an idea whose time has come."
>
> J. Peter Geerlofs, MD
> Family Physician
> Chief Medical Officer, Allscripts Healthcare Solutions, Inc.

Only as physicians are properly equipped to envision new possibilities and to collaborate in bringing about such possibilities will we experience significant and sustainable improvements in the quality, access, and cost-effectiveness of healthcare. It is not enough to *demand* that physicians be *willing* to lead the way. We must *equip* physicians with the insights, attitudes, and skills to be *able* to lead the way.

> "Physicians focus on serving the immediate interests of the individual patient – often in the context of a specific encounter. Leaders focus on serving the long-term interests of the collective. That duality can be disorienting. The unlearning it requires is often difficult, even painful. And yet, the duality has its advantages as well. When frustrated by the challenges associated with either of those roles, physician leaders can find re-invigoration and renewal by focusing on the other."
>
> Deborah S. McPherson, MD, FAAFP
> Family Physician
> Associate Director, Family Medicine Residency Program,
> Kansas University Medical Center

Physician leaders are needed to guide and promote a healthcare system that meets the needs of everyone – including the poor, disenfranchised, illiterate, and otherwise underserved. Physician leaders are needed to bring clinical insights and professional ethics to the operational side of the healthcare industry. Physician leaders are needed to bring context, restraint, and perspective to the business decisions made within healthcare that have unanticipated consequences. Physician leaders are needed to understand healthcare delivery from "the trenches" and do something with that understanding. Physician leaders are needed to challenge the inadequacies of our current healthcare system, inspire shared vision of a better future, and enable others to act in ways that transform vision into reality.

We're convinced that many physicians truly desire to help lead the way toward higher quality, more accessible, more cost-effective healthcare. We believe many physicians are eager to gain the insights, attitudes, and skills needed to do so. And we're confident that most physicians who want to help lead the way have the capacity to become effective and fulfilled leaders, if properly equipped to take the necessary steps. Do you see yourself among these people we're calling physician leaders? If so, you have our blessings and support! We don't pretend your journey will be easy. We do believe it will be rewarding.

Three Powerful Principles for Physician Leaders

We believe three principles for success will serve you well in your quest to become an effective physician leader. Conceptually each is relatively simple and straightforward, but applying them consistently may be challenging. What three powerful principles are we suggesting?

- Identify role models and learn from them.
- "Show up."
- Get involved.

Identify Role Models and Learn From Them

The importance of identifying and learning from role models cannot be overemphasized for anyone aspiring to be an effective and fulfilled physician leader. In today's complex society, being a physician and being a leader are each extremely challenging in their own right! Those able to successfully do both have found ways of balancing multiple responsibilities, even multiple identities. Much can be learned from those who do so successfully. It simply requires a conscious determination to do so – an attitude of openness and a commitment of effort.

Begin by identifying several individuals who are role models for you. Study their attributes and achievements, observing them in action (if possible), and perhaps even getting to know them.

Learn as much about your chosen role models as possible. What career paths have they followed? How did they come to be leaders? What background elements influenced their journey toward leadership? What drives and sustains them, both personally and professionally? Identify many role models and learn from the "best" of each. We assure you great dividends will come from the time and energy invested in doing this.

Points to Ponder

1 Do you, at this point in your professional journey, have one or more role models? If so, who are they, and what career paths have they followed?
2 What background elements influenced your role models' journey toward leadership?
3 What drives and sustains them, personally and professionally?
4 What aspects of your role models' example do you want to emulate?

"Show Up"

For people in general and physicians in particular, opportunities to lead come along regularly. Students can take the lead by becoming involved in various special interest groups within and beyond their educational institutions. Practicing physicians have opportunities to influence their workplaces and their medical specialties through active involvement in committees and task groups. Each of us can take the lead in improving some aspect of our communities through participation on school boards, churches, and municipalities.

To seize these opportunities, we must first and foremost simply "show up." We may find these opportunities to practice and hone our leadership skills by attending meetings or get-togethers involving people who share our interests. Most of us would be well-served, especially early on in our development, by investigating a number of opportunities. Explore each possibility and evaluate them to identify which are best suited to your personal priorities.

A word of caution: Those who become "professional joiners" – becoming members of as many groups as possible but not actually making an impact with any of them – may build a lengthy curriculum vitae, but are unlikely to build a lasting legacy. Sometimes less is more. So anticipate learning to live with the paradox of continually scanning for new opportunities to lead, yet screening the possibilities to focus your energies and talents judiciously.

By being "out there," active, involved, ever mindful of unmet needs and opportunities to make an impact, you'll encounter plenty of opportunities to lead. Be ready to "catch them" as they present themselves. How? By being clear about the leadership skills you want to develop or use. That way, you'll be able to "choose" the opportunities of greatest benefit – to you and to those you lead.

Points to Ponder

1 Are you involved in too few or too many organizations?
2 If so, how is that impacting your ability to reach your full capacity as a physician leader?

Get Involved

No one in the history of humankind was born with all the knowledge and experience they need to be a great leader. Leaders are "made, not born." True, some individuals are blessed with extraordinary gifts and capacities, natural traits and characteristics that make leadership effectiveness easier for them to attain. But the reality is that leading requires attitudes, insights, and skills that are learned and refined with practice and experience. Tiger Woods has a gift for golf. And he practices golf diligently. So, too, must leaders practice the skills of effective leadership.

Leaders lead. Leaders lead others to do things that wouldn't otherwise happen. Leading is an action verb. Do you aspire to lead? If so, you must be "active" and "interactive" with those you seek to lead.

That's why it is so important to identify groups (collections of individuals with whom you share some common interest – be it employment in the same organization, or membership in the same medical specialty, or shared passion for a cause – perhaps a problem you collectively want to solve, or a vision you collectively want to achieve).

Imagine how improbable it would be for any of us to wake up one day and find ourselves – without any previous leadership experience – suddenly leading thousands of people toward the realization of magnificent achievements. The reality is, we lead well when we are successful in attracting others to collaborate with us toward the attainment of a shared vision. Being talented and seeing what needs to happen is necessary but insufficient for successful leadership. Leading well involves trust; and engaging others to make things happen.

Start by "blooming where you are planted." Look at the opportunities around you in the groups with which you're already aware or associated. Lead a few individuals to complete a defined task as a great beginning step. By doing so, you'll gain proficiency in the attitudes, insights, and skills you'll need to lead larger scale change. Books such as this one can illuminate key concepts. Books can expose us to "lessons learned" by those who've gone before us. But books cannot substitute for actual experience. Why? Because experience, especially when reflected upon thoughtfully and with an openness to learn, helps us identify who we want to lead, what we want to lead them to achieve, and how to lead successfully. Even more importantly, experience gets us involved with others, bringing us into contact with more role models, more ideas, and more opportunities to lead.

Regardless of your point of view on universal coverage, healthcare tort reform, or a host of other medically-related, societally-embedded issues, odds are you'll agree on this: healthcare is badly broken, we can and must do better. Physicians must contribute to the search for new solutions, rather than contribute to the problems. We trust you believe, as we do, that these times of chaos and complexity call for more than simply solid management; they call for transformational healthcare leadership.

We are surely faced with many challenges in healthcare – declining reimbursement rates, declining incomes, declining professional autonomy. We do not, however, face a decline in the number of patients who need and deserve excellent care. We do not face a decline in the need for physician leaders. Quite the opposite, in fact. We need physician leaders – now more than ever. Are you willing and able to count yourself among the ranks of the world's leading physicians?

Points to Ponder

1 Do you continually scan for opportunities to lead?
2 Do you screen the various leadership opportunities that come your way – saying no to some, in order to focus your talents and energies on those that are the highest priority?
3 In what situations or settings would you like to become involved? What positive impact might you be able to have?

Reference

Watson L. (1992) *The Dreams of Dragons: an exploration and celebration of the mysteries of nature.* Rochester, VT: Destiny Books.

Chapter 1

Good News: Physicians Can Be Well-Suited to Lead

"What makes physician leaders effective? Many of the same attributes that drive people to become physicians in the first place. Caring about the healthcare system and what happens to it; caring about and advocating for patients; an insider's knowledge of what is wrong with healthcare and what could work to transform it."

J. Peter Geerlofs, MD
Family Physician
Chief Medical Officer, Allscripts Healthcare Solutions, Inc.

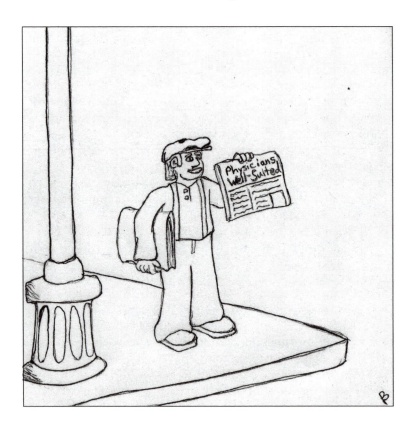

One of the main forces that compelled us to write this book was the observation and belief that physicians are particularly well-suited for many types of leadership. In their day-to-day lives, in their local communities, in nations around the world and throughout history, most physicians are conspicuously visible in leadership roles. Why is that? Why do those whose inclination, education, and training are oriented toward *helping* others, seem particularly well suited for *leading* others? We believe several personal characteristics appear congruent with practicing medicine and practicing leadership.

Characteristics Conducive to Both Medicine and Leadership

External Focus

Physicians, by the very nature of the work, are demonstrably focused external to themselves. Helping others, meeting patients' needs, relieving pain and suffering, mending broken bodies and minds. The view of physicians is externally focused – focused on patient care, patients' well-being, and helping patients overcome illness to attain and maintain full health. Is being rich your goal? There are many easier ways to achieve wealth than through the practice of medicine. Is being famous what you want out of life? A career in theater or politics will help you achieve fame far more reliably than will the practice of medicine. No, being a physician is not about being rich or famous. Being a physician is about meeting patients' needs, making patients' needs a priority, even above your own personal needs.

Unfortunately, an external focus is a two-edged sword. It often poses one of the more insidious challenges to physicians' personal lives. This external focus on patients and their needs too often becomes a stumbling block in physicians' personal lives, with negative consequences. Inadequate attention to one's family, inadequate attention to one's personal health, inadequate balance of one's personal and professional identities are commonly occurring adverse consequences of physicians' inclination to focus so persistently on patients and patients' illnesses. This may, in fact, be one of the most difficult challenges encountered by anyone in medicine.

A Selection Process

To become a physician, one must possess certain characteristics for sustaining the prolonged educational process and intellectual challenges associated with the profession. Natural curiosity, the capacity to learn, and the ability to retain large amounts of information are necessary to complete the many years of education, training, and testing required before physicians are permitted to practice medicine. And yet, it takes more than intellectual capacity to become a physician. To become a physician, one must be sufficiently goal-oriented and willing to work hard for that goal over an extended period of time. These characteristics are absolutely essential to the completion of the medical degree and the postgraduate training required of physicians today. Aren't these characteristics – curiosity, capacity to learn, disciplined thinking, and goal-directed thinking – many of the characteristics we want in those individuals whose lead we're willing to follow?

Social and Behavioral Skills

Both physicians and leaders must be skilled in the capacity to gather information, to process it in highly functional ways, and to communicate conclusions or opinions effectively. Medical training demands skill in communicating with people on a personal and individual basis. Physicians who lack such skills can expect to face constant challenges in their careers. They will find it difficult to achieve success in medicine or leadership.

Other Characteristics

Many other characteristics associated with medical practice resonate well with the work of a leader:

- The capacity to develop trusting relationships with others, even when they may not be "at their best."
- The capacity to work with and lead teams of individuals with differing roles and skills toward the achievement of a single shared goal, be it the completion of a complicated operative procedure or the achievement of a mutually shared vision.
- Acceptance of accountability for one's decisions and the actions that flow from those decisions.

Do healthcare organizations benefit from physician leadership? Yes, according to Richard Birrer, MD, MPH, MMM, CPE. In one of his two articles published recently in *Health Progress*, Dr. Birrer reported that " . . . in a recent survey of the more than 6,200 U.S. hospitals that have 25 or more beds, all of those judged to be among the top 100 had physician leaders at every level of their organizations" (Birrer 2002).

As a population, physicians generally hold themselves to very high standards. In fact, many physicians view human error as personal inadequacy, thus engendering substantial guilt and self-criticism. The standard of "never make a mistake, someone's life may be depending on you" is, of course, impossible to achieve in reality. Nevertheless, accountability for actions and high standards for success serve physicians well in the clinical environment and serve leaders well in society at large.

Points to Ponder

---

1 Why do you suppose some, but not all, physicians are motivated to assume leadership responsibility?
2 Do you believe most physician leaders are functioning at their peak potential?
3 If not, what do you believe is preventing those physicians from reaching their full potential?
4 How are physicians whose aptitudes are underutilized different from those who truly make a significant impact in healthcare?
5 Reflect back on a time when you found great satisfaction from leading. How was the experience meaningful to you?

Communication Skills

Patient satisfaction surveys indicate substantial diversity among physicians' capacity to "talk to patients." Some are certainly better communicators than others. Yet the reality is that few physicians would survive in the marketplace if they were not quite good at communicating with patients, employees, and colleagues. It is difficult to make accurate diagnoses without listening well – taking into account not only what is being said but also what is not being said through non-verbal cues. Physicians who are good at explaining unfamiliar, complex, and emotionally laden information to patients should be similarly skilled communicators in non-clinical interactions.

Of course, not all physicians are good communicators, but we would like to believe that the vast majority understand its importance. Sadly, this is not always the case. In a communication skill workshop led by Barbara Linney for the American College of Physician Executives (ACPE), participating physicians were taught to increase the effectiveness of communication with patients or colleagues by remembering to look at them while speaking. Ms. Linney suggested that physicians should make eye contact when others speak, and should nod affirmatively in order to convey interest to the person speaking. Although some might reasonably assume that physicians would know this, the majority of people in the room were actually taking notes as Ms. Linney gave that practical advice.

Leading Teams

Few physicians personally provide the entirety of care to their patients. With the exception of a physician assigned to the South Pole, for example, most interface regularly with nurses, medical assistants, technicians, clerks, and others who support and facilitate the care of their patients. The responsibility for providing direction to each member of the healthcare team usually falls to the physician. Certainly, the operating room setting is a good example where the physician (surgeon) can be clearly identified as the leader of a team of people who are working together toward a common goal.

Providing clear direction for a team, setting its course, and evaluating its progress are all behaviors and skills that can directly translate into non-clinical settings. There, too, physicians may be identified as team leaders. Taking responsibility for directing the activities of others is often comfortable for most physicians in the clinical setting. What works there can often be applied to other settings where groups need direction.

Sometimes, physicians are not the team leaders, but are one of several colleagues who are working together to care for a patient. Being an effective team member is equally important as being an effective team leader. Most physicians have substantial experience in both roles.

Managing Information

The care of a patient often involves the gathering of large amounts of information, identifying, and seeking other needed information, weighing available information for importance and pertinence to the situation at hand, then making the best possible decision for the patient. Making a diagnosis demands that sufficient information is gathered to support or refute an initial hypothesis. Frequently, a differential diagnosis is developed based upon the statistical likelihood of various options, despite information that may at times be insufficient or inconclusive. The skill involved in sorting through large amounts of information to make the optimal decision is directly applicable to non-clinical decision making as well. In fact, non-clinical decisions seldom demand the standard of "zero error tolerance" that must be applied in most clinical decisions. It should reassure physicians to know that a higher tolerance for suboptimal decisions will often be the norm in administrative settings.

Adaptive Learning, by Dr. Perry Pugno

I recall with fondness one of the first lectures I heard in medical school. An older physician with an excellent clinical reputation stood before us and said: "Today, you must make peace with the fact that at least 25 percent of what we are going to teach you over the course of the next four years is dead wrong. The challenge for your career in medicine is to identify that 25 percent, discern the correct answer and apply it in your practice."

As I look back on my own career, I realize how very true that statement was. In fact, it was recently brought home to me when my family and I were packing our possessions, preparing to relocate halfway across the country. On that memorable Saturday morning, my wife, **Terry**, said to me: "Today is the day you need to go out into the garage, pull out all of your old medical school notes and throw most of them away. We shouldn't be paying movers to carry them halfway across the country." Indignant with the thought of discarding several years' work which I had carefully preserved (but never looked at) in a filing cabinet in the garage, I immediately expressed my reluctance to do so. Her response to me was: "I'll tell you what. Pull a few files from that cabinet at random, sit down and read them. If you think the information is still important for you to keep, then you can take the whole batch with you."

Rising to her challenge, I immediately went out to the garage, pulled open a drawer, reached in and pulled out a file I had prepared some 25 years earlier on the care of patients with peptic ulcer disease. Fate was apparently trying to make the point to me, because as I read the contents of the folder, I realized that nearly every single piece of information I had carefully catalogued in those medical school notes is appreciated by every medical student today to be absolutely wrong. Assuming just poor luck, I pulled a handful of other folders on cardiology, neurology, and endocrine disorders. Following that confrontation with reality, I agreed my wife was right after all. So other than saving a few particularly glaring examples, I lightened my moving load (and the bill that accompanied it) by more than 300 pounds of paper.

The fact is medical knowledge is expanding and changing at an ever-increasing rate and a key challenge for physicians today is "keeping up." To be effective in that kind of environment, physicians must be adaptive learners, questioning what they have been taught to believe is true and identifying the resources necessary to update their information base on an ongoing basis. Searching for new solutions to old problems is a clinical skill that finds substantial applicability in the administrative setting. In the management literature, we might refer to this as creative problem solving or "thinking out of the box." For the clinician, this is simply one of many "difficult cases" that require an organized approach to its investigation and the identification of resources to aid that process.

Comfort with Complexity and Ambiguity

Thinking back across my career as a clinician, it becomes very apparent that I have seen very few "classic cases" of any particular diagnosis. The vast majority of my experience in the clinical setting has been the identification of illnesses that have afflicted my patients but produced complaints and symptom complexes quite different from the descriptions I read in my medical textbooks. Physicians are faced with patients presenting a constellation of signs and symptoms, the cause of which is often not readily apparent. Sorting through complex (and often conflicting) information coupled with the appropriate application of "watchful waiting" and therapeutic trials, most clinicians eventually come to the point where they can say: "Yes, I believe that is the diagnosis in this case." It seems that few cases are simple and straightforward, and few patients have only one thing going on at any one given time. Having a comfort with complexity and ambiguity is, in my opinion, one of the absolute survival skills for success in clinical medicine. Why, then, when physicians are in an administrative setting where the next step is not readily apparent, do many feel unprepared to deal with the situation? Weighing both information and options is no different in the two settings; the discipline applied to conscientious decision making in both is exactly the same.

Physicians in administrative roles and faced with leadership or management challenges need to remind themselves that many of the skills and approaches used by a good clinician can be similarly applied in the non-clinical setting. When faced with an administrative challenge, don't forget to look in your clinical toolbox – you just might find something you can use.

Points to Ponder

1 How well are you currently managing your time, energy, information, and other resources?
2 How comfortable are you with each key aspect of your role and responsibilities?
3 In what ways do you believe clinical and administrative leadership can be synergistic?
4 What are the rewards to be expected from developing both clinical and administrative physician leaders in healthcare?
5 Why are clinicians and administrators often at odds with one another in healthcare organizations?
6 In what situations could clinical and administrative leadership work together to improve patient outcomes (or increase professional incomes)?

Clinical and Administrative Leadership: A "Case Report" by Dr. Perry Pugno

In the late 1990s while serving as a faculty member and mentor for a physician training program in management and leadership skills targeted toward medical directors, I received a phone call from one of the participants. As the director of a large multi-specialty medical group, this program participant called to say that he had been assigned the task of developing an intra-organizational referral policy for use among several of the sub-specialties. He related to me that despite a number of meetings, the individual personalities and priorities for each sub-specialty were creating conflicts to such an extent that the group was unable to achieve consensus. This medical director asked me to provide him with some guidance for managing this group and facilitating their achieving consensus on a policy statement. He remarked that the arguing among the members of this committee reminded him of the petty disagreements he saw occurring between his own teenage children.

Realizing that the physician who called me was a physician with substantial training in behavioral science, I recommended to him that he reframe his views of the committee members and their working relationships. Specifically, I said:

> "This is an opportunity for you to draw from your family counseling skills. Look at the members of this committee as if they were members of a large family predominated by adolescent children. How would you help that family come to consensus? Apply the same communication and relationship building skills as you facilitate this group of sub-specialists to help them achieve consensus on a policy statement with which they can all live."

I could hear the skeptical tone of his voice as he agreed to try what I had suggested. However, approximately two weeks later, the physician called me back. He admitted having been somewhat skeptical at first, but had tried my suggestion and found, to his amazement, that it worked! He had helped that diverse group of individuals (with no lack of ego strength among them) craft a policy statement that addressed each member's needs and priorities, and established standards with which they were all reasonably comfortable. The medical director said: "Once I started looking at this group from a clinical perspective, I found that I seemed to know just what to say."

Physicians' training is naturally oriented toward preparation for clinical work. So the challenges faced in administrative leadership roles may at first seem daunting. Without formal education in business management or leadership, physicians can sometimes feel unprepared for dealing with administrative problems. Fortunately, many of the skills taught in clinical training are applicable in non-clinical settings as well. Physicians benefit by recognizing the connections between interpersonal dynamics in clinical and non-clinical settings.

Even physicians who mostly work in clinical roles develop some administrative knowledge over time. For example, physicians in many specialties and settings are often involved in periodic hospital reviews by the Joint Commission on Accreditation of Health Care Organizations (JCAHO). In our observation and experience, physicians typically learn both clinical and administrative skills which can, upon reflection, have applicability for leadership endeavors of various types.

References and Further Reading

Birrer R.B. (2002) The physician leader in health care: What qualities does a doctor need to be an effective organizational leader? *Health Progress* **83**(6): 27–30.

Birrer R.B. (2003) Becoming a physician executive: To be effective leaders, clinicians must first adopt a new mind-set. *Health Progress* **84**(1): 16–20.

Linney G.E., Jr. (1995) Comunication skills: a prerequisite for leadership. *Physician Executive* **21**(7): 48–9.

Chapter 2

Overcoming Special Challenges Often Faced by Physician Leaders

"Our lives are not determined by what happens to us, but by how we react to what happens; not by what life brings to us, but by the attitude we bring to life. A positive attitude causes a chain reaction of positive thoughts, events, and outcomes. It is a catalyst ... a spark that creates extraordinary results."

Successories

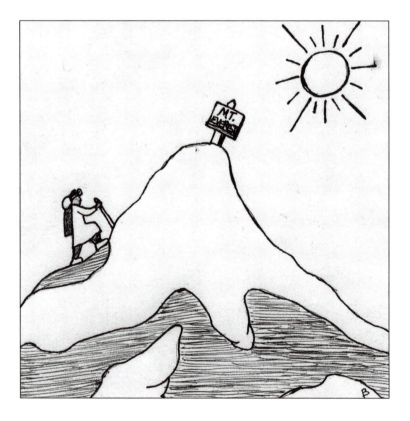

Many of the skills that make physicians "*good doctors*" (and good *managers*) include values – such as autonomy and personal responsibility. These values, however, can work against physicians who aspire to lead because teamwork and shared responsibility are primary values in that domain. As **Norman Kahn,** MD has said, "To equip physicians to become effective leaders we should send them to Mars and deprogram them from the cult of medicine."

While there is some truth to that viewpoint, the development of an emerging physician leader is not unlike that of a parent, for example, whose role must evolve as children grow. When raising young children, parents must be directive, supportive and proactively guide their children toward functional development. As children grow into adults, parents must change their approach and shift their emphasis toward positive role modeling, advising and encouraging the independence and self-development of their children. Similarly, as the physician leader moves from the clinical setting to that of the leadership role, change must occur.

> "Physicians cannot escape noticing how broken healthcare is. I'm not referring to medical advances. Health science isn't broken. Healthcare delivery is broken. Ambulatory care has been organized around the convenience of the doctors, not the patients."
>
> J. Peter Geerlofs, MD
> Family Physician
> Chief Medical Officer, Allscripts Healthcare Solutions, Inc.

In fact, as pointed out by Donald Lurye, MD, MMM "Management is neither more nor less difficult than practicing medicine, it's just different." Dr. Lurye further explains:

> "Being an executive and practicing medicine require completely different sets of skills. To lead well, we must enjoy the process as much as, if not more than, the outcome.
>
> When physicians address patient health issues, we try one approach. If it doesn't have a positive impact, we try another approach. In contrast, managers often deal with multi-faceted issues that are ambiguous or at least not as straightforward in the short term. Managers must invent unique new approaches for unique situations. Years may pass before we are able to assess the effectiveness of our managerial decisions.
>
> Another difference between leadership and medical practice involves the breadth of focus required for each role. Physicians, by training and necessity, focus on the health and well-being of one patient at a time. Managers deal with collective concerns of defined populations at an organization-wide or system-wide level.
>
> And there is a distinct behavioral dimension to leadership. Successful executives understand that governance does not involve yelling, whining, or overtly directing other professionals. Persuasion is important – particularly persuasion of colleagues to accept representational governance – where a subset of a physician organization is empowered to make decisions on behalf of the whole. This is counterintuitive for many physicians who equate professionalism with complete autonomy.
>
> Physicians often think medical background and general knowledge somehow equip us to lead fellow professionals effectively. However, in most cases, additional education and training are necessary. If we are open to new ideas and attitudes; committed to listening and observing; and willing to adapt our behavior, we can

make the transition to effective leadership. But many physicians won't, and that's OK. Not all physicians need to be organizational leaders."

Donald R. Lurye, MD, MMM
Family Physician
Chief Medical Officer, Welborn Clinic

Changes in Healthcare Delivery

"Most physicians are leaders by nature. The difficulty is when the doctrines we learn on the path to becoming a physician conflict with the business and market realities of leading an organization. I frequently see physician leaders, early in their management careers attack all problems as if they were an illness to 'cure.' Unfortunately, this often results in hastily made decisions. Taking a moment to look over all management options and searching for possible 'win–win' solutions is most prudent. I have grown to appreciate the axiom, 'There are almost no management problems so emergent that time cannot be spent reviewing all related factors and issues.'"

Roland Goertz, MD, MBA
Family Physician
President, McLennan County Medical Education and Research
Foundation

Fundamental shifts have occurred in recent years in the way that healthcare is delivered, according to Kathleen Montgomery, PhD. She points out that changes have come about in the way healthcare decisions are *determined* (from physicians' experience to clinical protocols and evidence-based medicine) and *accessed* (from patient self-referrals to gate-keeping). Changes have also occurred in the way healthcare is *organized* (from solo-practice to multi-specialty groups) and *monitored* (from self-regulated codes of ethics to externally-controlled utilization review). Changes have certainly come about in the way healthcare is *paid for* (from fee-for-service to capitated prospective payments) and *financed* (from individual and private indemnity plans to government and employer sponsored managed care plans). (Montgomery 2001).

Current political and economic pressures in healthcare are challenging physicians' long-cherished claims to professional dominance, autonomy, and self-regulation. Professional autonomy is being impacted by increased use of guidelines for care decisions. Self-regulation is being impacted by increased oversight of resource utilization in healthcare. According to Montgomery (2001), some perceive that one of the most important roles of contemporary physician leaders involves the protection of their profession from those pressures.

"There exist two very different cultures in medicine and management. Ministers and policemen are two other professionals with such a unique set of stresses placed upon them by individuals and society. Ministers, policemen and doctors are always expected to have instantaneous, perfect judgment in very challenging situations. People who don't understand that phenomenon don't understand what some-times seems like irrational behavior on the part of the professionals who must bear that stress.

The key that differentiates physicians from pharmacists or nurses is primarily the degree of independence. There also exists among physicians a level of paranoia and skepticism you don't see in many other professions. It makes doctors very difficult to lead. It stems from the realization that people's long-term well-being is impacted with life and death decisions.

It's a tremendous burden that creates a level of stress others simply cannot understand. Effective physician leaders can see both the laymen's perspective *and* can see the physician's perspective."

Randall Oates, MD

Family Physician

Founder and President, Docs, Inc.

According to a published article by Dr. Richard Birrer, MD, MPH, MMM, CPE, in *Health Progress* "Autonomy – the essence of professional status – actually works against physicians seeking to turn themselves into effective leaders" (Birrer 2003). Dr. Birrer goes on in the article to recommend that physician clinicians who want to become physician executives should:

* Create relationships based on shared principles and purposes.
* Commit to measured accountability.
* Learn to work differently. The fact that an executive has a title and power will not, in itself, compel others to respect and willingly follow him or her.
* Don't try to please everyone. Go with those who buy into the program early on.
* Think systemically.

These attitudes and behaviors are not necessarily easy to adopt, given the fact that they are not typically encouraged through traditional medical education or training. In fact, some physicians find it quite challenging to move beyond self-defeating mindsets and behavioral habits that impede them from making their full contribution toward improvement in the practice of medicine.

Moving from *Persecution* to *New Solutions*

Have you heard physicians described as whiners, victims, or egotists by other professionals or even by patients? It is easy to understand why, when weary of such destructive labels, physicians sometimes respond just as unproductively, with sarcasm or cynicism about managed care bureaucracy, pharmaceutical industry greed, hospital administration incompetence, or patient laziness. Stereotyping is never justified. And yet, we can perhaps glean insight from the labels ascribed to our profession or peer group.

Say, for example, you hear someone say that too few physicians possess busi-ness acumen or that too few physicians demonstrate leadership in healthcare. Would you react defensively and irritably to such comments? Or would you wonder why such statements had been made and ask yourself whether the stereotype might yield any insights for you personally?

> "Physicians can expect to face challenges in their quest to become effective leaders if they don't have the passion to explore innovative new ways to do business, or, worse, remain in denial about their own contributions to the problems in healthcare.
>
> Many physicians have difficulty thinking from a systems perspective. Often people who go into medicine are by nature single-minded, and then are trained to focus on one patient at a time. Many physicians are much more inclined to focus on improving their individual work or working conditions, rather than searching for ways to benefit the healthcare system overall."
>
> J. Peter Geerlofs, MD
> Family Physician
> Chief Medical Officer, Allscripts Healthcare Solutions, Inc.

Until just a few years ago, many people believed that physicians did not need business acumen or leadership skills. Few would make that claim today. In these contemporary times, physicians need leadership skills to deal with an increasingly challenging environment.

> "Most physicians go into medicine, and stay in medicine, because they truly want to serve people – to help their patients. Unfortunately, the situation in healthcare these days is tough. People become weary. We need malpractice tort reform. We need universal coverage. Those things are important. But they pale in comparison to the essence of medicine, which is about caring for people."
>
> Gary Morsch, MD
> Family and Emergency Medicine Physician,
> U.S. Army Reservist
> Founder, Heart to Heart International, Physicians Who Care and
> Priority Physician Placement

Challenges Faced by Physician Leaders

Imagine this scenario: The monthly staff meeting of the large multi-specialty medical group is just ending. The medical director has just finished pleading with other physicians to assist administration in controlling costs by minimizing unnecessary overtime for the medical assistants. Colleagues with whom the director previously had a good working relationship began to grumble. "He has forgotten what it is like to try to manage so many patients each day without adequate support from the medical assistants of the practice. He has turned in his white coat for a suit, and now he's become just like all the other directors we've had – demanding and insensitive to our needs and those of our patients."

When entering the realm of leadership positions, physicians often face challenges not encountered by leaders in other fields. The sad reality is that physicians who function as leaders in healthcare and other environments can expect to face special challenges simply by being physicians. Those challenges often fall into several categories:

"Just another whiny doc"

When physicians enter positions of leadership within the administrative structure of a healthcare institution, they may interface on a regular basis with administrators and other leaders who are not physicians. Preconceived notions and stereotypic beliefs by those individuals may "pigeonhole" the physician leader as simply another "doc."

Physicians are often characterized as individuals who routinely "pester" administrators for resources they feel they deserve. Physician leaders who are attempting to convince administrators to address unmet needs of the medical community may be blocked by stereotyping that hinders their credibility with administrators. Physicians can help to dispel, or at least overcome, such stereotypes by accepting a sense of shared responsibility and accountability for the current state of affairs in healthcare. This notion is explained by Jeffrey Kramer, MD, a cardiothoracic surgeon who is currently earning an MBA degree in healthcare leadership while still in full-time practice.

> "It seems, perhaps, to many of us that issues which are vital to our professional lives and the lives of our patients are impacted by forces over which we have little knowledge and even less control. This has led to an undercurrent of dissatisfaction with the practice of medicine.
>
> What are the roots of the problem? Surely many of the factors are beyond physicians' control, such as the medical liability system and the skyrocketing costs of healthcare. As a consequence, there is also increasing involvement of governmental agencies.
>
> Still, as physicians, we need to take an inward look to make a balanced assessment of the origins of this predicament. There is a great tendency to blame external forces for our misfortunes, but this is probably not accurate, nor particularly helpful, if we are to navigate our way out of this difficult conundrum.
>
> Only through an evenhanded examination of the issue can we effect changes in physician behavior that might positively impact medical care in the future. In fact, much of our profession's powerlessness is self-induced, either through benign neglect of important aspects of healthcare delivery, or through actual disdain for the non-clinical (i.e., socio-economic or political) aspects of medical care.
>
> **Apathy Toward Non-Clinical Issues**
> Most hospital-affiliated physicians would agree that the scale of control for medical policy has sharply tipped toward non-medical professionals. Not all may recognize, however, our own contribution to that trend. Physicians have traditionally assigned low priority to affairs not directly related to patients' medical care, such as committee work that affects hospital operations. Too often, we have left these important tasks to a handful of interested individuals – for example, not attending scheduled meetings or participating merely on a perfunctory level. Certainly, doctors are very busy in the care of patients, but these non-clinical activities are also of crucial importance. They are vital to the health and viability of the medical system,

and therefore ultimately to the well-being of our patients. Our apathy has often been interpreted by administrators as an indication that physicians' involvement in such decision making is not necessary. Physicians have largely failed to recognize the connection between their ineffective team involvement and the subsequent disenfranchisement from the healthcare system.

Language Barriers

Medicine's increased complexity and cost have necessitated the entry of 'third parties' into the traditional doctor–patient paradigm; a relationship which, on its own, is no longer sufficient to provide adequacy of healthcare coverage. These 'third parties,' with their specialized financial and organizational skills, are responsible for supporting the financial viability of our current system of care; they allow our doctor–patient relationships to exist.

Unfortunately, physicians have come late to the realization that in order to effect changes with the institutions responsible for the system's financial solvency, we must learn to speak their language. Imagine a team composed of mostly English-speaking members but with a handful of members who speak only Chinese. Very little would be accomplished – without good translators, at least!

Most physicians do not welcome intrusion of 'business people' into the medical realm. Similarly, most of the people charged with maintaining healthcare's financial viability have little utility for physicians who cannot appreciate the nuances of financial matters. There simply is no mechanism to address the concerns of both medical and non-medical healthcare professionals without common ground on which meaningful discussion can take place. Unfortunately, both parties suffer by the lack of dialogue. Neither party can perform its mission without the other.

As physicians, we must make the effort to learn this language and participate in a meaningful way. If not, we in effect abdicate our responsibility to influence decisions that directly impact us. Gone are the days when physicians can comfortably concentrate on clinical affairs and leave the business of medicine to others."

Jeffrey B. Kramer, MD
Cardiothoracic Surgeon
Kansas University Medical Center

"You've become a suit"

Physicians in administrative roles may be accused – or may anticipate being accused – of having abdicated their clinical responsibilities, leaving colleagues in the trenches to deal with clinical cases while they assume new administrative priorities. In extreme instances, clinicians may be accused of building "alliances with the enemy." This risk is particularly likely in environments where resources are scarce and the demands for productivity are increasing. Collegial trust may erode when one or more physicians challenge the status quo. These physician leaders may no longer be viewed as a member of the professional community and may even be accused of having "lost their souls" as physicians. If patients make remarks such as "Oh, what a shame that you're not a doctor anymore" the pain can be almost palpable.

Physicians have often measured colleagues according to perceived clinical skills, inviting or electing them into leadership roles based upon a reputation for clinical excellence. Why? Physicians have traditionally tended to *assume* that anyone who is a good doctor must be equally good at managing others. This, however, sets up a situation of pressure and conflict for physician leaders because the more time and energy we apply toward leadership responsibilities, the less time we have for maintaining and improving our professional skills.

Decreasing the time spent in clinical activities to increase one's impact as a leader can trigger a sense of mourning for the loss of clinical skills. In fact, many physician leaders' personal identities and self-esteem are partially dependent upon their capacity to continue seeing themselves as physician-healers. It is important for physician leaders to carefully evaluate any role change that has a material impact on their capacity to maintain clinical skills.

> **"When Management Meets Science: A Review of Particle Physics**
> A major research institution recently announced the discovery of the heaviest element yet known to science. This new element has been tentatively named 'Administratium.' Administratium has one neutron, 12 assistant neutrons, 75 deputy neutrons, and 111 assistant deputy neutrons, giving it an atomic mass of 312. These 312 particles are held together by a force called morons, which are surrounded by vast quantities of particles called peons. Because Administratium has no electrons, it is inert. However, it can be detected as it impedes every reaction with which it comes into contact. A minute amount of Administratium causes one reaction to take over four days to complete, when it would normally take less than a second. Administratium has a normal half-life of three years; it does not decay but instead undergoes reorganization via which a portion of the assistant neutrons and deputy neutrons exchange places. In fact, Administratium's mass will actually increase over time, because each reorganization causes some morons to become neutrons, forming isodopes. This characteristic of moron-promotion leads some scientists to speculate that Administratium forms whenever morons reach a certain quantity in concentration. This hypothetical quantity is referred to as 'Critical Morass.' You will know it when you see it."
>
> Source unknown

Shifting Gears

When functioning in leadership positions, physicians frequently find themselves challenged by the need to move back and forth from the clinical to administrative realm many times each day. The roles and priorities demanded in the two different environments are sometimes in opposition. This can create a sense of instability and stress resulting from the need to move among differing priorities while attempting to maintain equilibrium among them. This instability drives some physician leaders to inappropriately "second-guess" themselves, causing them to appear to have difficulty making decisions or to be ambivalent about the ones they do make.

> "Physicians focus on serving the immediate interests of the individual patient, often in the context of a specific encounter. Leaders focus on serving the long-term interests of the collective. That duality can be disorienting. The unlearning it requires is often difficult, even painful. And yet, the duality has its advantages as well. When frustrated by the challenges associated with either of those roles, physician leaders can find re-invigoration and renewal by focusing on the other."
>
> Deborah S. McPherson, MD, FAAFP
> Family Physician
> Associate Director, Family Medicine Residency Program
> University of Kansas School of Medicine

Concern that time spent in medical school was wasted

When physician leaders move away from their clinical roles into full-time administrative responsibilities, a question they must often face is, "Was my time in medical school wasted?" Whether having had just a short career in clinical medicine, or having practiced for many years, the question can be troubling. Many physicians experience a sense of mourning when no longer seeing patients. Some are bothered by the decision and may require substantial subsequent investment of time and effort acquiring education, skills, and credentials.

It is important for physician leaders to utilize their experiences from having been "in the trenches," and to recognize those they lead may be dealing with similar challenges and pressures. This clinical experience provides a perspective and context for decision making that are not accessible by non-physician leaders.

Points to Ponder

1 Have you closed the door or in some other way limited your medical practice? If so, is that a career direction you are comfortable with having made?

Reflections from Dr. Pugno

While writing this section of the book, I was struck by the fact that just talking about these challenges caused me to begin to second-guess myself. I found my self wondering, "Who am I to be telling other people, who are obviously more qualified than I, how to go about being a physician leader? Maybe I wasted my medical education by moving into administrative roles. Have I abdicated the value system that brought me to a medical career in the first place?"

Other Settings in Which to Practice Medicine

One physician leader who actively addresses the unmet health needs of the underserved is Bridget McCandless, MD. Whether working as Medical Director at a free clinic, serving on the Board of Directors of a Healthcare Foundation, giving lectures at local medical schools, or leading initiatives to help community citizens eat healthier and exercise more, Dr. McCandless continuously exhibits leadership in her quest to make health and healthcare accessible to all. And yet she recognizes the very real challenges experienced by some physicians when seeking to live out their professional or personal aspirations. In fact, Dr. McCandless points out several practical reasons that can cause physicians to forego leadership opportunities.

Insights from Bridget M. McCandless, MD

"Physicians often hold assumptions or perspectives that prevent us from identifying with the notion of physicians as leaders. For example, we may think that if we do a good job on a project or committee, we will be tasked with more to do.

We aren't inclined to see 'leadership' as desirable, partly because we like what is measurable, provable, and concrete, but leadership seems intangible. We may be ambivalent about leading others because we tend to be resistant to being led ourselves – we prefer instead to be the 'captains of our own ships.'

Because physicians have vastly different jobs, we have very different perspectives, needs, and priorities. This makes cohesiveness of purpose among physicians seem nearly impossible to us.

We have worked for years and made great sacrifice to get where we are. It is difficult to consider threatening our definition of self by making a change in our role identity. And we were raised to be loyal to our fellow residents and to our institutions. It would be very difficult to change our standing in the medical group without risking loss of respect from partners and colleagues, as well as risk of placing increased demands on their time through our own shift in focus.

So many things are decided without our consent regarding our patients, the care we provide them, and the compensation we earn for providing that care. Many of us feel powerless to impact the enormity of issues in medicine.

Most of us were confident in our ability to excel in medicine, and it is human nature to enjoy what we excel in. The notion of expanding far outside our comfort zone – learning or conducting business, finance, and advocacy – can be threatening and therefore unappealing. Physicians are trained to excel in short-term, case by case, crisis management. But most of us were not trained to develop long-term strategic plans.

There is great seduction in the idea of being needed and walking the journey of life with our patients. Physicians typically believe that no one could care for our patients as well as we do. We struggle to imagine chang-

Continued

ing our focus if it seems in doing so, we would be abandoning that precious trust."

> Bridget M. McCandless, MD
> Internist
> Medical Director, Jackson County Free Health Clinic

Other Challenges to Overcome

James Reinertsen, MD has also noted the special challenges often faced by physician leaders, pointing out five challenges in particular that must be addressed if a physician is to lead successfully. Those include the long-cherished custom of "professional autonomy" (referred to by those outside the profession as unexplained variation), the tendency toward cautious judgment – what Dr. Reinertsen (1998) refers to as "black hat thinking," the inherent tension between administrators and physicians due to the disparity of responsibilities held by each position, the specialized training that tends to encourage focus on the compartment rather than the whole, and the extreme reluctance of physicians to violate the autonomy of colleagues.

Drs. David Fairchild, Evan Benjamin, David Gifford, and Stephen Huot (2004) have written about challenges often faced by physician leaders in academic medical center settings. They point out, for example, that external funding of scholarly activities on topics pertaining to management, quality improvement, or finance may be more difficult to secure or may come from non-traditional sources such as industry or foundations. Furthermore, because promotion review committee members may be unfamiliar with the types of journals in which such research is likely to be published, physician leaders may be disadvantaged if evaluated by traditional criteria that is more clinically or scientifically oriented.

Points to Ponder

1 Do you know physicians who feel "professionally persecuted" or hold a "victim mentality"? If so, why do you suppose that happens?
2 Do you know many physicians who are actively searching for new solutions to the challenges faced in healthcare today?
3 What obstacles are hindering physicians from becoming involved in the search for new solutions to improving healthcare delivery?
4 How would healthcare be different if all physicians were to become more effective leaders?

The Issues are Real

The number of uninsured and underinsured citizens in this country is alarming. The incidence of preventable medical errors is tragic. The shortage of skilled clinical and administrative staff has reached crisis levels in some states, exacerbated in many instances by skyrocketing professional liability (malpractice insurance) premiums. That's why we need physician leaders now, more than ever before in the history of modern medicine – clinically trained professionals who are passionate about patient care and equipped with the leadership insights, attitudes, skills, and experiences to mobilize that passion toward significant, sustainable improvement.

> "There are no desperate situations; there are only desperate people."
> Heinz Wilhelm Guderian

The Difference is Leadership

Not all physicians are discouraged, cynical, or exhausted by the complex issues inherent in our current healthcare system. Some are actually energized by the challenges, and invigorated by the possibilities.

> "It has always fascinated me why one practice in a community could thrive and grow, whereas, another in the same geographic area, with the same patient and insurance mix, could struggle to survive. Or why one individual can become successful in any realm of activity, be it politics, business, or academe, and another from the same background struggles to get by.
>
> What is the difference? I think that the difference is *leadership*. In this context physician leadership is an admixture of several parts: vision to conceptualize what can be; energy to bring together the seemingly disparate parts; intuitiveness to surround themselves with others who can see the vision and take ownership; understanding that the sum is greater than any of its parts; and, an unshakable conviction that the vision can accomplish a greater good."
> Michael O. Fleming, MD
> Family Physician
> 2003–2004 President, American Academy of Family Physicians

Keep Things In Perspective

> "It's OK to fight for tort reform, but keep it in perspective. A lot of doctors are very unhappy because the practice of medicine doesn't align with their expectations. They're focused on their loss of control, the loss of money, the loss of prestige. But you know what? We haven't lost the opportunity to serve others! We still, more than ever, have patients who need us to serve them through excellent clinical care. Students still need us to serve through academic medicine. Employees still need us to help them do clinical research, or healthcare administration.
>
> The most important thing is that we serve others and make a difference in their lives, so we can go to our graves knowing that we lived and died doing the right thing. Sure, we can learn techniques

to improve our effectiveness, but we must start at the core, by improving ourselves first."

Gary B. Morsch, MD
Family and Emergency Medicine Physician, U.S. Army Reserves
Founder, Heart to Heart International

Points to Ponder

1 What challenges do you believe hinder many physicians from becoming more successful as leaders?
2 What sacrifices do you believe physicians must make to become successful leaders in healthcare?
3 What tips would you give other physicians for overcoming the challenges often faced by physician leaders?

Insights from William F. Jessee, MD, FACMPE

"I became interested in medical management back when I was in medical school at the University of California – San Diego. Hal Simon, the Associate Dean of Student Affairs, had a big influence on me. While in school, I served on a couple of national committees of the Student American Medical Association (SAMA). After going into the United States Public Health Services to give my two years service to my country, I became even more interested in medical management. Having partially completed a residency in pediatrics, I was assigned to an agency to improve quality in Medicare. That became my first real introduction to government and to management. I found to my surprise that I took to it quickly, perhaps because success in leadership is based upon good people skills – skills that are also essential for pediatricians.

After staying an extra year in Public Health Services, I accepted an invitation to join the University of Maryland as Assistant Dean of Continuing Medical Education and Assistant Professor of Social and Preventive Medicine while completing my residency in Preventive Medicine. My final project involved development of a state-wide CME Grand Rounds program for outlying (rural) hospitals which were referral sources for the medical center.

I then worked as a practicing pediatrician and emergency physician, and later held a faculty appointment in health policy and administration at the University of North Carolina – School of Public Health. As American Medical Association's Vice President for quality and managed care standards, I led the development and implementation of the American Medical Accreditation Program. I was also a founding board member of the International Society for Quality in Health Care and served as its President from 1989 to 1991. I've been President of the Medical Group Management Association since.

Throughout all of these experiences, I've a list of eight 'rules of leadership' that I believe are applicable for physicians; applicable, in fact, for people of any profession:.

1 No whining. Leaders are not victims.
2 Inspire followership. Don't command and demand it. Set the example that others want to follow. Be trustworthy.
3 Know where you're going. People follow those who offer clear and compelling direction.
4 Do things for the right reason. Self-serving leadership is a contradiction in terms. Serve a higher purpose and stick to your moral compass.
5 Be a change agent. The larger the group you wish to influence, the tougher this will be.
6 Communicate clearly, concisely, correctly. Verbally and in writing.
7 Listen well – without stereotyping or predicting. Reflect back what you heard, to clarify or confirm understanding.
8 See others' point of view. It's OK to have strong convictions, if you respect others' convictions too."

William F. Jessee, MD, FACMPE
Pediatric, Preventive and Emergency Medicine Physician
President, Medical Group Management Association

References and Further Reading

Birrer R.B. (2002) The physician leader in health care: What qualities does a doctor need to be an effective organizational leader? *Health Progress* **83**(6): 27–30.

Birrer R.B. (2003) Becoming a physician executive: To be effective leaders, clinicians must first adopt a new mind-set. *Health Progress* **84**(1): 16–20.

Fairchild D.G., Benjamin, E.M., Gifford D.R. and Huot, S.J. (2004) Physician leadership: Enhancing the career development of academic physician leaders and administrators. *Academic Medicine* **79**(3): 214–18.

Montgomery, K. (2001) Physician executives: The evolution and impact of a hybrid profession. *Advances in Health Care Management* **2**: 215–41.

Reinertsen, J.L. (1998) Physicians as leaders in the improvement of health care systems. *Annals of Internal Medicine* **128**: 833–8.

Chapter 3

Leadership Concepts and Competencies

"Leadership is the capacity to translate vision into reality."
Warren Bennis, PhD

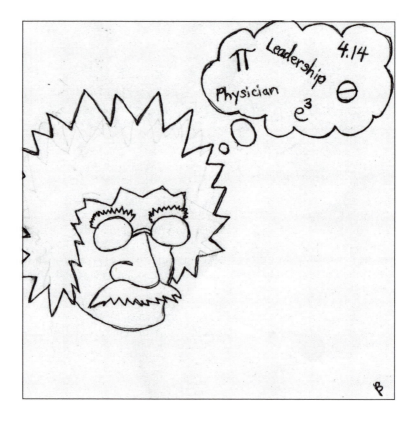

Perhaps you aren't yet certain that you want to "be a leader," or you aren't yet clear about what "being a leader" entails. As a physician, you are, of course, well-educated in medical science. Perhaps you've also received some education or training in related fields such as technology, law, or public health administration. Yet, if you are like most of your colleagues in medicine, you have invested little time and effort to study the field of business, the science of management, or the art of leadership.

Is that true of your situation? If so, before embarking on a journey to become an effective physician leader, you'll benefit from gaining a clear understanding of who leaders really are, what they do, and how some leaders (though certainly not all) lead well. That's why, without delving too deeply into the theoretical underpinnings of the subject, we offer you a bit of background.

Leading vs. Managing

Before deciding whether to embrace the mantra of '*physician* leader' you'll first want to have a clear understanding of what leaders *are* and what they *do* – not in medicine, particularly, but in general. We know, for instance, that leaders tend to have very personal and powerful attitudes toward the goals they set for themselves and others. Leaders champion change, often creating controversy with their out-of-the-box ideas and approaches to solving problems. Such leaders contrast sharply with conventional managers – who tend to view themselves as agents of their organization, encouraging people to accept the realities of their current situation and pursue accomplishment within the context of those realities. Leaders are often described as visionaries or change agents, people who get results by inspiring or provoking people to do what's never been done before. Managers, on the other hand, are usually acknowledged for their ability to generate predictable results through coordination of resources and processes.

Even the language used to describe leaders and managers reflects the distinction. We've all heard about great humanitarian leaders, spiritual leaders, world leaders – certainly not world managers. And yet, managers have their place. Who among us doesn't want a competent manager to serve as our project manager, budget manager, or facilities manager?

Managers help us deal with complexity by producing order. They organize processes and allocate resources in order to achieve predictable results on time and within budget. Leaders help us deal with chaos by producing change. They develop a vision for a new and better future, then inspire and guide others to achieve that vision.

Consider an analogy that illuminates the contrast between the role of a manager versus the role of a leader. We've all used a road map when seeking guidance for navigating through unknown territory, right? Or more precisely – territory that is known to our map-maker, but unknown to us. We benefit from seeing the situation described by one who previously encountered and assessed the place in which we now find ourselves, or perhaps the place where we intend to go. In those instances, maps are very helpful. Maps help us when we know where we're going, and want to follow the path of one who has gone before. Managers provide us with road maps for navigating through complex situations. However when times are changing, and we need to go somewhere that no one has ever gone before, there are no maps available to help. In times of change, we need a compass – a directional guide, a means of staying "on track." Leaders provide people a compass for staying "on track" in uncharted terrain.

In fact, many leaders have experience as managers. Such experience often brings helpful insight and perspective, and yet it sometimes makes the conversion to a leadership role somewhat more difficult when it causes the individual to want to "do it all." Peter McGinn, in his book *Leading Others, Managing Yourself*

(2004), describes well the importance of attaining a level of self-mastery before attempting to influence anyone else.

As you reflect back on the people you've worked for or with, odds are you would describe some of them as strong leaders and others as strong managers. We hope you've not had the misfortune of working closely with someone who neither leads nor manages well, although it does happen more often than any of us would like. In our many years of experience working with people of all professional backgrounds, we've observed that the people who exhibit strong leadership *and* strong management abilities are rare indeed. And yet, both leadership and management skills are needed for the consistent achievement of remarkable results.

Insight

To illustrate explicitly just how rare it is for individuals to be blessed with extraordinary abilities in both managing and leading, we tell you this: we have been working in healthcare, collectively, for well over 50 years. We've known a lot of managers and leaders. Suppose we decided to count on our fingers and toes, the number of people we've known who were truly exceptional at both managing and leading. Well, let's just say ... we're pretty sure we wouldn't need to take off our shoes and socks.

We emphasize this point to spare you the futility of striving for the often-elusive dream of excelling at medicine, and management, and leadership. Many of those who govern successfully take a pragmatic approach to deal with this phenomenon. They surround themselves with colleagues who excel in the areas for which they have neither the gifts nor the inclination (e.g., time and energy) to develop proficiency.

It's common sense, really, which we all know is uncommonly found in organizations.

The world needs managers. Managing brings order in the midst of complexity; it maximizes efficiency. Effective managers oversee tasks; providing the discipline of standardization, the systems and processes to deliver predictable results, on time and within budget. Managers use "maps" to help us follow the "rules of the road" and to keep us from "re-inventing the wheel." Effective managers preserve the status quo and keep things running smoothly. When benchmarks can be identified, best practices can be adopted, and milestones can be measured – evidenced-based management is vital!

And yet, in this Age of Uncertainty, the world needs leaders. Leading brings change in the midst of chaos; it enables attainment of the previously unattainable. Effective leaders are catalysts; providing vision, enthusiasm, commitment, and collaboration to bring about a better future. With unprecedented quantities of available information and a relentlessly increasing pace of change, the use of "road maps" is inadequate for navigating uncharted territory. We need leaders who use "moral compasses" to help us blaze new trails. In times like these, preserving the status quo is unacceptable, for our best practices are not good enough. In times like these, there are no benchmarks or milestones for our new and rapidly changing endeavors. In times like these, we have no evidence on which to base the appropriateness of our decisions or the effectiveness of our actions. In times like these – credible, clear leadership is imperative!

Points to Ponder

1 How do you believe leading is similar and dissimilar to managing?
2 What attributes do you consider to be characteristic of effective (and by contrast, ineffective) physician leaders?
3 Do you believe most physicians exhibit effective leadership – from the perspective of attributes exhibited and from the perspective of accomplishments achieved? If so, why? If not, why not?
4 Why do you suppose so few people are exceptional at leading people *and* at managing processes?

Are You an Effective Leader?

Glance through this tongue-in-cheek list of the *"Top Ten* signs that you may be an effective leader." How well are you doing at this point in time?
10 You may be an effective leader if you ... *Focus on both tasks and relationships*
9 You may be an effective leader if you ... *Can envision a better future for all involved*
8 You may be an effective leader if you ... *Notice what's needed and take the initiative to address it*
7 You may be an effective leader if you ... *Focus on helping everyone achieve their individual goals, so that collectively the group meets its overall goals*
6 You may be an effective leader if you ... *Use a variety of approaches to – motivate others, communicate, set goals, make decisions, and solve problems*
5 You may be an effective leader if you ... *Address both short-term and long-term challenges*
4 You may be an effective leader if ... *Teams you're on get results*
3 You may be an effective leader if ... *People follow your lead*
2 You may be an effective leader if you ... *Devote a significant amount of your time and energy to developing other leaders*
1 You may be an effective leader if ... *Those you work with become highly effective leaders*

Source unknown

Do you agree that managing and leading are complementary but distinct activities? Have you noticed that most people are relatively more inclined to enjoy (and be gifted in) one significantly more than the other? A few unfortunate souls find both managing and leading to be elusive; even fewer of us are blessed with the extraordinary capacity to excel at both.

"Managing" is the work done by administrators, supervisors, executives –

when governing the operations of an organization (or a department within an organization). The term "manager" has traditionally been used to refer to people in positions of authority for overseeing the work of other people – by hiring (and sometimes firing), training, supervising, and rewarding people, and for providing people with the direction and support they need to accomplish their tasks. Managers also oversee the utilization of funds and other resources – by setting budgets and controlling expenditures, and by coordinating use of supplies, equipment, facilities, and information. The world needs people who are good at managing things. We need people who are willing and able to manage meetings and projects, budgets and schedules, facilities and campaigns. Perhaps that is why most of the twentieth-century research into business and human behavior focused on the scientific management of organizations.

With the more recent interest in leadership models, we're intrigued to explore what exactly is involved in the act of "leading." While definitions vary, dramatically in some cases, several notions seem to be embedded within nearly all of them. Leading, it seems clear, essentially involves the act of envisioning a better future and inspiring collaboration to bring that future about. Leading can be done by anyone; it is not necessarily associated with a position of authority, nor is it always framed within the context of an organizational setting. We discern who the leaders are, not by their roles, but by their relationships. Leaders always attract followers.

Consider the world's great leaders – humanitarian leaders, diplomatic leaders, thought leaders, spiritual leaders, and inspirational leaders. We measure the success of leaders, not by their efficient oversight of tasks, but by their transformational impact on people.

"Yeah, right" you may be thinking to yourself. "I'm just trying to make it through each day, delivering the best care I can for my patients without incurring a frivolous malpractice charge, and making it home in time for dinner with the kids, and now I'm supposed to be thinking about world leaders? Let's get real!" We know, we know! Your work is exhausting, demanding, at times even demoralizing. That's *exactly* why you "need to lead" – so you can envision and bring about a better future, for yourself and others who matter to you. As you read the description provided below by Dr. Francine Gaillour, you may begin to glimpse the exciting possibilities available to you if you are willing to "follow your heart" – responding to your innermost yearnings and to the opportunities that arise throughout your professional journey.

Insights from Francine R. Gaillour, MD, MBA, FACPE

"I don't often think of myself as a 'physician leader' per se, though certainly my professional focus involves a great deal of coaching and advising physicians on how to be more effective, authentic leaders. My own professional experience spans over 18 years in healthcare delivery and healthcare technology business management, as a former practicing Internist, then healthcare technology executive, and now business consultant and coach.

My undergraduate studies were in biomedical engineering at the

University of New Mexico; my medical training was also at the University Of New Mexico School Of Medicine, where I was elected to Alpha Omega Alpha Medical Honor Society. I then completed residency training at the University of Washington. I am board certified in Internal Medicine and spent over 10 years in clinical practice.

In those years of practicing on the front lines of care delivery, I witnessed the whole spectrum of patient care: fee for service, managed care, private practice, staff-model-HMO; consumer-driven care, point-of-service evolution, and continuous break-through in pharmaceuticals and technology.

During that time I had always observed and was keenly interested in the spectrum of responses by physicians and providers to healthcare change (me included!). What led some to lead, some to follow? Some to innovate, and some to resist? And still others to courageously forge a non-traditional path? What were the underlying talents, passions, values, and needs of the physicians, executives, and clinicians in each camp? What inspired them to move forward, rather than hold back?

My own inspiration to become a leader and innovator came when I developed a preventative medicine program for my private practice patients. When I discovered that I could break out of my routine and become an innovative teacher of patient groups, it was a revelation: 'Wow! Even with a 100 percent full clinical practice, I am tapping into only a fraction of my full potential! If this is true for me, it's true for all of us in healthcare.' I was witnessing first hand the tremendous capacity of my patients to tap into their potential and transform their lives, families, work, and community.

So in 1998 I earned a Masters degree in Business Administration from the University of Tennessee and became a Fellow and Board Member of the American College of Physician Executives, the leading organization of health system medical officers and leaders. I transitioned into the business world, serving first as Medical Director for PHAMIS/IDX, where I was responsible for electronic medical record development and market strategy for the integrated delivery system market. Later, at HBS International, I held the position of Medical Director and Sr. Vice President of Research and Development, overseeing new product development, healthcare outcomes research, and clinical effectiveness programs.

Eventually I decided to complete my executive coach training through the Academy for Coach Training and the Graduate School of Corporate Coaching. I then went on to launch my consulting and coaching firm, Creative Strategies in Physician Leadership™, an organization that serves as a forum for the provision of executive coaching and strategic consulting resources for healthcare leaders in a variety of professional endeavors.

Officially, I suppose one would say that I am a certified Executive Coach, leadership consultant, and professional speaker. However, I consider myself a 'holistic' *advisor*, because I help physicians and other professionals and executives – within and outside of healthcare – discover and develop their unique gifts, talents, and strengths; leverage these to

Continued

improve their effectiveness; and ultimately, achieve extraordinary results for their organization and themselves. As a *business and leadership strategist*, I help executive teams and entrepreneurs understand what their organization does best and how to communicate their vision with power and authenticity. In healthcare delivery organizations, my focus is helping physician and executive leaders *manage and lead the cultural change* being driven by technology, evidence-based practice, and the growing sophistication of patients and consumers. I often speak and write for organizations across the United States, striving to lay a foundation for adaptive change in order to usher in the new era of professional accountability in healthcare.

As I have continued to develop myself as an educator, communicator, then technology product manager and health industry executive, my professional mission has become clearer:

- **My mission:** I am a 'holistic' advisor dedicated to transforming healthcare through my fearless leadership, laser insights, and creative communication.
- **My purpose:** I help healthcare leaders, emerging leaders, innovators, and entrepreneurs develop their full potential as business executives leading the way into the new era of possibility and accountability.
- **My approach:** I am a partner, ally, spiritual advisor, and co-strategist for my clients, helping them making their vision for themselves and their organizations become reality.

That is why, in all the work that I do – whether coaching or advising, speaking or writing, I encourage physicians and other leaders to live the authentic life you alone were created to enjoy. Tap into your potential – you have so much to offer! Don't settle for anything less. The benefits of expanding, exploring, and venturing out of your comfort zone are huge!"

Francine R. Gaillour, MD, MBA, FACPE
Internist
Founder and Director of Creative Strategies in Physician Leadership™
President and CEO, The Gaillour Group

Points to Ponder

1 How clear are you – right this minute – about your professional mission?
2 Can you articulate your "reason for being" (or at least your "reason for working") in a way that inspires others to join you in the journey?
3 Suppose you were to ask three colleagues to describe your professional mission. What would they say? Would you receive three vague and varied responses, or one response from all three colleagues?
4 The clearer we are about our mission and purpose, the easier it is to "know what to say no to." How clear are you about what really matters in your work – about what to accept and what to "say no to" in the myriad of opportunities (and distractions) that come your way?

A Brief Recap of the "Classics"

As the Industrial Age triggered work on assembly lines, experts Taylor and Drucker advocated use of scientific management techniques, while Deming and Duran championed total quality management (TQM) and continuous quality improvement (CQI). Behavioral scientists explored the mediating impacts of needs and traits on motivation and job satisfaction. Maslow proclaimed that people seek to address a universal hierarchy of needs, while Myers and Briggs developed a self-assessment instrument for classifying individual's work styles and thus their relative "fit" for various work environments. Yukl's description of nine tactics for influencing others and MacGregor's contrast of Theory X and Theory Y managers took into account the individual differences among managers and employees.

Organizations grew in size and complexity over the years, leading to a shift in focus toward the study of change (e.g., change experts such as Bennis, Beckhard and Beer). Peters championed service excellence, Porter identified three key bases for competitive advantage, Mintzberg offered insights on strategy, and Senge advocated the importance of learning organizations while Wheatley authored new insights regarding chaos theory and complexity science, synthesizing research from the natural and behavioral sciences, which have been applied to organizational effectiveness by Shelton and others.

Meanwhile, another trend emerged – dramatically increased interest in the study of leadership models, each with distinct frameworks and flavors. Hersey and Blanchard advocated situational leadership. Greenleaf emphasized the need for servant leadership, while Block championed stewardship as a framework for leading. Burns encouraged transformational leadership, while Weber and Conger investigated the power and perils of charismatic leadership. Covey advocated principled leadership and seven habits for personal mastery.

Leadership is clearly something distinct from the administrative executive role. Leadership includes any activity in which someone is inspiring collaboration toward a better, changed future. Leaders can be found inside and outside healthcare, from the world of "work" and also community leadership in community boards, government, church, athletics, neighborhood and school programs. Most people would agree with experts such as Jack Canfield and John Maxwell that successful performance stems from successful leadership on a personal level, regardless of the job we hold.

In fact, some might claim the key indicators of successful leadership include the ability to make a positive first impression, disarming demeanor, rapport building, empathy, trustworthiness, and perceived respectability, while organizational influences on leadership success include strategy, culture, values, and operating guidelines. To effectively lead teams of individuals, leaders are well-served to establish the team's purpose, set challenging, clear, specific goals, understand the team's norms, establish team roles, and direct the team through all of its natural stages of development.

Contemporary Leadership Models

In contemporary times, Jim Kouzes, PhD and Barry Pozner, PhD have long been respected for their research and expertise in the field of leadership. They developed the widely used Leadership Practices Inventory (LPI) and have co-authored several books, including the best selling book and workbook entitled *The Leadership Challenge*.

Kouzes and Pozner (2002) have been surveying thousands of people from around the world for the past several decades in order to understand the traits people look for in a leader. They've found that four characteristics are universally acknowledged as demonstrative of effective leaders. Specifically, their research has shown that people from all nationalities, cultures and industries view successful leaders as honest, competent, forward-looking, and inspiring. Furthermore, they have found that nearly all great leaders are consistent in their practice of five behaviors:

- modeling the way
- challenging the status quo
- inspiring a shared vision
- enabling others to act
- encouraging the heart.

Another contemporary leadership expert addresses the special nuances associated with physician leadership. Michael Guthrie, MD, MBA, points out that the art and act of leading physicians is unique in several important ways. He observes that leadership of physicians is unique because of social and cultural differences; that leading other physicians is challenging due to the professional selection, socialization, and training of physicians; and that much physician talent exists untapped and underdeveloped. Fortunately, he also claims that steps can be taken by individual physicians and by healthcare organizations to improve the quality of physician leadership.

Points to Ponder

1 How are the findings and recommendations of leadership experts relevant and helpful for physicians today?
2 What can we learn from the example of the world's great leaders – both inside and outside the profession of medicine?
3 In what ways have you been personally transformed by someone's leadership?
4 What additional leadership expertise would you like to learn about, or gain exposure to?
5 How can you make that happen?

Competencies as a Framework for Effectiveness

"Certainly a leader needs a clear vision of the organization and where it is going, but a vision is of little value unless it is shared in a way so as to generate enthusiasm and commitment. Leadership and communication are inseparable."

Claude I. Taylor
Chairman of the Board
Air Canada

Effectiveness in performance, or the attainment of an envisioned future, has been central to higher education since at least the early twentieth century. Educators seek to help learners expand their knowledge, yes, but also their abilities. This is true whether the educational experience is academically oriented toward the achievement of a formal degree; professionally oriented toward the achievement of licensure, certification; or practically oriented toward the application of developmental experiences. Why? Expert performance requires far more than knowledge alone. Expert performance requires integration of knowledge, analysis, evaluation, reflection, and affective changes in beliefs, attitudes and emotions.

Many if not all of the accrediting bodies for various fields of medicine and management currently use the assessment of competencies as a framework to assure learning and change are achieved. Competencies are most often construed as the knowledge, skills, and abilities (KSAs) that enable people to know and do tasks proficiently. It is not easy to identify the competencies that may reasonably be expected from incumbents in various roles. And identification of the KSAs is just the beginning. To assess individuals' attainment of competencies we must be able to measure demonstration of the competencies against some universal, or at least generalizable, standard.

Six core competencies have been identified (by the Accreditation Council for Graduate Medical Education and the American Boards of Medical Specialties) as being essential to the practice of medicine. Those core competencies range from conventional domains such as medical knowledge and patient care, to somewhat more subjective domains such as systems-based practice and practice-based learning and improvement. Various organizations have identified competencies pertaining to healthcare administration and general management. Those competencies include functional proficiency in fields such as accounting and economics, as well as interpersonal behaviors such as teamwork and communication skills.

Competency assessment and development moved to the forefront of management research during the late 1980s. That trend permeated all industries, including healthcare. Studies have been conducted, for example, to identify the management competencies required in both ambulatory and acute care delivery settings.

The use of competencies as a framework for assessing and developing effectiveness in performance eventually diffused into the practice of medicine as well. Physicians began being evaluated not only through professional peer review and recertification, but also through organization-based performance assessment. Physician executive positions emerged in provider organizations and in pharmaceutical, medical device, managed care, and technology companies. And those naturally led to the emergence of physician leadership competency assessment.

Leadership effectiveness is mediated by use of various technical or functional knowledge and skills: intellectual, cognitive, analytical abilities; attitudes, motives, values; interpersonal behaviors; and personal characteristics. Specifically, effective leadership typically requires proficiency in forming and sustaining strong interpersonal relationships – built upon a framework of communication, teamwork, decision making, negotiation, problem solving, and conflict resolution. Though some of the characteristics associated with leadership tend to include innate traits – such as charisma, and various other know-them-when-you-spot-them aptitudes – many leadership practices involve acquired abilities such as business acumen involving accounting, finance, quantitative measurement, operational management, and deep understanding of key stakeholders' markets or industries.

Physician Core Competencies

So, you may be wondering, what does competency assessment and development have to do with physician leaders? In late 1999, the Accreditation Council for Graduate Medical Education (ACGME) approved new minimum requirements for medical residency programs. These changes resulted from an *Outcome Project* in which the Council began mandating that medical residency programs assess participants' competencies in six core areas and demonstrate provision of educational experiences that enable medical residents to develop those competencies. There are six core competencies, which apply to all 26 allopathic and osteopathic medical specialties in the United States:

1 **Patient Care:** "Residents must be able to provide patient care that is compassionate, appropriate and effective for the treatment of health problems and the promotion of health."
2 **Medical Knowledge:** "Residents must demonstrate knowledge about established and evolving biomedical, clinical and cognitive (e.g., epidemiological and social-behavioral) sciences and the application of this knowledge to patient care."
3 **Practice-based Learning and Improvement:** "Residents must be able to investigate and evaluate their patient care practices, appraise and assimilate scientific evidence, improve their patient care practices."
4 **Interpersonal and Communication Skills:** "Residents must be able to demonstrate interpersonal and communication skills that result in effective information exchange and teaming with patients, their patients' families and professional associates."
5 **Professionalism:** "Residents must demonstrate a commitment to carrying out professional responsibilities, adherence to ethical principles and sensitivity to a diverse patient population."
6 **System-Based Practice:** "Residents must demonstrate an awareness of and responsiveness to the larger context and system of healthcare, and the ability to call on system resources to provide care that is of optimal value."

Assessment of those six core competencies typically involves use of self-scored ratings, expert observation, and standardized measurements. Regardless of the method used, residency programs must now demonstrate use of dependable measures to assess residents' competence in the six core areas. Furthermore, programs must have in place specific mechanisms for providing regular and timely performance feedback to residents. And finally, assessment findings must be applied toward residents' achievement of progressively improving proficiency. Assessment instruments and approaches should allow sound inferences regarding what the learners know, believe and can do in defined contexts. Assisting physicians-in-training to achieve these competencies is one of the most important interventions that teaching institutions can contribute to their education. The development of a proficient medical staff with strong communication skills is an exceptionally powerful marketing strategy for any hospital (McKenna and Pugno 2002).

Other Competency Models in Healthcare

Of significance to note, once the ACGME published its list of competencies, the American Boards of Medical Specialties (ABMS) adopted the ACGME's core competencies as a framework for certification and the LCME adopted it for pre-doctoral education. We also understand that competencies are being considered for incorporation in the MCAT exam though this has not yet been confirmed.

The Accreditation Council for Graduate Medical Education (ACGME) is certainly not alone in its focus on competencies. Many if not most of the organizations and associations responsible for leadership development – within and beyond healthcare – have identified skill domains, bodies of knowledge, or other competency-based designations to describe the essential capabilities their members or participants should exhibit.

The American College of Medical Practice Executives (ACMPE) is the organization responsible for board certification of medical practice professionals – most often those in medical group practice positions such as office manager or group administrator. The ACMPE has identified eight core competencies as necessary for effective performance. Calling the competencies 'bodies of knowledge', the ACMPE focuses on:

1 financial management
2 human resources management
3 planning and marketing
4 information management
5 risk management skills
6 governance and organizational dynamics
7 business and clinical operations skills
8 professional responsibility skills.

The American College of Healthcare Executives (ACHE) has also identified competencies for leaders in healthcare, focusing on these 10 areas:

1 governance and organization
2 planning and marketing
3 human resources
4 financial and assets management
5 plant and facility management

 6 healthcare financial information management
 7 management
 8 quality assessment and improvement
 9 government regulations and the law
10 organizational arrangements and relationships.

The Healthcare Financial Management Association (HFMA) has identified eight competency domains:

1 strategic thinking
2 systems thinking
3 results orientation
4 collaborative decision making
5 action orientation
6 champion of business thinking
7 coaching and mentoring
8 influence.

Similarly, the Council on Linkage Between Academic and Public Health Practice (CLAPHP) has identified eight competency domains:

1 analytic assessment skills
2 policy development/program
3 communication skills
4 cultural competency skills
5 community dimensions of practice
6 basic public health skills
7 financial planning and management
8 leadership and systems thinking.

Health Care Leadership Competencies have also been developed by the Association of University Programs in Health Administration (AUPHA)/Commission on Accreditation of Health Management Education (CAHME, formerly known as the Accreditation Council on Education in Health Services Administration – ACEHSA), the AAMA, ACHCA, ACMPE, and various other healthcare organizations.

Notice the similarities among these lists? So did Counte and Newman (2002). Their research indicated a high level of agreement among practitioners and academicians concerning the competencies that are addressed in health management education, but also revealed many concerns regarding how competencies should be applied.

Despite a relatively high level of agreement regarding the competencies needed for leadership in healthcare, minimal evidence that such competencies do, in fact, lead to improved outcomes has been published to date. Montgomery (2001) mentions this and then points out that, "Nevertheless, the promise and potential of physician executives continue to be described in glowing terms, with physician executives hailed as a change agent for new models of health-care delivery. Data suggest that healthcare organizations are responding to these optimistic predictions with attractive compensation packages for physician executives that meet or exceed compensation for clinicians, especially those in primary care."

Points to Ponder

1 How would healthcare delivery be better if competencies were truly assessed and developed?
2 Which of the ACGME's core competencies do you have greatest strength in?
3 Which are you least comfortable with understanding or consistently exhibiting?
4 Which do you develop in those you seek to lead?
5 How do you believe physician leadership competencies are best developed or assessed?
6 If your answer is 'it depends' – what does it depend upon?
7 What competencies do you believe are most urgently needed by physician leaders?
8 Why do you believe that to be true?

"The Association of American Medical Colleges (AAMC) recently issued a report expressing concern about the information overload that medical students face today. In reading the report, I thought to myself, 'They could have written that report 30 years ago when I was in medical school!'

The fact is, despite the ever-increasing volume of medical information being published, most medical schools still use the nearly 100 year old Flexner model for education – two years of basic science and two years of clinical rotations. This needs to change fundamentally. We must quit trying to force vast quantities of information into students' brains, while ignoring the development of critical skills such as teamwork, finance, and organizational governance. We expect physicians to play crucial roles in quality and safety improvement, yet we do little to equip them with the skills or insights needed to do so. Most physicians realize that the situation must change.

The six core competencies required by the Accreditation Council for Graduate Medical Education (ACGME) hold great potential because they define the desired outcome. It is a step in the right direction. Unfortunately, there exists a long-cherished tradition of 'academic freedom' that allows faculty to teach what they want how they want. Bringing about change is very difficult in medical education.

That's one reason we need physician leaders. Perhaps, given the rapid rise in dual degree programs, and the increasing focus on leadership competency development and assessment by many organizations – ACGME certainly, and also ACMPE, NHCL, ACEHSA, AACSB, and others – the tide will turn and medical education will reinvent itself to meet the needs of today's medical professionals."

William F. Jessee, MD, FACMPE
Pediatric, Preventive and Emergency Medicine Physician
President
Medical Group Management Association

References and Further Reading

Canfield J. and Switzer J. (2005) *The Success Principles: how to get from where you are to where you want to be*. New York: HarperCollins Publishing.

Counte M.A. and Newman J.F. (2002) Competency-based health services management education: Contemporary issues and emerging challenges. *Journal of Health Administration Education* **20**(2): 113–22.

Guthrie M.B. (1999) Challenges in developing physician leadership and management. *Frontiers of Health Services Management* **15**(4): 3–26.

Kouzes J.M. and Posner B.Z. (2002) *The Leadership Challenge: how to keep getting extraordinary things done in organizations*. San Francisco: Jossey-Bass.

Maxwell J.C. (1993) *Developing the Leader Within You*. Nashville, TN: Injoy, Inc.

McGinn P. (2004) *Leading Others, Managing Yourself*. Chicago: Health Administration Press.

McKenna M.K. and Pugno P.A. (2002) Strengthen physician relations by helping residents develop ACGME-mandated competencies. *The Society for Healthcare Strategy and Market Development Spectrum*.

Montgomery K. (2001) Physician executives: The evolution and impact of a hybrid profession. *Advances in Health Care Management* **2**: 215–41.

Chapter 4

Our Research Findings About Physician Leadership

"Encouraging physician leaders is never more critical than during the undergraduate medical school experience. It is during these years that future physicians and leaders of the profession are open to ideas, challenges, and insight into what awaits them during the practice years.

It is unfortunate that there is a paucity of physician leaders to guide them during these times. Physicians in the academic setting have, for the most part, chosen comfortable invisibility. With few role models to

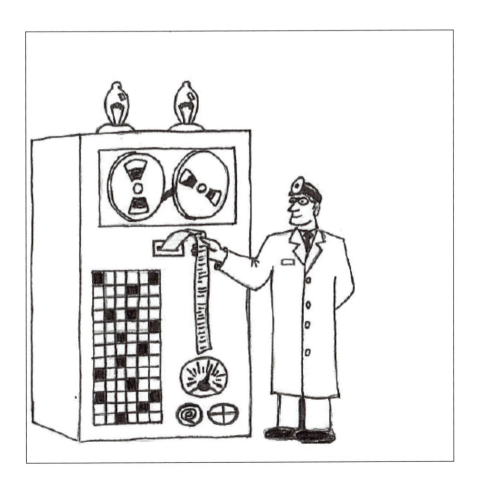

emulate, our medical students are left to their own devices. Later in their medical lives, when the need for leadership arises, they cannot answer the call and feel someone else should take the reins.

It is primarily for reasons such as these that the medical profession is left without sufficient effective leadership when it becomes necessary. A way must be found to encourage leadership from a very early time in the medical years."

Burt N. Routman, DO, FACOFP
Family Physician
Chair, Department of Family Medicine
Western University

Research Regarding Physician Leaders' Work Styles and Motivational Values

Despite a growing awareness of the need for physician leaders, we discovered not too long ago that minimal research had been done to understand the work styles, motivational values, or perceptions of physician leaders. Most people would readily agree that ever-increasing cost pressures and complexity in healthcare service delivery are fueling *the need for effective physician leaders* to guide policy level and organization-specific decision making. And yet, few benchmarks or best practices have been identified in regards to physician leadership abilities, activities, or attitudes. Physicians are being urged to help lead improvements in healthcare quality, access, and cost-effectiveness, *yet few physicians are properly trained or equipped to be leaders.*

Research Objectives

Because we were concerned about the lack of research regarding physician leadership development in medical education, we conducted research, along with colleague Myles P. Gartland, PhD, MBA to investigate the matter (McKenna *et al.*, 2004a,b).

We wanted to understand the work styles and values of physician leaders. We also wanted to know what perceptions are held by physician leaders, physician educators, and physicians in training (medical students) regarding:

- the *importance* of various *competencies* for effective physician leadership
- the extent to which various *activities* are *indicators* of effective physician leadership and
- the *effectiveness* of various *methods for developing* physician leadership competencies among *physician leaders, physician educators,* and *medical students.*

Research Methodology

Participation in the research was solicited from several organizations whose members include physician leaders, medical residency program directors, physicians in academic medical institutions, and medical students. Data was collected between May and September of 2002 via an electronically distributed self-administered survey including three brief assessments. We solicited 721 study participants from the convenience sample, including 172 physician leaders, 499 physician educators, and 50 medical students, achieving 110 study participants for an overall response rate of 15.3 percent. Though not an atypical response rate, we readily acknowledge that the relatively small sample size could pose a risk of selection bias, could limit the generalizability of the study, and may not reliably represent the population. Our research was exploratory, intended simply to begin to delve into these previously unasked questions.

Measurement Instruments Used

The assessments we used included two highly regarded behavioral and motivational assessments. These instruments are distributed by The KENNA Company for the developer, Target Training International Inc. The "DISC Work Styles" instrument is now called "Success Insights." It is used to measure study participants' natural and adapted behavioral styles. The "PIAV Motivational Values" instrument is now called "Workplace Motivators." It is used to measure study participants' primary and secondary values – those deeply held attitudes, beliefs, and commitments that explain why we do what we do. Extensive research has been done to verify reliability and validity of both of those instruments. See Tables 4.1 and 4.2 for a description of the instruments and the characteristics they measure or refer to the full description of their research in the article published by the American College of Physician Executives.

To grow and succeed, leaders need a realistic understanding of their behaviors, motivators, and competencies. If you would like to learn more about yourself, we suggest you complete the assessments referred to in this research. For more information, call The KENNA Company at (816) 943-0868 or visit www.kennacompany.com/physicians.pdf for special pricing available to physicians who read this book. KENNA Company also provides interpretation and executive coaching. Its President, Joe McKenna, is married to Mindi McKenna, and has over 30 years' experience working with professionals inside and outside of healthcare.

Table 4.1 Managing For Success (now known as "Success Insights.") Preferred work style descriptions.

Variable	Descriptions of Variables, Including Strengths and Weaknesses
Dominance	How one responds to problems, decisions, and challenges. • Likes challenging assignments, driven to attain results. • Poor listener, lacks diplomacy.
Influencing	How one influences others. • Optimistic, persuasive. • Impulsive, unrealistic, disorganized.
Steadiness	How one responds to the pace of the environment. • Patient, loyal, values the importance of listening. • Resistant to change, desires task completion.

Continued

Table 4.1 *Continued*

Variable	Descriptions of Variables, Including Strengths and Weaknesses
Compliance	How one responds to rules and procedures. • Well disciplined; adheres to high standards. • Bound by procedures and traditions; avoids controversy.

Table 4.2 Managing For Success PIAV (now known as "Workplace Motivators.") Primary motivational value descriptions.

Variable	Description
Social (SOC)	Values kindness and selflessness; seeks to help those in need.
Traditional (TRA)	Values unity, order, and tradition; seeks a system for living often found in religion or rules.
Individualistic (IND)	Values power; seeks influence and renown.
Theoretical (THE)	Driven by the pursuit of rational, objective truth; seeks intellectual knowledge.
Utilitarian (UTI)	Interested in practical business matters; seeks security and the accumulation of wealth.
Aesthetic (AES)	Interested in artistic aspects of life; seeks symmetry, fitness, and harmony.

Research Findings Regarding Physician Leaders' Preferred Work Styles

Results of our investigation regarding physician leaders' preferred work styles revealed that under normal conditions, *dominant* or *compliant* work styles are the most prevalent preferred styles among all three sample groups – physician leaders, physician educators, and medical students. However, the pattern does not hold true under stressful conditions. When under stress, the majority of study participants indicated a preference for *compliant* or *influencing* work styles, while *dominance* became the least prevalent style. Study participants' preferred work styles are presented in Table 4.3.

Table 4.3 Managing for Success DISC ("Success Insights.") Preferred work style questionnaire responses.

Context	n: Predominant Work Styles			
	Dominance	Influencing	Steadiness	Compliance
Normal Conditions	40	22	26	33
Stressful Conditions	25	32	28	36

Note: Some participants exhibit two preferred work styles, thus totals exceed the total sample size.

Research Findings Regarding Physician Leaders' Motivational Values

Results from our research regarding physician leaders' primary motivational values found *theoretical* and *social* values to be the most prevalent motivational values. In contrast, a*esthetic* and *traditional* values were those least prevalent among study participants. Participants' primary motivational values are presented in Table 4.4.

Table 4.4 Managing for Success PIAV ("Workplace Motivators.") Primary motivational value questionnaire responses.

Value	N	%
Theoretical	42	38.2%
Social	36	32.7%
Utilitarian	13	11.8%
Individualistic	8	7.2%
Traditional	3	2.7%
Aesthetic	2	1.8%
Unusable Responses	6	5.4%

Note: A total of 104 usable responses were received from the 110 study participants.

Conclusions Regarding Physician Leader Attributes

Our research indicates that many physician leaders, physician educators, and medical students are likely to perform best in structured roles, and may find the non-specific nature of leadership to be uncomfortable. This finding needs to be understood by those involved in the mentoring or development of physician leaders. While the growing availability in recent years of physician-tailored leadership development programs is encouraging, we are concerned that such programs have not necessarily been designed in accordance with the work styles or motivational values of the physicians whose needs they are intended to address.

Research Regarding Physician Leader Competencies

Given the marked increase in recent years on the use of competencies as a framework for assessing and developing physicians' and healthcare leaders' effectiveness, would you expect to find extensive research regarding the competencies needed by physician leaders? If so, you would be disappointed. For despite rapidly escalating interest in the topic of physician leadership, not much had been published regarding the competencies associated with physician *leadership*, or how those competencies are best developed.

Historically, physician leadership research has focused primarily on the physicians who hold executive positions – their attributes and the tasks they perform while in those positions. Only within the past few years has the scope of attention on clinical leadership begun expanding. At the present time, interest is rapidly growing in notions of physician leadership that fall outside the traditional administrative responsibilities held by physician executives in large healthcare organizations. For example, a growing number of physicians are helping lead the commercialization and adoption of information systems technologies, helping shape health policy pertaining to accessibility and funding of care, and helping reform medical education to better equip future generations of physicians for success in complex practice environments.

Research Objectives

We explored the beliefs held by physician leaders, physician educators, and physicians in training regarding the extent to which various competencies are perceived as important for or indicative of effective physician leadership, and perceptions regarding the methods by which those competencies are best developed.

Dr. McKenna designed a "Physician Leadership Competency" (PLC) questionnaire that was used to explore our study participants' perceptions regarding the relative:

- importance of various physician leadership competencies
- extent to which various activities are indicators of physician leadership
- effectiveness of various methods for physician leadership competency development.

Research Methodology

The "Physician Leadership Competency" (PLC) questionnaire that was developed specifically for this research asked respondents to indicate the relative importance of nine competencies for effective physician leadership, the extent to which 10 activities are indicative of effective physician leadership, and the relative effectiveness of seven methods for the development of physician leadership competencies.

The research was not designed to collect and analyze comprehensive, conclusive empirical data. Rather, it was designed to advance the field of physician leadership development – a field that is still in very early stages of development. By illuminating the beliefs and perceptions about physician leadership that are currently held by physician leaders, physician educators, and medical students, the investigators seek to encourage additional research in this important field.

Specifically, we wanted to understand study participants' beliefs regarding the extent to which nine competencies are important for effective physician leadership. Those results are summarized in Table 4.5. A full description of the research summarized in Tables 4.5–4.7 was published by the *Journal of Healthcare Administration Education*.

Points to Ponder

1 If you were to design a research project regarding physician leadership, what would you want to determine?
2 How would you design a study to answer that question?

Table 4.5 Physician Leadership Competencies: Questionnaire Responses. Extent to which each competency is *important* for effective physician leadership.

Code	Mean	SD	Competency Description
ICS	1.02	.157	Interpersonal and communication skills
ESR	1.10	.301	Professional ethics and social responsibility
CLI	1.33	.537	Continuous learning and improvement
CC	1.41	.527	Ability to build coalitions of support for change
CE1	1.46	.564	Clinical excellence
VIS	1.48	.580	Ability to convey a clear, compelling vision for the future
SYS	1.62	.624	System-based decision making and problem solving
MS	1.63	.699	Ability to address the needs of multiple stakeholders
FIN	1.83	.665	Financial acumen and resource management

Research Findings Regarding Physician Leader Competencies

We found that our study participants perceive numerous competencies to be important for effective physician leadership. Results revealed that respondents perceive "interpersonal and communication skills" to be the most important competency domain for effective physician leadership. Respondents identified "professional ethics and social responsibility" as the second most important competency domain. The competency ranked lowest by study participants was that of "financial acumen and resource management." (However, it should be noted that the average rankings of *all* nine of the competency domains indicated that they are perceived to be of relatively high importance to physician leaders, physician educators, and medical students.) We believe these findings demonstrate the perceived value of non-quantitative skills for leadership success in healthcare.

Research Findings Regarding Physician Leader Competency Indicators

When exploring the extent to which various types of activities are indicators of physician leadership, we found that our study participants perceive a wide range of activities to be indicative of it. Their responses indicate that a broadly delineated definition of physician leadership is emerging.

The notion of physician leadership appears to now encompass physicians who are engaged in a variety of roles and activities. In fact, there appears to be growing recognition that the term "physician leader" appropriately refers to any medically trained professional whose vision and influence are making a positive difference in the quality, cost-effectiveness, or accessibility of healthcare. In that context, physician leadership is occurring more often than explicitly acknowledged, perhaps in part because physicians are leading healthcare enhancement through a variety of methods – some of which are distinctly unconventional. Such methods may include, but do not necessarily involve, administrative responsibilities (e.g., sizable budget and staff) within a formal employment context.

We also asked participants to indicate the extent to which they consider 10 activities as being indicative of effective physician leadership. A summary of the responses are presented in Table 4.6.

Table 4.6 Physician Leadership Competencies: Questionnaire responses. Extent to which each activity is *indicative* of effective physician leadership.

Code	Mean	SD	Activity Description
IP	1.66	.655	Influencing peers to adopt new approaches in medicine
ADM	1.75	.725	Administrative responsibility in a healthcare organization
CE2	1.87	.755	Clinical excellence (exceptional patient outcomes)
VL1	1.92	.740	Volunteerism (e.g., leadership within a medical society)
TCH	2.04	.749	Teaching (medical school, residency programs or CME)
LBY	2.05	.818	Lobbying for policy, legislative or regulatory changes
PRE	2.11	.754	Presentations (CME or non-accredited programs)
WP	2.42	.774	Writing and publication (of studies or articles)
CR	2.63	.798	Clinical research
ENT	2.65	.944	Entrepreneurship (e.g., commercialize new medical devices)

Results revealed that participants perceive "influencing peers to adopt new approaches in medicine" to be the activity most indicative of effective physician leadership. The second most indicative activity, according to study participants, is "administrative responsibility in a healthcare organization." Conversely, "entrepreneurship such as commercialization of new medical procedures or devices" was ranked lowest of the 10 activities included on the questionnaire as being potentially indicative of physician leadership. Overall, results revealed that a majority of study participants perceive many of the competencies included in the questionnaire to be important for effective physician leadership and perceive many of the activities included in the questionnaire to be indicative of effective physician leadership.

Finally, we asked study participants to indicate their perceptions regarding the relative effectiveness of seven methods used to develop physicians' leadership competencies. Their responses are summarized in Table 4.7.

Table 4.7 Physician Leadership Competencies: Questionnaire responses. Extent to which each method is effective for the *development* of physician leadership competencies.

Code	Mean	SD	Development Method Description
MNT	1.35	.560	Coaching or mentoring from an experienced leader
EXP	1.48	.534	On-job experience (e.g., management position)
T$	1.78	.704	Time or funding (to support leadership activities)
LP	1.84	.664	Leadership programs (e.g., skill building workshops)
ED	1.94	.665	Formal education (e.g., MBA, MPH, MHA degree)
VL2	1.98	.692	Volunteerism (e.g., leadership role in a medical society)
SS	2.14	.737	Self-study (e.g., books, audiotapes, videotapes)

Research Findings Regarding Physician Leadership Development Methods

We explored perceptions and beliefs held by physician leaders, physician educators and medical students with regard to the relative effectiveness of various methods used to develop leadership competencies. We did so in recognition of the currently strong interest in using competencies as a framework for assessing and developing healthcare leaders' effectiveness. We believed the research was needed because, despite the fact that competency frameworks have been developed for physicians and healthcare leaders, there do not yet exist clearly agreed upon definitions of healthcare leadership effectiveness nor of the competencies associated with such effectiveness. Nor does much research exist to reveal the means by which physician leaders best gain the skills, knowledge, and attitudes they need in order to successfully affect positive change in healthcare. One thing is certain. Physicians are by no means assured of gaining such competencies through traditional medical education! Thus we anticipated that our investigation might yield useful insights for those involved with physician leadership development.

Results revealed that respondents believe "coaching or mentoring from an experienced leader" to be the most effective method for developing physicians' leadership competencies. This is not surprising, given the extensive use of mentoring in the current medical education model that all physicians are accustomed to. The second most effective method for development of physician leadership competencies, according to study participants, is "on-job experience via a management position." In contrast, the development method that received the lowest average ranking was "self-study resources such as books, audiotapes, or videotapes."

Conclusions Regarding Physician Leader Competency Research

Our research findings suggest several implications for those responsible for the development of physician leaders. Though the development of leadership competencies among physicians is now generally deemed to be important, minimal evidence has been published illuminating approaches that may reasonably be construed as "best practices" in this emerging field. The research findings reported here confirm other experts' recognition of the utility of mentoring and on-the-job experience for development of physician leadership competencies.

The fact is, traditional academic approaches that emphasize knowledge transfer may be appropriate for the acquisition of certain technical and functional skills such as quantitative analysis but contextually embedded, personally relevant, behaviorally-based experiential learning is essential for the successful development of physician leadership competencies. Time will reveal whether such learning will be mediated most frequently or most effectively through academic institutions or by the organizations that employee substantial numbers of physician leaders.

Note: Portions of the research were first presented at a Scientific Poster Session entitled "Physician Leadership Competencies: Survey Research Results" at the National Conference of the Medical Group Management Association in

Philadelphia October 12–15, 2003. The research is also cited in the following articles by McKenna, Gartland, and Pugno as listed below.

Points to Ponder

1 How do you and your colleagues define physician leadership?
2 In what ways are your colleagues' definitions similar to or different from your own?
3 What does this research imply to you about the need to develop physician leaders and the methods most suitable for doing so?
4 Do these research findings alter your beliefs and perceptions? If so, in what way?
5 If you were to design a research project to explore or advance physician leadership, what would you want to find out or determine? How would you design the study to answer your research question?

References and Further Reading

Bonnstetter B.J., Suiter J.I., and Widrick R.J. (2001) *DISC: A reference manual.* Scottsdale, AZ: Target Training International, Ltd.

Counte M.A. and Newman J.F. (2002) Competency-based health services management education: Contemporary issues and emerging challenges. *Journal of Health Administration Education* **20**(2): 113–22.

McKenna M.K., Gartland M.P. and Pugno P.A. (2004a) Development of physician leadership competencies: Perceptions of physician leaders, physician educators and medical students. *The Journal of Healthcare Administration Education* **21**(3): 343–54.

McKenna M.K., Gartland M.P., and Pugno P.A. (2004b) Defining and developing physician leadership competencies. *The American College of Physician Executives Click Online Journal for Medical Management.* Posted online 1/27/04 at www.acpe.org.

Section II

Physician Leadership Pathways and Outcomes

"It is tough to come up with names of widely recognized physician leaders. The fact that I can't immediately list recognizable physician leaders is in itself telling. We physicians lack leaders who can influence, thus raising the bar for the profession. Leadership is needed – individual or through professional organizations."

Randall Oates, MD
Family Physician
Founder and President,
Docs, Inc.

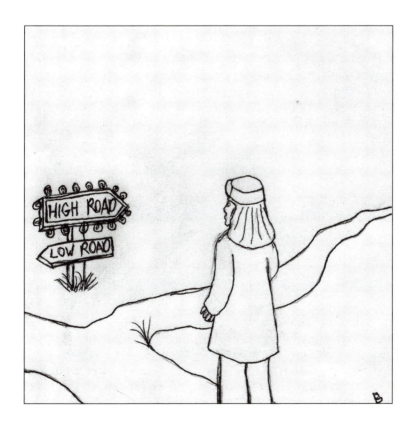

Given the strong cry for physician leadership, and the fact that physicians often assume leadership in community roles outside their profession, why isn't more physician leadership visible in healthcare? One typical explanation is the badly tarnished image of physician leadership roles. Some believe that no one in their right mind would voluntarily choose to suspend themselves in the vast crevasse between the fraternity of clinicians and the equally cohesive but distinct realm of administrators.

Another possible explanation is the apparent lack of definition regarding what physician leaders do, who they are, what they achieve, and how. This view holds that physicians may be willing to accept the challenge, but lack clarity in how to do so.

A third possibility concerns the scarcity of role models, the lack of reinforcing and supportive mechanisms to increase the likelihood that such a vocation will be rewarded extrinsically, with, for example, attractive compensation levels. Perhaps more importantly, physicians may not be attracted to seeing themselves as "leaders" because the notion has not traditionally been perceived as offering the intrinsic gratification that can come from the practice of medicine when it can be known with certainty that the effort made has truly had a significant impact.

> "Some of us are driven to improve the healthcare system. It's hard to know where that motivation comes from. Others derive satisfaction from helping individual patients.
>
> Pioneers don't worry about status quo. They're interested in what's new that could make a difference – perhaps a new technology or financing innovation. Executives, on the other hand, are primarily responsible for helping their organizations be financially successful in the next quarter. So they're under a lot of pressure to be conservative. But they, too, make an important contribution because they can help their organizations take bite-sized steps toward innovation and transformation. They are in a position to put the innovations into action.
>
> Sometimes unrecognized as physician leaders are the 'nuts and bolts' action takers; those physicians (and others) who by themselves won't change the world, but are open to taking the necessary small steps, one after another, to move us forward. Organizations would do well to identify these practical pioneers and find a way to mentor some of them into future leadership roles."
>
> J. Peter Geerlofs, MD
> Family Physician
> Chief Medical Officer
> Allscripts Healthcare Solutions, Inc.

We want to dispel the misconceptions that deter some physicians from pursuing a path of leadership in healthcare. We have no magic solutions, but do offer ideas to consider. We provide a model or framework for exploring several key types of physician leadership and include success stories from several role models who are making contributions within each of those realms. This information is intended to help you identify your abilities, define your aspirations, and determine the actions you will need to take in order to achieve your aspirations. This book does not provide a clear road map, for no such map exists. Rather, it offers a compass of sorts, a perspective-enriching experience and toolkit to help guide your development and strengthen your effectiveness as a physician leader.

> "Must physicians continue practicing medicine to successfully govern other physicians? It's an age-old debate. I do not believe continuation of patient care responsibility is essential, but it does strengthen our credibility with other physicians. And there is something to be said for living in your own laboratory."
>
> Donald R. Lurye, MD, MMM
> Chief Medical Officer
> Welborn Clinic

Experts and Executives

Conventional wisdom among clinicians holds that to attain a "position of leadership," physicians must first "prove themselves" through demonstrated clinical excellence. People who hold this traditional viewpoint believe that only upon being recognized as a clinical expert can physicians gain the respect of peers that is vital for earning the right to lead.

Some physicians aspire to become executives in healthcare – with sizable staffs and budgets and other responsibilities associated with positions of administrative responsibility. Not all do so because of a passion for organizational excellence. Too often in the past, physicians who were burned out and weary of the pressures associated with patient care transitioned into administrative leadership roles. This was sometimes fueled by a misperception that non-clinical roles would be less stressful or less discouraging. Rarely is that the case. When performing a role that feels foreign, the focus turns to career survival – hardly an environment for organizational excellence. And yet, some physicians have moved successfully into governance roles and gone on to guide their organizations to remarkably heightened levels of effectiveness.

> "One of the wonderful aspects of medicine is that it offers so many options for people. Some doctors love to do research; others focus on clinical care. Different directions may require different skills. Some of us gravitate to administration where other unique qualities are required. I've seen a few spectacular failures after such transitions which made me realize the importance of cultivating leadership skills as early as possible. And of course, we all specialize in our particular field of medicine. Doctors are well served by knowing our particular talents and by pursuing whatever fills us with passion."
>
> Monte L. Anderson, MD
> Gastroenterologist and Hepatologist
> Mayo Clinic Scottsdale

Two commonly held assumptions about physician leadership warrant examination. First, there is often an assumption that leadership is situated within the context of a "position" or role within organizations. Such a definition of leadership is quite narrow. In fact, many of the world's leading physicians are making a difference in the lives of untold numbers of patients without reliance upon a large staff or departmental budget. Second, there is also a commonly held assumption that the competencies needed for *clinical excellence* are positively correlated with the competencies necessary for *organizational effectiveness*. Some traits associated with clinical excellence can be applicable to the work of leadership. And yet, there are many differences between the work of clinicians and the work of administrators.

Innovators and Activists

Leadership to enhance clinical excellence and leadership to enhance organizational effectiveness are just two of the many types of physician leadership that are needed in healthcare today. A third type is leadership to advance medical knowledge and clinical care by championing, commercializing, and accelerating the adoption of evidence-based innovations. Physician leaders engaged in this type of activity are pioneers. They lead discovery or invention, or they help refine or disseminate new medical knowledge, procedures, practices or technologies.

A fourth type of physician leadership, less often acknowledged for its impact on healthcare, but certainly no less important, involves advocacy for reform of healthcare policy, laws or regulations. Physician leaders who serve as advocates for various causes or constituencies can often be found working in or with governmental agencies; in legislative or policy-making roles; as heads of patient advocacy groups; or as vocal spokespeople on behalf of various groups of stakeholders including healthcare professionals or patients, in particular, various underserved populations. Although activists may be underappreciated by those who view physician leadership as belonging within clinical and organizational boundaries, the path of the reform catalyst is as important for the enhancement of healthcare as are all other types of physician leadership.

The following chart depicts these various types of physician leaders, including the achievements they make, the actions they take, and the competencies they need in order to do so.

Suppose the Awards Committee of a leading medical society convened to review candidates and select a winner for the *physician leader of the year* annual awards ceremony. Imagine the conversation went something like this. "I believe LaTanya Williams, MD, deserves the highest honors this year. She exemplifies clinical excellence – serving as the standard bearer for her specialty. She is prolific in publishing outcomes from use of evidence-based protocols and serves on her hospital's clinical quality improvement task force. Dr. Williams tirelessly mentors medical residents; she has a reputation for being demanding but fair in her determination. I believe she is making a difference in healthcare by increasing the adoption of best practices among physicians in her own organization and in her specialty all across the country."

One of the other committee members quickly responded "Yes, LaTanya is a great role model, and an excellent clinician. However I would prefer to recognize the accomplishments of Carlos Rodriguez, MD, CEO of ABC Medical System, whose organization proves that it is possible to offer high quality

Figure II.1 Achievements made, actions taken, and competencies needed by four types of physician leaders.

	Focus: Organization-Specific	Focus: Non-Organization specific
Focus: Administrative	Type of Physician Leader: EXECUTIVE Achievements: ORGANIZATIONAL EXCELLENCE Actions: MANAGE STAFF AND RESOURCES Key Competencies Needed: SYSTEM-BASED PRACTICE & FUNCTIONAL SKILLS	Type of Physician Leader: ACTIVIST Achievements: HEALTHCARE REFORM Actions: ADVOCATE POLICY AND REGULATORY CHANGES Key Competencies Needed: INTERPERSONAL & COMMUNICATION SKILLS
Focus: Clinical	Type of Physician Leader: EXPERT Achievements: CLINICAL EXCELLENCE Actions: TEACH AND TRAIN CLINICIANS, PUBLISH AND SPEAK IN FIELD Key Competencies Needed: PATIENT CARE AND MEDICAL KNOWLEDGE	Type of Physician Leader: PIONEER Achievements: MEDICAL ADVANCES Actions: ACCELERATE DISCOVERY, INVENTION OR DIFFUSION OF INNOVATION Key Competencies Needed: CUTTING-EDGE KNOWLEDGE & CHANGE INTERVENTION

patient care while remaining fiscally viable, despite turbulent marketplace dynamics. This country needs more physician leaders who are respected both by their colleagues in the medical profession and by the administrators who run the operational side of healthcare. Dr. Rodriguez has proven that physicians can be effective executives, providing a compelling vision and aligning resources to significantly improve patient safety and operational efficiency."

As if the debate weren't already complex enough, a third committee member pipes up. "That's all well and good, but what we really need to do is show, by our physician leader of the year award, that we recognize and respect those who aren't content to simply continue on our current course. Healthcare is broken. We need radical change. Sam Hudson, D.O. is the best physician leader I've seen when it comes to serving as a catalyst for healthcare reform. He has done more to impact the laws and regulations that constrain our field than any other physician in the country. Not only has he generated huge media visibility for key healthcare policy issues, he has led our lobbying efforts with Congress and mobilized thousands of other physicians to take a stand on important issues so our voice is heard in Washington. Dr. Hudson envisions a dramatically improved healthcare system for our country, and through his leadership that vision just may be possible. He's made a believer out of me!"

Another committee member quickly replied, "I agree that we want our physician leader of the year award to symbolize our respect for change. But rather than bestowing our highest honors on someone who focuses on the economic, regulatory, and policy aspects of healthcare, I believe we should bring visibility to the accomplishments of a physician whose leadership is driving significant medical advances – breakthroughs in the science and clinical care process. Kim Lee, MD, has contributed groundbreaking discoveries through application of clinical informatics to the fields of epidemiology, genomics, and pharmacology. Dr. Lee is a clinical pioneer whose discoveries, inventions, and entrepreneurial endeavors will have far-reaching impact on healthcare for decades to come."

Torn between which of these physicians should be deemed "most deserving" of the top honor? If so, you're not alone. Most of us would find it difficult to select the physician leader of the year award winner from among these individuals. Why the dilemma? For one thing, we lack a commonly agreed upon definition of physician leadership. Many of us hold not just one, but several profiles in our mind's eye of the traits, competencies, and achievements – the profile, you might say – of an effective physician leader.

In fact, all of these fictitious characters represent an aspect of effective physician leadership. Together, they embody four distinct yet equally important notions of physician leadership – clinical excellence, organizational excellence, healthcare reform, and medical advancement. Our hope is that by more clearly understanding each type of physician leadership, you will develop a crisper conceptual framework from which you can make concrete decisions and take concrete actions to become an effective physician leader or to enhance your effectiveness as a physician leader.

Perhaps by now you are reaching some level of clarity about the type of results you aspire to achieve – the type of physician leader you are or hope to one day become. You may be wondering, "So what exactly would I do, or do differently, if I were in fact a successful physician leader?"

Points to Ponder

1 What are you interested in and passionate about – willing and able to do exceptionally well?
2 Which of these types of physician leader – clinical experts, organizational executives, reform activists, and innovators – do you most closely identify with? Why?
3 Who do you aspire to lead? What, exactly, do you aspire to lead them to be, or to achieve?

Chapter 5

Physicians as Experts: Leading Clinical Excellence

"Physicians face a level of complexity you don't see in many professions, and we've got to get out of the mindset of being superhuman. Technology offers great potential. Larry Weed, MD offers an insight. He says, 'if travel agents worked like doctors they'd try to keep all the flight schedules in their head.' The expectations of superhuman perfection aren't just held by doctors. Patients often expect it as well. I can recall patients who were shocked when I needed to look up the contra-indications for a medication – despite the fact that there is no way anyone could keep up with them all. Physician leaders know docs must now take advantage of tools and resources available to them."

Randall Oates, MD
Family Physician
Founder and President
Docs, Inc.

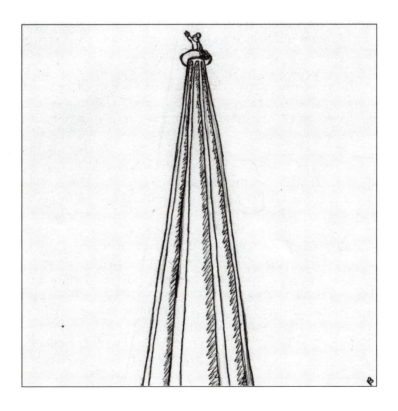

Some attributes that tend to serve physicians well are also likely to serve leaders well. However, the activities of clinicians are altogether different than the activities involved in leading other physicians to excel clinically. Physician leaders who aspire to enhance clinical excellence typically devote some portion of their time to maintaining their own clinical expertise – in part by providing patient care. And they are likely to devote as much or more of their time and attention to helping other physicians more accurately, quickly, cost-effectively, and appropriately diagnose and treat patients. These standard bearers are passionate about "raising the bar" in regards to the quality of care delivered and the clinical outcomes attained.

Leading Clinical Excellence Through Research and Education

Physician leaders who pursue the path of championing clinical excellence are typically involved in research and publishing, teaching, and training. Their influence on other physicians may be accomplished through informal mentorship of junior colleagues or through some type of formal responsibility such as a faculty appointment at an academic medical center. They may contribute to advances in their specialty by serving as clinical trial investigators and subject matter experts at new product approval reviews conducted by the Food and Drug Administration.

"I'm a history buff so I enjoy reading about physicians from years gone by. There are so many upon whose shoulders we stand! Understanding their accomplishments shows us how easy we have it today. For example, **Icgnaz Semmelweiss**, who discovered a way to prevent childbed fever, was ridiculed mercilessly throughout his career. When I began training as a gastroenterologist, none of us really knew what caused ulcers nor did we have any very effective treatment. An Australian physician, **Barry Marshall**, announced that he concluded from his studies that bacteria can cause ulcers. To say that some of our leaders were skeptical is an understatement. Now we know his insights to be true, and that took place in the 1970s.

The 1988 book *Doctors: The Biography of Medicine* by **Sherwin Nuland, MD** – Professor of Surgery at Yale – profiles over a dozen doctors. The book is not exhaustive, but it illustrates clearly what I've been saying. For example, the book features a French military surgeon named **Ambroise Paré** who worked with Napoleon's Army back when the accepted treatment of large wounds consisted of cauterizing them with hot oil. The patients would spend their nights in agony. One day the supply of oil was exhausted, and Paré noticed that his patients fared better. So he became a 'minimalist surgeon,' performing only necessary interventions. Another good book is *The Doctors Mayo* written by Helen Clapesattle. I am inspired by reading about these people and their great contributions to the tradition of medicine."

Monte L. Anderson, MD
Gastroenterologist and Hepatologist
Mayo Clinic Scottsdale

Evidence-Based Management for Evidence-Based Medicine

Physician leaders who apply their abilities and passions toward the advancement of clinical excellence often invest considerable effort in supporting the development, dissemination and utilization of best practice guidelines, seeking to ensure new medical knowledge makes its way into mainstream practice. They are likely to be strong advocates of evidence-based medicine and evidence-based management. As Atul Gawande, MD, points out, "Overall, physician compliance with various evidence-based guidelines ranges from over 80 percent . . . to less than 20 percent in others. Much of medicine still lacks the basic organization and commitment to make sure we do what we know how to do." (Gawande 2002: 236).

Physician leaders whose passions and abilities are focused on clinical excellence find this unacceptable, and actively work to address the underlying issues. One of those issues is the misplaced confidence that many physicians have in their own abilities. Gawande cites research that indicates " . . . the vast majority of surgeons believed the mortality rate for their own patients to be lower than the average" and another study that " . . . examined not just the accuracy but also the confidence of physicians' judgments – and found no connection between them." (Gawande 2002: 238).

Howard Smith *et al.* (2001), have suggested five evidence-based methods for increasing physician compliance with medical practice guidelines. Specifically, they recommend making the guidelines easy to access and understand, instituting a peer review process, offering immediate reminders and feedback, stabilizing guidelines, and educating providers about use of the guidelines.

> "A few years ago, while speaking at the Academy of Management, **William Jessee**, MD, FACMPE offered the following hypothesis: 'Management decision making in healthcare organizations, if based on external research and internally gathered evidence, can increase the likelihood of positive organizational outcomes as measured by financial performance, satisfaction (among patients, employees, and physicians) and clinical results.'
>
> **Dr. Jessee** then explained that evidence-based medicine began 30 years ago and has had a long torturous path to acceptance. Too often, physicians would say 'I've seen . . . therefore I believe . . . '. The concept of randomized trials, meta-analysis, and other tools of evidence-based medicine came from non-medical fields. More research is needed regarding the reasons underlying the gap between the existence of evidence and real shifts in clinical practice – say, for example, the use of beta blockers after myocardial infarction or retinal exams for diabetics. Why are some innovations quickly accepted, yet others are not? Evidence-based medicine is still not universally applied, but it has become the generally accepted mode for clinical decision making. Most healthcare professionals believe in evidence-based medicine, but don't practice evidence-based management.
>
> Referring to the work of **Tony Kouner**, PhD (Kouner 2000), **Dr. Jessee** described several barriers that hinder the adoption of evidence-based management. First, the author had written, managers often resist because there is too little evidence about best practices, and such

evidence isn't shared widely enough. Too often, healthcare organizations lack size and critical mass to conduct and assess applied research, except for the Veteran's Hospital Administration and the Department of Defense. Healthcare organizations focus on operating margins, and are thus unwilling or unable to fund needed research. Healthcare administrators typically lack training and experience in collaborating with researchers, and lack the commitment to applied research.

Too often, MPH and MHA programs have focused on knowledge transfer to students, rather than on helping students build the skills they need for lifelong knowledge acquisition. Not-for-profit healthcare organizations sometimes lack direct accountability for doing and demonstrating best practices.

To that list, **Dr. Jessee** adds three additional barriers that have inhibited progress toward evidence-based management. First, it requires too much work. Busy professionals prefer to act on instinct whenever possible. Second, leaders like to lead – seeking evidence, especially evidence published by others, can threaten our self-image as pioneers. It isn't trendy enough. Few books or articles are being published on the topic. Management education too seldom emphasizes the importance of evidence-based decision making.

In this realm, physician leaders may have an advantage over non-clinically trained professionals. Clinicians are becoming more aware of the value of evidence-based decision making. And when solid evidence is lacking, we bring experts together to develop a consensus. Perhaps then, as clinically-trained leaders, we can help our administrative colleagues develop respect for the concepts we have come to appreciate in medical science. I believe it is high time for both evidence-based medicine and evidence-based management."

William F. Jessee, MD, FACMPE
Pediatric, Preventive and Emergency Medicine Physician
President
Medical Group Management Association

Leadership for Quality Improvement

"Those on the cutting edge, planning the future of medicine, recognize that survival and successful growth demand an integrated partnership between hospital administration and medical staff leadership. As the Computer Age enters the hospital and evidence-based medicine readies healthcare for best practice outcomes, success in the hospital will be unlikely unless there are physician champions."

Andrew M. Schwartz, MD
Cardiac Surgeon
Vice President, Medical Staff
Shawnee Mission Medical Center

"Nursing doesn't have a lot of career advancement or trajectory like medicine does. It is important for nurses and doctors to work together.

Nurses are often good facilitators of teams given their clinical background. Some nurses co-lead quality improvement teams with doctors. To address quality we must begin by seeing the problems for what they are. Many doctors don't see it."

David G. Fairchild, MD, MPH
Internist
Chief of General Medicine,
Tufts – New England Medical Center

Leadership for Quality Improvement

Physicians' misplaced confidence in their own clinical judgment can be deadly. Gawande (2002: 198) cites studies that investigated how often autopsies reveal a major misdiagnosis in the cause of death. Studies conducted in 1938 and 1998 both revealed a misdiagnosis rate of 40 percent. Do you find it disturbing that the misdiagnosis rate is so high? Or are you more troubled by the fact that the misdiagnosis rate has remained constant for 60 years, despite significant advances in diagnostic equipment and procedures?

> "I meet with hundreds of physicians each month, and I believe deep in my heart that the majority of physicians have a lifelong passion for medicine. For most physicians, it's not a job, it is a calling. Most physicians have a deep love for patients; they genuinely care about quality and outcomes."

J. Peter Geerlofs, MD
Family Physician
Chief Medical Officer
Allscripts Healthcare Solutions, Inc.

Lack of standardized protocols and misplaced confidence aren't the only causes of medical errors. Inexperience, inadequately designed technology and techniques, and insufficient staffing and teamwork also contribute. Physician leaders who advocate clinical excellence among colleagues are often at the forefront of quality improvement movements and other initiatives designed to address these concerns.

An example of such leadership can be found in the field of anesthesiology, as described by Dr. Gawande (2002: 64–8). In 1982, anesthesiologist Ellison (Jeep) Pierce, MD was elected vice president of the American Society of Anesthesiologists and turned for help to Jeffrey Cooper, a bio-engineer at Massachusetts General Hospital. By analyzing mishaps and identifying methods to reduce the problems that led to them, then publishing the findings and sponsoring conferences to address the issues, they enabled remarkable improvements in anesthesiology success rates. Anesthesiology residents' hours were shortened, machines were redesigned to be more "goof-proof," procedures were modified, and anesthesiologists were trained to adopt those new "best practices." Physician leaders who will champion initiatives like this are needed in every medical specialty.

> "If you have knowledge, let others light their candles at it."

Thomas Fuller

Physician Leaders as Standard Bearers

Some physicians remain focused throughout their professional lives on maintaining a level of clinical excellence that enables them to care for their own patients with the utmost quality. This is a noble path and all of us who are "patients" at various points in our lives must be grateful for their devotion.

Clinical Experts as Leaders

Physician *leaders* who serve as standard bearers for clinical excellence take the passion for excellence a step further. These leaders find ways to enhance clinical excellence across their specialty, their organization, or in cross-disciplinary fields. These leaders accept responsibility for focusing, day in and day out, on helping colleagues enhance their clinical acumen.

Physician leaders are committed to the achievement of positive health outcomes – not only for their own patients, but for patients overall. This involves the investment of time and effort to understand and address the barriers that are preventing physicians from adopting the best practices in any given field. Physicians who are serious about improving clinical excellence across their specialty or across all specialties are likely to be vocal champions of evidence-based management and all other techniques by which best practice protocols are developed and widely adopted.

> "A physician whose leadership I respect is **Paul Farmer, MD**. In the book *Mountains Beyond Mountains: Healing the World – the Quest of Dr. Paul Farmer*, author **Tracy Kidder** wrote about Dr. Farmer's work at the **Partners in Health** hospital he founded in Haiti. **Dr. Farmer's passion** is treatment of tuberculosis in places where drug-resistant TB is emerging such as jails and underdeveloped countries within Africa and South America. **Dr. Farmer** earned a large grant from the Bill Gates Foundation and has received publicity in the *New York Times* for his work in infectious diseases."
>
> David G. Fairchild, MD, MPH
> Internist
> Chief of General Medicine
> Tufts – New England Medical Center

What competencies are required for successful leadership of clinical programs in particular? According to Joseph Spallina, FACHE, FAAHC, (2002) effective clinical leadership requires:

- operational and clinical research expertise
- service and technology evaluation and design
- organizational management
- financial and business planning, evaluation, and management
- quality assessment process design and management
- information systems management
- strategic planning
- physician relations management

- marketing and promotions
- facility programming and planning.

A physician who understands the power of collaboration and applies it toward advancing the emerging field of sleep disorders is Steven Hull, MD, FCCP, FAASM. Whether overseeing clinical trials, seeing patients of his own, giving presentations to physicians or the public, Dr. Hull seeks out every opportunity to advocate greater emphasis on what he believes to be an underemphasized field of medicine. Given his passion and dedication to the specialty, Dr. Hull could rightly be described as "a man with a mission."

Insights from Steven G. Hull, MD, FCCP, FAASM

"When I entered medical school, it didn't occur to me that I'd end up specializing in sleep disorders. I'd grown up in a small town in Illinois (Pinckneyville, total population of 3,000). I went to **Southern Illinois University School of Medicine**, then to the **University of Illinois** for my internship and residency, and **Kansas University Medical Center** for Pulmonary and Critical Care.

I began working at **Kaiser Permanente** in Kansas City following my fellowship training and within six months I became Chief of Internal Medicine. Kaiser was committed to the development of its leaders, and funded my participation in an **'Advanced Leadership Program' at the University of North Carolina**, which was an intensive executive education program consisting of three two-week blocks in residence and project work between those blocks, all completed during an eight month time period. Through that program I learned about the human side of leadership and governance. I also learned about the business of medicine, and gained skills in marketing, finance, operations, and strategy – all of which contribute to my effectiveness as a leader and as a clinician. Later, I became the Director of Quality and Risk Management at **Kaiser**, followed by my last position as Associate Medical Director.

When **Kaiser** was sold locally to **Coventry Health Care** my job was eliminated, and I was recruited to be the Medical Director for **somniTech, Inc.** – an organization that specializes in the research, treatment, and prevention of sleep disorders. I oversee large-scale clinical trials and oversee the day-to-day operations of our sleep labs located around the country. The work includes a great deal of variety, which I enjoy, and allows me to see patients without feeling pressure to rush the encounters that many physicians must face these days. I also spend a significant portion of my time educating other clinicians and consumers/patients about sleep disorders.

I am self-taught in the field of sleep disorders, with supplemental training from the **Stanford School of Sleep Medicine** and the **Atlanta School of Sleep Medicine**. I became a 'Diplomat' (board certified) in the specialty partly because it was a way of continuously developing my clinical expertise, and partly because I believe I have a responsibility to be a good role model for

Continued

deep medical knowledge in one's specialty. Just 2300 physicians worldwide are board certified in sleep disorders. That number does not remotely begin to meet the demand of the field.

Not all physicians aspire to be 'leaders' in their specialty. Some are simply focused on the excellent delivery of high quality care for their patients. The world needs physicians like that. But those of us who want to contribute significant advances in medical research and in healthcare delivery must invest extra time and effort to gain a variety of skills and insights beyond the traditional clinical role. We can do that by reading the medical and management literature, by being actively involved in our medical specialty associations, and by conducting research and sharing our findings through publications, speaking and mentoring others in our field.

My passion encompasses the provision of great care for my own patients, and the enhancement of healthcare in ways that benefit far more patients than any one physician could ever personally treat."

Steven G. Hull, MD, FCCP, FAASM
Internist and sleep medicine specialist
Medical Director, somniTech, Inc.

Dr. Hull offers us insights through his example. He demonstrates how a leading physician can make an impact in healthcare through the application of clinical expertise. While Dr. Hull has a very clear clinical focus, he's invested extra effort to equip himself with additional skills beyond those used in traditional clinical care. Such is the path of the "clinical expert" physician leader. Their skills are, of necessity, quite broad – ranging from strategic decision making to operational management, from public speaking to scientific research.

Reverend Harris, MD, tells about another physician whose leadership has advanced clinical excellence and improved outcomes for patients:

"**Paul Brand,** MD, was a physician missionary to India until he passed away in 2003. He was a true pioneer in medicine. As a surgeon, he restored hand function. Dr. Brand significantly advanced our understanding of the pathophysiology of leprosy. In his book *The Gift of Pain* with co-author **Philip Yancey**, Dr. Brand explained that pain is good by sharing an example from his work with lepers in India. Because the patients were unable to feel pain, they didn't realize when rats ate off their fingers and toes in the middle of the night. So Dr. Brand hit upon a practical alternative. He used kittens to ward off the rats, an approach now referred to as 'kitten therapy.' That approach, combined with visual inspection to identify infection, enabled earlier treatment and helped many leprosy patients avoid preventable loss of digits."

Reverend Pamela S. Harris, MD
Physical Medicine and Rehabilitation Physician
Kansas City Veteran's Administration Hospital
and Minister of Health
United Methodist Church of the Resurrection

Physician leaders who promote clinical excellence are often characterized by a clinical curiosity that is both intense and sustained. Such leaders respect the value of board certification and other mechanisms by which expertise is assured within their specialty or within all clinical specialties.

Highly effective physician leaders are distinguished by their focus on continuously monitoring, evaluating and improving the clinical effectiveness of other physicians. In doing so, they improve the clinical outcomes of many patients, not just those they personally treat. Sometimes clinical excellence is advanced simply by exposing physicians to new and better clinical procedures, protocols or pathways. Often, however, clinical leadership involves helping physicians change their suboptimal behaviors in order to improve their effectiveness. At times that is not easy.

Points to Ponder

1 What are you interested in and passionate about?
2 What are you willing and able to do exceptionally well?
3 Which of the types of physician leaders described here – clinical experts, organizational executives, reform activists, or innovators – do you most closely identify with? Why?
4 Which of the four types of contribution described here – clinical excellence, organizational excellence, healthcare reform, or advances in medicine – do you aspire to achieve?
5 Who exactly do you lead, or aspire to lead, one day?
6 What exactly do you or will you lead those people to be, to do, or to achieve?
7 How can comparing ourselves to others impede our likelihood of fulfilling our own unique capacity for contributions in healthcare?
8 To whom do you compare yourself?
9 How does comparing yourself to others help or hinder your progress toward becoming a more successful physician leader?

References and Further Reading

Anonymous (2002) Physician leadership: More than clinical excellence. *Health Leaders* Sponsored Supplement, October. RT2–RT15.

Berwick D.M. (1994) Eleven worthy aims for clinical leadership of health systems reform. *Journal of the American Medical Association* **272**: 797–802.

Brand P.W. and Yancey P. (1993) *The Gift of Pain*. Grand Rapids, MI: Zondervan Publishing House.

Clapesattle H. (2003) *The Doctor's Mayo*. Minneapolis, MN: Mayo Clinic Health Management.

Gawande A. (2002) *Complications: a surgeon's note on an imperfect science*. New York: Picador, Henry Holt and Company.

Kidder T. (2003) *Mountains Beyond Mountains: Healing the World. The Quest of Dr. Paul Farmer*. New York: Random House.

Kouner T., *et al.* (2000) *Frontiers of Health Services Management* **16**(4): 3–24 as quoted by William F. Jessee, FACMPE, FACPM, in his presentation *Does Management Affect Healthcare*

Outcomes? What's the Evidence? at the Health Care Management Division session of the Academy of Management annual conference in Washington, D.C. on August 12, 2002.

Nuland S.B. (1988) *Doctors: The biography of medicine*. New York: Random House.

Smith H.L., Yourstone S., Lorber D. and Mann B. (2001) Managed care and medical practice guidelines: The thorny problem of attaining physician compliance. *Advances in Health Care Management* **2**: 93–118.

Spallina J.M. (2002) Organizing clinical programs: Requirements for contemporary leaders and successful organizations. *Spectrum* 8–9.

Chapter 6

Physicians as Executives: Leading Organizational Excellence

"A recent survey of workers across the United States revealed that nearly 85 percent of those interviewed said they could work harder on the job. More than half claimed they could double their effectiveness 'if they wanted to.'"

John Maxwell

Organizational Leadership

While some physician leaders apply their abilities and interests toward the advancement of clinical excellence, others focus on the organizational processes that are necessary for the consistent delivery of accessible, affordable, quality

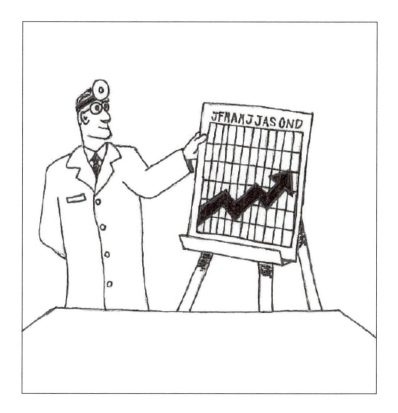

care. They recognize that healthcare providers must generate enough revenue to sustain operations, as indicated by the often-used phrase "No margin, no mission." Physicians who aspire to lead through organizational governance must grasp the intertwined aspects of clinical and administrative activity – the fact that improved patient outcomes and increased professional incomes are not contradictory but are, in fact, synergistic.

> "Since I started in practice in 1978, I have always been puzzled by the way medicine has chosen leaders. An example is how hospital medical staff leadership has been chosen. If you have been on the staff for a long time and you are a person who has not been in a leadership role, you will be nominated to be on a committee first as vice-chairman, then as chairman, not because you are good at it or you want to do it. It is just 'your time has come.' We need more professional ways to choose our leaders. We need people who want to lead in these important positions and who want to 'run for' the office and train for it. It would be more prestigious, and should be a paid position. Frequently, leadership is thrust upon physicians whether they seek it or not, or whether they are any good at it or not. This last bothers me even more – continuity in leadership is so important as policy decisions are made and carried out. We certainly don't have businesses that just rotate through each of the employees and everyone takes a turn at being chairman. I think we need a better way to ensure that the right people are leading at the right time.
>
> Hospital leadership is quite important, but there are many aspects for which physicians are generally not well trained – cost issues, managed care, access to care. They also must represent a very broad base of physicians, from pathologists and radiologists, who are facility-based, to physicians with their own practices.
>
> Most physicians are also small-business owners and they need to understand how to run a small business – whether they delegate that to their office manager, or a partner, they need to understand relationships of small business, and at the same time, they have to manage their costs as employers. The cost of healthcare not only is an issue for us as providers, but as small-business owners or part of a business entity, there is a need to understand what the effects of increasing healthcare costs are on their businesses."
>
> Daniel S. Durrie, MD
> Opthamalogist
> President
> Durrie Vision Center

The Need for Physician Leaders in Organizations

> "My organization [The Riner Group, a business strategy and management consulting firm] offers strategy, new business development, and performance improvement services for hospitals, health systems, large medical groups, and healthcare companies. Sometimes we

temporarily manage their organizations during transition. The medical practices we work with clearly have a tremendous need for strong leadership – particularly leadership in an organizational context. The nuance of medical practice leadership is a distinct entity worthy of consideration.

Most clinicians perceive themselves as being good clinical leaders, but not necessarily good business leaders. Business experience, the right values, communication skills, and relationships with people are essential."

Ronald N. Riner, MD
Cardiologist
President
The Riner Group

Defining the Role of the Physician Executive

Although there is not yet a universally accepted definition of the physician executive's role, a working definition has been proposed by Schneller, Greenwald, Richardson, and Orr (1997):

"We propose that the term physician executive be applied to individuals who (1) are employed in formal managerial positions to design, manage and sustain system of care (including networks and alliances), clinical work teams, clinical environments, (2) provide advice to non-clinical and clinical constituents, (including payers, purchasers, and patients) regarding the implication of managerial decisions for clinical processes and outcomes, and (3) negotiate or contract for settlements that sustain the profession's role to 'reconcile, integrate, or choose among conflicting applications of a solution within the context and culture of a given delivery system.'"

Being Selected is Just the Beginning

"It isn't uncommon for healthcare organizations to rotate physicians through medical staff leadership roles every couple of years. Thus physicians end up in the role whether they're good at it or not, whether they're interested in it or not. That doesn't make much sense to me."

Daniel S. Durrie, MD
Ophthalmologist
President,
Durrie Vision Center

Do you want to lead an organization toward enhanced effectiveness in caring for patients? Perhaps you are called to the role of physician executive involving governance of a healthcare delivery organization. If so, attaining an administrative leadership position is simply the first and perhaps easiest step on your journey. Making good decisions and taking appropriate actions day after day is, you will find, far tougher. And even tougher still are the relationship building and resource allocation decisions required of organizational executives.

"The key to making any organization successful is for its leader(s) to inspire followership – get people pulling together to accomplish something they all see as important and meaningful. At MGMA, for example, our organizational culture places a high priority on service – to our customers, members, and to each other. Because we value service, we measure it. We measure customer, member, and employee satisfaction every year. The metrics help us know where to strengthen our efforts. We've built a sense of camaraderie that is quite strong. In fact, the majority of our employees tell us they actually like coming to work each day. Unfortunately, that's not always the case in healthcare, or in any industry, for that matter.

Open communication is essential for establishing that kind of a positive work environment. When I joined MGMA in 1997, the organization employed 170 people. We had to downsize by approximately 30 positions. That can alienate and discourage people! But we shared the facts with our staff. We talked openly about our financial challenges. We achieved as much of the staff reduction as possible through natural attrition. Then when we had attained the 'right size' for our organization, we let people know we didn't expect any more layoffs. That enabled everyone to refocus on their responsibilities, on making a contribution for the future.

We also believe it is important to treat others as you want to be treated. All of us want to be respected as adults. We want to be trusted, and kept informed. When leaders are candid, honest, and straightforward, people tend to be very loyal to the organization and its leaders. For example, I hold bi-weekly staff meetings with our senior management team. They know that I expect them to immediately go back and share the decisions and information from those meetings with their employees.

Strong leaders also provide clear direction for others. When we told our employees about the financial challenges our organization was facing, we also let them know their help was needed. We set clear, actionable, measurable objectives, and committed to share the success for achieving our budgeted revenue numbers and operating bottom line. I'm pleased to say this is the third year we've been able to pay annual bonuses. What a great way to help people see that their hard work is not only appreciated, it is rewarded!"

William F. Jessee, MD, FACMPE
Pediatric, Preventive and Emergency Medicine Physician
President
Medical Group Management Association

Physician Executive Responsibilities

Despite significant changes in the healthcare delivery environment in recent decades, the core role and responsibilities of physician executives have remained relatively constant. According to research cited by Kathleen Montgomery, PhD, (2001) the hybrid role is primarily intended to merge clinical interests with managerial ones by its boundary-spanning representation of two constituencies – the organization and the medical profession. Montgomery explains that physician executives' reported responsibilities include three broad categories of tasks – quality assurance, communication, and relationship building/negotiation. Quality assurance includes clinical education, oversight, and accreditation. Communication includes information flow between medical staff and administration. Relationship building/negotiation includes clarification of goals, agreement regarding priorities, and mediation of conflicts between physicians and non-physicians.

> "How are clinical versus administrative leaders different? It's subtle. You're expected as a physician to be a broader thinker. Right or wrong – people defer to you. Good leaders recognize that phenomenon and make extra effort to gain insights from pharmacists, nurses, etc. But when medical groups organize themselves, nine times out of 10 the leader is a doctor."
>
> Monte L. Anderson, MD
> Gastroenterologist and Hepatologist
> Mayo Clinic Scottsdale

Physician Leadership: A Hybrid Profession

Do you know anyone who presumes that physicians who pursue administrative leadership responsibilities must be weak clinically? Research indicates that this is not true. Rather than physician leaders having been *pushed out* of their clinical roles, they seem to have been *pulled into* their broader governance roles – often by the desire to have a policy-making voice and an impact on large numbers of people. (Montgomery 2001: 224)

In fact, research indicates that physician executives who are, by definition, members of a hybrid profession have not replaced their clinical identity with one emphasizing management. Rather, they have enlarged their self-identity to include management along with clinical practice (Montgomery 2001: 224). Bodenheimer and Casalino (1999) describe this phenomenon rather colorfully, reporting that for these physician executives "the distinction between the suit and white coat is negligible."

Organizational Excellence Supports Good Clinical Outcomes

The Mayo brothers offer an instructive example of the way in which physicians' passion for organizational excellence in healthcare delivery can be applied toward the enablement of exceptionally favorable clinical outcomes. As Dr. Monte Anderson explains:

> "Physician leaders have the ability to visualize a problem from multiple perspectives. **Will** and **Charles Mayo** were certainly pioneers! Really great men! They were truly concerned with patient care, teaching and research. Their writings from the early 1900s remain applicable today.

Here at Mayo Clinic – Scottsdale we recognize that physician leadership is very important. We have two or three programs for leadership development. One is for administrators. Another is for physician leaders. All of Mayo's CEOs are physicians. We have some superb administrative people as well. We physicians may be starting out with a handicap – many people feel, and I think it is often true, that doctors are poor money managers. We go so long without any money while we're in medical school, then suddenly we have substantial incomes, but we don't know how to use money appropriately. So doctors who run a clinic, for example, must learn how to use resources well."

Monte L. Anderson, MD
Gastroenterologist and Hepatologist
Mayo Clinic Scottsdale

Leading Healthcare Organizations

Are you interested in the organizational aspects of healthcare delivery? Perhaps you're intrigued by the possibilities you can imagine when you envision truly outstanding operational excellence within your organization. Alternatively, your interest may stem from a desire to tackle the frustrating, problematic, burdensome aspects of administration in medicine. Perhaps you've been pulled into an administrative role or had operational responsibilities thrust upon you. You may be drawn toward the business of medicine or you may be motivated to "fix" it. Either way, if you believe that your leadership contributions to healthcare may be applied in the realm of organizational governance, there are a few points you'll want to consider.

As evidenced from research conducted by Kouzes and Posner (2002), effective leaders – in every industry – demonstrate several fundamental practices. Effective leaders nearly always challenge the status quo – inspiring a shared vision for a better future, and enabling others to achieve that vision. Effective leaders earn the right to do so by modeling the way, or personally setting the example. They're not task masters; they "encourage the hearts" of those they lead.

From "Physician" to "Physician Leader"

Having been the Chief Executive Officer of a University Medical Center, and now helping many organizations accomplish 'turnaround' scenarios through his consulting work, Dr. Richard Birrer, MD, MPH, MMM, CPE, clearly understands what it takes to lead and lead successfully in a healthcare organization. Dr. Birrer shared his perspective on the evolution from "physician" to "physician leader" in a recent article (2003).

"Physician leaders are not born. Some physicians may have a certain capacity for leading, or be committed to it, but the fact is that leaders are grown and trained. Physician leaders must understand finance, legal, and regulatory matters, human resources. They must set the mission, be ethical, and clinically credible. Physician leaders can expect to be judged by their peers (clinicians) and by administrators – who may be jealous of them. Physicians become leaders when an opportunity presents itself and they embrace it.

I punched through the glass ceiling by being immersed in situations that required leadership. I'm watched every day in my current role as interim CEO of this medical center. The responsibility involves a steep learning curve, but I'm doing the job, knocking down big issues, building a track record of accomplishments.

There is a big difference between various leadership roles. Being chairman, versus chief of staff, versus program director, are very different in several important ways. Many would say that physicians are 'de facto leaders' – but not in the sense that most other fields would describe leadership. How can we know whether a physician has the capacity to lead? By considering whether they can move away from the bedside; whether they can shepherd cats.

Physician executives have traditionally held roles such as Vice President for Medical Affairs, Chief Medical Officer, or Chief of Staff. Some then evolve into broader operational roles by becoming Chief Operating Officer or Chief Executive Officer of their organizations. Currently, less than 10 percent of hospital executives are medical doctors.

I've written two articles for *Health Progress* in which I've described the glass ceiling often faced by physician leaders, and identified the skills, knowledge, attitudes and competencies needed to break through that ceiling. I like the four physician leadership categories you've mentioned – clinical experts, pioneers, activists, and organizational executives. I believe there are other categories as well.

Executives usually lead with an autocratic style. Evidence indicates that an autocratic style is typically most effective in the long run, though such a style is more or less well-received at various points in history and various organizational contexts.

Medical staff leaders are typically most effective when they're good at cheerleading, even while raising the bar (standards of excellence) among their colleagues.

Role models of effective physician leadership include **Tom Royer, MD,** who is CEO of **Christus Health System** in Texas. He is a former trauma surgeon, and is now doing fantastic work in his organization. Tom previously worked at **Geisinger**, then **Hopkins**, then **Henry Ford Health System**. Other role models include **Joe Bushak,** MD, **Larry Green,** MD, **Mike Fleming,** MD, **Bernadine Healey,** MD, and **Bill Frist,** MD.

I've noticed that many physician leaders are *not* located on the East Coast of the U.S. (perhaps east coasters tend to be too crusty). More are located in the Midwest or on the West Coast.

Examples from further back in history include the **Mayo brothers** – two physicians who influenced the role of physicians in hospitals.

'Administrator time' and 'doctor time' are quite different. For example, when administrators say to physicians 'Be patient, I'll get to it soon' they might be thinking in terms of days or even weeks. When physicians hear "I'll get to it soon" they likely expect action to be taken within just a few minutes or hours.

Chief Medical Officers are sometimes put in the awkward position of being expected to represent the medical staff AND the executive team. This can be dangerous.

Who do I consider to be effective physician leaders? The American College of Physician Executives (ACPE) does a lot of work on physician leadership development. Trends evolve in physician leadership development. Traditionally, most of the help for doctors aspiring to become leaders has come from non-medically trained healthcare professionals, including PhDs and various types of administrators. For example, **Barbara and George Linney**, a husband and wife team, have written several books and articles for publication by the **ACPE**. In recent times, there has been an increased trend in physicians helping other physicians."

Richard B. Birrer, MD, MPH, MMM, CPE
Family, Emergency, and Sports Medicine Physician

Physician Leader in Academic Medical Centers

To successfully lead an organization – inside or outside of healthcare – you'll need strong decision-making skills, an understanding of how to select, train, motivate, and reward talented clinicians and administrative staff, and a means of addressing "problem performers."

"You're only as good as the people you hire."

Ray Kroc
Founder, McDonalds

Successful organizational leadership also requires the ability to establish or adapt the systems and processes that are required for efficient, effective service delivery. According to an article by Fairchild *et al.* (2004), "Success as an academic physician administrator/leader requires additional expertise beyond the typical skills of an academic internist. Strategic planning, finance, leadership, negotiation and other management skills are often necessary for advancement in these positions."

Dr. Fairchild expands in more detail on this subject:

> "In my paper 'Physician leadership: Enhancing the career development of academic physician leaders and administrators' I explain the change that is occurring in physician leadership selection patterns. Traditionally, physicians were placed into administrative leadership roles because they were great clinicians or researchers. More recently, physicians are promoted into leadership because they're effective leaders. This broadens the profile and acknowledges the importance of leadership in its own right.
>
> There are many other physician leaders for whom I have great respect. Some of those physician leaders include, for example, **Tom**

Lee, MD, who is the Medical Director for **Partners Healthcare**. He is on the editorial board for the *New England Journal of Medicine*.

Another well-respected physician leader is **Sam Their,** MD, who is a Former Chairman of Medicine at **Yale University** and President of **Babson College. Dr. Their** was at the **Institute of Medicine** and then served as Chairman of **Partners Healthcare**. He led with an iron fist – a traditional-style leader who blended roles as a researcher, department chair, and administrator By contrast, **James Mongan,** MD, the current CEO of **Partners Healthcare**, has a totally different leadership style – more inclusive, less authoritarian. **Sam's** style was a good fit for the organization at the stage when he was in the lead. Now the organization needs Jim's style and his focus on quality."

David G. Fairchild, MD, MPH
Internist and Chief of General Medicine
Tufts – New England Medical Center

Physician Leadership Competencies

Dr. Birrer describes in further detail the competencies required by physician executives, stating in another article that:
"To perform effectively, physician executives must be familiar with:

- management of medical staff relations (including conflict resolution, the issuing of credentials and privileges, network management, and recruitment and retention)
- efficiency practices (including those involved in informatics, staff perform-ance and compensation, and managed care/insurance)
- quality management (including quality assurance, clinical benchmarking, outcomes and disease management, resource utilization, risk management)
- legal and regulatory issues
- liaison functions (including mergers/affiliations and operations)
- cost management (including finances, cost accounting, cost containment, profit/loss statements)
- technology assessment
- decision making in uncertain situations
- clinical medicine
- organizational issues (including sales/marketing analysis, negotiation of contracts, strategic planning, governance)."

Dr. Birrer went on in that article to recommend that executives routinely "Communicate, be accountable, enhance information technology, develop mission and vision, work with committees, lead rather than managing, mentor and model."

Rather than being intimidated or threatened by the successes of those around them, effective physician leaders are pleased to be surrounded by the best possi-ble resources – including human resources. They seek out individuals with diverse backgrounds, perspectives, and capabilities, recognizing that such diversity will strengthen their organization and enable it to adapt quickly and nimbly to emerging opportunities and threats.

> "Administrators operate on a different time frame. Administrators say 'I'll get right on it' meaning sometime during the next quarter. Docs hear 'I'll get right on it' and expect it to be done that afternoon. The physician's reference model involves time frames that are much more immediate."
>
> Randall Oates, MD
> Family Physician
> Founder and President
> Docs, Inc.

Not only do effective organizational leaders focus on hiring top talent; they also work hard to offer job security and stability, recognizing that constant downsizings and reorganizations take a toll on individuals that impact organizational effectiveness far beyond the financial transaction seen on the organization's balance sheet.

An example of physician leadership in an organizational setting is provided by Reverend Pam Harris, MD. Dr. Harris explains how she provides leadership as a physician – through her work at a VA Hospital and her role as Minister of Health at her church.

Insights from Reverend Pamela S. Harris, MD

"During the hospital's reorganization, I functioned in the role of Service Chief of Clinical Support, a new grouping of nine departments created during the reorganization. I didn't want the job at all, but I had proposed the VA keep some of those departments being placed in that service line together under common supervision to balance the demands among them. After all, the departments are actually each others' key customers. The hospital administrators recognized the value in what I was proposing, and asked me to accept the responsibility for 120 days, giving them time to 'hire me a boss.' Of course, 120 days passed quickly, and they said they needed me to keep doing the job. For three years prior, I'd been head of the 25-person Rehabilitation Department, so it was quite an adjustment.

I believe in servant leadership. I believe leaders have to really want to serve those we want to lead. Leaders must be seriously interested in our employees – I mean, to know if they've recently lost a parent, to throw a baby shower for them, and celebrate their successes over meals. When we share in one another's lives, we convey that we truly care about their needs. Otherwise, claiming to be a servant leader is just empty words.

From a management standpoint, you gain the ability to understand employees' jobs by doing those jobs. I've learned to place orders that purchasing agents usually place. I'm on rotation for cleaning the microwave. Experiencing what the employees do lets me know how long the processes take, and what difficulties the employees are likely to face. That way, I can demonstrate clearly to my bosses when limitations prevent us from meeting their requests.

I've sat the Hospital Director and Chief of Staff down and showed them how a new computer menu could be used by clinicians for documentation and ordering particular devices – how doing so streamlines patient flow and improves productivity. Leaders who know what they're talking about reduce the 'it's not my job' grumbling. When people see their Department Head doing a task, they're less likely to refuse doing it themselves. Great leaders clearly define the essential duties that people are hired and trained to do, and yet grow a culture in which people don't stay within those clearly defined roles. They create an environment in which people see what needs to be done and do it.

People ask me how I keep up with such varied responsibilities. Perhaps juggling and prioritizing comes more naturally for me than for some people. Or perhaps I learned to be resourceful and view things broadly by growing up in a small town. It's natural for me to want to understand processes and fix them, to make things as efficient as possible. For example, I've written computer templates with pick menus to simplify documentation so it meets quality assurance requirements but isn't redundant. I've set up our systems to be as 'goof-proof' as possible, so our employees have fewer chances to fail.

Training is important. Good leaders ensure people understand why something is important, rather than just telling them to do it. For example, I realize that protecting against Medicare Fraud and Abuse is important, and yet many doctors don't naturally have much interest in addressing that issue. I have helped them see how billing and revenue maximization directly impacts the number of employees we're able to hire. Now that's something people can get excited about! Documentation has improved markedly once people realized it enables us to secure the funding we need to hire more staff.

At the **VA Hospital**, I work with a professional union and a non-professional union. I'm trying to change the culture by holding monthly meetings in which I give updates about the hospital and explain 'how we do things around here.' I listen to people's concerns and guide them in addressing specific situations. Some of our staff lack computer skills, so I build time into their weekly schedule to take courses in the computer lab. It will expand their career options by giving them new job skills.

I help managers get above the frenzy of responding to daily issues so they can see how improvements may be made. I get all stakeholders together to understand what each needs, then work out solutions amongst themselves."

Reverend Pamela S. Harris, MD
Physical Medicine and Rehabilitation Physician
Kansas City Veteran's Administration Hospital
Minister of Health, United Methodist Church of the Resurrection

Organizational Leadership Responsibilities May Vary

Leaders can be found in a variety of governing roles inside and outside of healthcare organizations. Some serve on governing boards, others on executive management teams – as Chief Executive Officer (CEO), Chief Operating Officer (COO), Chief Financial Officer (CFO), or Chief Information Officer (CIO). The acronym CMO can be confusing because it may refer to Chief Medical Officer (in healthcare organizations, of course) or to Chief Marketing Officer (usually not inside healthcare, where marketing has until recently been undervalued at best, or seen as inappropriate at worst). Leaders also serve as department heads, committee chairs, and in various other clinical and administrative positions.

When fulfilling a role within a medium to large organization, physician leaders' job responsibilities may involve any or all of the following:

- **human resource management:** recruiting, selecting, orienting, training, supervising, compensating, rewarding and handling disputes or performance issues among the staff
- **information systems technology:** overseeing the allocation of funds and the evaluation, selection, lease or purchase, implementation, training, maintenance, utilization and ongoing evaluation of computer hardware, software, networks, and other data and telecommunications services and equipment
- **financial management:** pricing or reimbursement policies, contract negotiations with health plans or other payers, collections, and the establishment and adherence to annual operating budgets as well as major capital investments
- **business development:** this can include a variety of functions such as strategic planning; market research and competitive analysis; new service line development, advertising, promotions, and publicity; and mergers, acquisitions, and other forms of alliance or partnership
- **quality improvement:** involving the evaluation and credentialing of clinicians; assessment and improvement of patient safety, satisfaction and outcomes; compliance with various laws, regulations, or industry standards; organizational procedures; utilization review; process improvement; and various other individual performance related and system-wide factors.

Inter-connectedness

One of the distinguishing characteristics of physician leaders whose passion is organizational excellence is their awareness of the extent to which healthcare delivery systems are truly interconnected. Marketplace competition may be a business reality, but collaboration is the means by which "all rise."

Working "In" the System and Working "On" the System

"A 'recipe' is needed for identifying and nurturing physicians who are innate leaders, but need help knowing how to apply their abilities. I know many physician executives who manage but do not lead. They're prevalent in health plans, integrated delivery networks, and large medical clinics. They're fulfilling their day-to-day roles, but not making innovative transformative change happen.

In fact, executive roles can actually incline people to be more conservative, so the most creative ideas often come from others who are working outside the context of large organizations.

Ambulatory care has been organized around the convenience of the doctors, not the patients. We need to help physicians and others catch a glimpse of what a transformed healthcare system can be; what it can mean to patients and the professionals who work within it. We need leaders with passion."

J. Peter Geerlofs, MD
Family Physician
Chief Medical Officer
Allscripts Healthcare Solutions, Inc.

Not all Physician Executives are True "Leaders"

As Dr. Belfer points out, simply being hired or promoted into an executive position within an organization does not necessarily make someone a leader. Conversely, some individuals exert a leadership influence on others despite the fact that they do not hold an official "management" position.

"Physician leaders and physician executives are not necessarily the same. Leaders are those we look up to and strive to be like, those who can bring people together for a common cause, and get others to come along.

Executives may or may not be good leaders. They may quietly get the job done (the work of administering within organizations), but their focus is more about working with systems than people. They bring about change in different ways.

Executives are managers in high level positions. Leaders can be found in any type of role or organizational level. Sometimes executives enable practitioners to do their work better, but a lot of them don't, because they aren't necessarily focused on practitioners' or patients' interests."

Mark H. Belfer, DO, FAAFP
Family Physician
Residency Program Director
Akron General Medical Center/NEOUCOM

References and Further Reading

Betson C. (1989) Physician managers: A description of their job in hospitals. *Hospital & Health Services Administration* **34**(3): 353–69.

Birrer R.B. (2002) The physician leader in health care: What qualities does a doctor need to be an effective organizational leader? *Health Progress* **83**(6): 27–30.

Birrer R.B. (2003) Becoming a physician executive: To be effective leaders, clinicians must first adopt a new mind-set. *Health Progress* **84**(1): 16–20.

Bodenheimer and Casalino (1999). The unintended consequences of measuring quality on the quality of medical care. *New England Journal of Medicine* **341**(15): 1147–50.

Brooks K. (1994) The hospital CEO: Meeting the conflicting demands of the board and physicians. *Hospital & Health Services Administration* **39**(4): 471–85.

Curry W. (1994) *New Leadership in Health Care Management: physician executive.* Tampa: American College of Physician Executives Press.

Dunham N., Kindig D. and Schulz R. (1994) The value of the physician executive's role to organizational effectiveness and performance. *Health Care Management Review* **19**(4): 56–63.

Fairchild D.G., Benjamin E.M., Gifford D.R. and Huot S.J. (2004) Physician leadership: Enhancing the career development of academic physician leaders and administrators. *Academic Medicine* **79**(3): 214–18.

Friedman E. (1986) Physicians as administrators. *Medical World News,* **June 23.**

Gauvreau E. (2002) On board: How a physician becomes an effective member of your medical group's board of Directors. *MGMA Connexion* **February**: 3839.

Hagland M. (1991) Physician execs bring insight to non-clinical challenges. *Hospitals & Health Networks* **September 20**: 42–8.

Kaufman A. (1998) Leadership and governance. *Academic Medicine* **73** (9 Suppl.): 11S–15S.

Kindig D.A. and Lastiri-Quiros S. (1989) The changing managerial role of physician executives. *Journal of Health Administration Education* **7**(1): 36–46.

Kirschman D. (1999) Leadership is the key to chief medical officer success. *Physician Executive* September/October: 34–6.

Kouzes J.M. and Posner B.Z. (2002) *The Leadership Challenge: how to keep getting extraordinary things done in organizations.* San Francisco: Jossey-Bass.

Linney G.E., Jr. (1995) Communication skills: a prerequisite for leadership. *Physician Executive* **21**(7): 48–9.

Matheson G. and Gill S. (1988) Good management for good medicine, the role of the vice president of medical affairs. *Healthcare Executive* **3**(5): 31–3.

Maxwell J.C. (1993) *Developing the Leader Within You.* Nashville, TN: Injoy, Inc. and Thomas Nelson Publishing.

Montgomery K. (2001) Physician executives: The evolution and impact of a hybrid profession. *Advances in Health Care Management* **2**: 215–41.

Ruelas E. and Leatt P. (1985) The roles of physician-executives in hospitals: A framework for management education. *Journal of Health Administration Education* **3**(2): 151–69.

Schenke R. (ed.) (1980) *The Physician in Management.* Washington, DC: American Academy of Medical Directors.

Schneller E., Greenwald H., Richardson M. and Orr J. (1997) The Physician Executive: Role in the adaptation of American medicine. *Health Care Management Review* **22**(2): 90–96.

Weil T. (1997) Physician executives: Additional factors impinging on their future success. *Frontiers of Health Services Management* **13**(3): 33–7.

Chapter 7

Physicians as Pioneers: Leading Innovation in Healthcare

"Not all executives are leaders. Not all physician executives are physician leaders. One of the characteristics of leaders is that they constantly test new and better processes that lead to improved quality and effectiveness."

J. Peter Geerlofs, MD
Family Physician
Chief Medical Officer
Allscripts Healthcare Solutions, Inc.

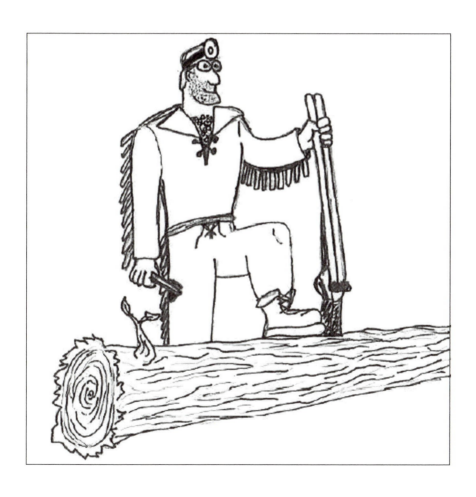

Physician leaders who serve as pioneers – champions of change, advocates for the adoption of new innovations – are experts in anticipating future implications of present realities, and guiding the discovery, invention, dissemination, and acceptance of new drugs and devices, new practices and procedures that create new possibilities for professionals to diagnose, treat, and manage the patients they serve.

Never before have the legal, regulatory, financial, and socio-political issues surrounding healthcare been so complex. And never before have such breathtaking advances been made in the life sciences that underpin the practice of medicine. Breakthroughs in molecular biology, genetics, stem cell research, and information technology are occurring at a dizzying pace.

Many physicians, in fact many people in general, find rapid change unsettling and sometimes quite stressful. But disequilibrium can also be a good thing. As explained in Christensen's book *The Innovator's Dilemma* (1997), disequilibrium can be a necessary catalyst for positive improvements to come about. Without disequilibrium, most of us would become too entrenched in the status quo to take risks and consider fundamentally new perspectives or, as some would say, to "think outside the box."

In her books and presentations, well known healthcare policy advisor Glenna Crooks, PhD attributes many of the issues faced in healthcare today to the broken covenants and misguided expectations that patients hold of healthcare professionals and professionals hold of themselves. Former President of the American Red Cross Bernadine Healy, MD (2004) claims the rapidly escalating costs of healthcare are simply a sign of the significant progress being made – the life-extending and sometimes quality-of-life-enhancing breakthroughs we complain about paying for but eagerly seek when we need them.

Author Barbara Starfield, MD, compares healthcare delivery in the U.S. realistically yet rather unfavorably to that of other countries. She does so in an attempt to help us identify ways to improve care quality, access, or cost-effectiveness. Fitzhugh Mullan's book entitled *Big Doctoring in America* (2002) illuminates these points, as does an article by Gruen *et al.* entitled "Physician-citizens: Public roles and professional obligations" (2004).

Physician Leadership in Healthcare Information Technology

A physician who applies his aptitude for clear thinking toward the diffusion of innovation in medicine is Randall Oates, MD. Naturally gifted in the natural sciences and in the use of information technology, Dr. Oates has for many years been using computers to improve patient care and patient communication. What began as a time saver and productivity enhancer for his own practice has grown to become a software system used by thousands of physicians on behalf of tens of thousands of patients. Dr. Oates believes his continued involvement in the practice of medicine is integral to his ability to offer clinically sound technology enhancements – for the benefit of patients seen in his own practice, and for the benefit of the practice of medicine overall.

Insights from Randall Oates, MD

"While growing up, I was always into science and electronics. I was the kid who built radios and gadgets of all kinds. Most people, including myself, expected that I'd become an electrical engineer. But in high school I discovered that I hated algebra – putting all that effort into abstractions didn't seem practical to me. About that time I also discovered a love for biology and decided to go into medicine.

Very quickly, I found that I loved medicine, but I hated charting. The turning point for me came one night during the flu season of 1988. I'd seen over 70 patients that day. Most had nearly the same history, findings, and treatment plan. Late into the evening, I was still documenting, and became convinced something had to change. All those people were really sick, hurting, and uncomfortable. None of us were really happy with the interaction with each other. There had to be a better way of giving information to them – helping them understand when it is really serious and when it is simply uncomfortable.

I was aware of publications that verified how little patients retain from what they've been told verbally. The patient's concerns were repetitive. I knew computers allow us to better manage repetition. More importantly, I knew that, using computers, I could better help patients know warning signs, what to expect, what to do next. The computer was the obvious way to do all that. So I used a word processor to create patient handouts on paper.

But keeping files of paper handouts was too labor-intensive – I couldn't keep up. I noticed that creation of prescriptions was also repetitive so figured if I wrote a simple software program that linked prescription writing with handouts and charting I'd save even more time. I haven't hand-written very many prescriptions since 1989. My writing is bad, and it is just too inefficient. This way, my patients leave my office with their prescription, and usually with a printout that explains what to expect and possible warning signs to watch out for.

By 1990, some of my peers who saw what I was doing wanted to do it themselves. At that year's Annual Scientific Assembly of the **American Academy of Family Physicians**, I demonstrated the work I was doing at a scientific exhibit. Approximately 30 docs had begun using my prototype by 1992. So that year I began hiring programmers to write good software code. I'm a physician not a programmer, so I prefer to focus on what I do best, and delegate other activities to others – such as programmers who are able to write tighter code.

I still see patients one or two days each week. If I were to quit seeing patients, I'd be unable to orchestrate software development. I believe strongly that a person must be in the culture and experience the day-to-day pressures in order to be effective at understanding and addressing the issues, to offer the functionality that is really needed."

Randall Oates, MD
Family Physician
Founder and President, Docs, Inc.

Another physician who exemplifies the leadership of innovation in healthcare is J. Peter Geerlofs. As you will discover, Dr. Geerlofs applies his passions and abilities toward the advocacy of fundamental transformative change across the entire healthcare system.

Insights from J. Peter Geerlofs, MD

"Physician leadership is a great topic to write about. Leadership happens at every level. Here at Allscripts, we're trying to help our customers deal with the human side of technology change, including process re-engineering and vision setting for organizations. An EMR project is not ultimately about the software. It's about an organization's willingness and ability to honestly assess itself and its processes, and then use software as an enabling tool to manage new, efficient and more effective processes. Ultimately, it's all about changing human behavior and, more specifically, changing physician behavior. The introduction of the EMR is as much art as science and provides wonderful opportunities for budding physician leaders to emerge as a catalyst for change in their organization.

My passion is healthcare information technology and its potential to enable and accelerate healthcare transformation. I recently attended a small gathering with **Newt Gingrich** to discuss his ideas on transforming healthcare. He has created the Center for Health Transformation, and although our politics couldn't be further apart, I believe he is exhibiting real leadership in promoting practical, often IT-based solutions to the dilemmas we're facing in healthcare. **Newt** believes healthcare is broken in a fundamental way and incremental change isn't sufficient. We need true transformation. I agree.

Many of the physicians I meet around the country feel overwhelmed. They are caught in the dilemma of having too little time and energy to find creative new processes that would give them more time and energy. The best way for healthcare to transform is from within. If, through appropriate physician leadership, rank and file clinicians could see a way out of the current mess and put their collective weight behind innovative process improvement, healthcare would transform overnight. There is a critical need for leaders whom physicians can relate to, and who can help those physicians past their resistance to change by painting a compelling step-by-step path towards a better, more rewarding system of care.

I'm participating on the Connecting for Healthcare steering committee sponsored by the **Markle Foundation** and **Robert Woods Johnson**. This is a public/private initiative to help enable the local and national health information infrastructure necessary for a fully interconnected and transformed healthcare system. This experience has taught me that clinicians and other leaders can get past what is only best for them or their organization, and work together for the benefit of the system as a whole.

Earlier today I received a call from venture capitalists in Raleigh who are exploring an interesting notion. Suppose venture capitalists buy the primary care practices in a region and help them establish a consumer-centric, informatics-driven model for the delivery of care, one that would be highly innovative and competitive. Once this model was perfected, then suppose those venture capitalists franchised it across the country. Imagine the possibilities!

Physician leaders must actively engage in discussion of new ideas. They must actively participate in projects that explore new ways of delivering care. Physician leadership is critical to getting healthcare organizations to change. If 'rank-and-file' doctors don't have a leader they can trust, it is nearly impossible to move them.

'Geek physicians' who love technology aren't always the best leaders to help an organization transform. The nature of early adopters is that they are sometimes more interested in the technology itself than the transformed processes the technology could enable. They tend to quickly move from one new technology to another, never pausing to discover what it could do for the organization. Most importantly, non-technological physicians cannot relate to them. 'Of course he can make an EMR work – he's really into computers.' And thus they aren't really helpful in accomplishing the mainstream adoption of technologies that offer real value for the practice of medicine. True physician leaders are not seen as 'technologists' but as respected clinicians who're interested in improving the underlying process of healthcare.

I decided to leave my practice because it wasn't possible to have a software business and still practice primary care one day a week. Family Medicine is all about continuity of care. I practiced medicine for 20 years. This is essential to my effectiveness now. Other doctors know that I've lived their life for many years. Doctors who practice for six months and then leave to earn an MBA may not seen as credible by their practicing peers.

Our system of healthcare is so complex it is very difficult to come up with a clear definitive strategy on how to change it. Where does one start? I've always been fascinated by the Federal Express story. It wasn't rocket science to figure out that businesses would pay for one day delivery of packages. The real genius was how to start with nothing and build a system which was capable of moving packages from anywhere to anywhere else. A partial solution wouldn't offer the value necessary to drive the business model. There are no shortage of ideas on what a transformed healthcare system might look like. What has been missing is a nuts and bolts strategy to get from here to there.

Catalysts such as **The Markle Foundation**, **Newt Gingrich**, and the **Electronic Health Initiative** are trying to 'get the ball rolling' now in healthcare. What are the practical steps which will lead to transformation? How can government participate in an appropriate and effective manner? What kinds of public/private partnerships can help? What are the practical, doable demonstration projects which get us to the tipping point? The opportunity for physician leaders in health organizations, insurance companies, government, pharmaceuticals, and academia to participate in

Continued

designing and implementing concrete steps is more real than it's ever been before.

Insights in the **Institute of Medicine's** *Crossing the Quality Chasm* report have the potential to impact significant change in healthcare. And yet, few doctors have read it, understand it, or have a forum to explore and build upon it. Most doctors have, however, read about patient safety in the popular press. So we need to use all available forums for exposing doctors to fresh insights and engaging them actively in discussing and tackling the issues.

Mentorship is an important way to grow physician leaders. One form of mentorship is to study the work of other physician leaders. I believe that's an important reason for the existence of this book. Some of the physician leaders for whom I have deep respect include **Donald Berwick,** MD who founded IHI, the **Institute for Health Improvement.** He has fostered a movement among participating organizations to think out of the box and make one small step at a time towards transformation. I respect him because he stands not only for transformation, but for making it doable by the average health organization.

Another favorite of mine is **Larry Weed,** MD. Larry is an iconoclast – always 10 to 15 years out in front of the rest of us. I think of him as the father of the problem-oriented medical record – a new way to document care which dramatically improved both the readability of the health record and the thought process of the clinician documenting care back in the 1970s. The whole concept of the problem list, which seems like a no-brainer now, came from that work. Over the past 15 years he has been championing something he calls problem-knowledge coupling. What if the clinician always had right at hand the evidence-based information needed to make correct decisions? What a novel thought.

Then there are leaders who have helped us define potentially new healthcare models. **Alain Enthoven,** PhD at **Stanford University** is an example. Alain and others in the **Jackson Hole Group** defined a model they called 'managed competition.' Blending the original concept of managed care, where the organization is incentivized to manage health and chronic disease rather than just react to acute illness, with competition, where market forces and consumers determine quality and cost, this model held promise of a system which was both affordable and appropriate to the needs of our population. Although, when proposed, its time hadn't come – I believe many of these ideas will eventually find their way into a transformed system of care delivery.

Another physician leader who comes to mind is **Mark Levitt,** MD, former founder and CEO of **Medicalogic, Inc.** One could argue that he was the first to create an EMR with enough clout to get the attention of the average physician. Before Medicalogic, EMR companies tended to be mom and pop shops or venture-funded flash in the pans. Mark created a product and company that was a leader in a new wave of products that actually had the potential to automate large numbers of practices. This played an important role in getting us to where we are today, where the EMR is no longer an 'if', it's just a 'when.'

Finally, I wanted to mention a physician who represents a different type of leader. He's not famous, but is part of an emerging breed of leaders who are having profound impact on individual health organizations. When I knew him, **Rick O'Neil** was a physician leader in a medium sized internal medicine practice near St. Louis. One day he read **The Goal** – an excellent book by **Eliyahu Goldratt** having to do with the science of improving efficiency through process engineering. He began wondering what constraints and bottlenecks were typical in the medical practice of internists and what might be done about them. He recognized that the most expensive resource is the clinician, but they often spend their time doing work which lower paid staff could do just as well. So using process re-engineering and information technology, he completely redesigned his practice. The last time we spoke, the group of internists at his practice were seeing almost 40 patients per day, patient satisfaction was never higher, and his physicians were happy, didn't feel overworked, and were getting home at a reasonable time every night. This is a microcosm of what we have to do system-wide.

In my own case, I had a wonderful family practice for 20 years in rural Washington State. Because of my passion and belief that health information technology was the key to transforming healthcare, I decided to create a software company called Medifor to try and make that dream come true. This was in 1994 when the notion of the EMR hadn't caught on, so we focused on a product which could provide much of the benefit of the EMR, but would be much easier for physicians at that time to accept. It focused on rapid creation of fully customized patient care plans. In seconds, the physician could write electronic prescriptions, document much of the encounter, and be able to hand the patient fully customized health information and instructions. We had one of the first health portals where these instructions could be transmitted to patient via a secure web site, and patients could communicate with their doctors using secure messaging. So we cherry-picked the EMR and came up with what we believed were the most important yet easily accepted components during that time. Medifor was acquired by Allscripts in 2000. At that time, almost 5000 physicians had used what we called The Patient Ed System. I had stopped practicing about four years after founding Medifor, but by the time the company was acquired, we had impacted hundreds of thousands of patients. For me, shifting away from day-to-day healthcare into clinical informatics was a way to leverage my years of practice experience, and have a beneficial impact on many more patients than I could possibly have seen personally. As rewarding as practice was, this phase of my career has been even more rewarding.

I have been struck by the extraordinary opportunity at this moment in time for physician leaders to play a huge role in some of the most profound changes healthcare has ever seen. I can think of no more satis-

Continued

fying time for physicians to move into a leadership and advocacy role to help drive the transformation. It's going to change with our without us – so let's be sure we're in the game and participate in the solution, rather than be seen as part of the problem.

To be an effective leader requires skills in listening, speaking, and writing. Physician leaders need to be good communicators as well as idea people. Thinking outside the box is not natural for many physicians, who spend years functioning within a fairly narrow confine. I believe many physicians have the innate ability to lead, but haven't nurtured or developed their ability to do so.

The 'elephant in the room' is looming larger than ever. Healthcare delivery simply doesn't work the way its consumers and payors need and want, but many physicians are too overwhelmed to do anything about it. That's a large part of why I'm so passionate about the potential for a new breed of physician leaders. Even with managed care and the advent of large practices and IDNs, healthcare remains largely a cottage industry – with each organization or clinic operating as though it were an island. Physician leaders must help physicians grasp how infinitely better healthcare could be if we changed our minds and decided to operate as regional and national teams on behalf of our mutual customer – patients!

The **American Academy of Family Physicians** has pointed out that a family physician who diligently reads three clinically relevant articles per night, would be 600 articles behind by the end of a year. The American College of Physicians estimates that primary care physicians have at least 12 unanswered questions each day. Clearly, human beings unaided by information technology have no chance of keeping up with rapid advances in knowledge and evidence. And yet physicians without the help of information tools make decisions each day that result in the majority of the healthcare costs borne by our country.

So any significant and sustainable transformation in healthcare requires finding ways to lead physicians towards better ways of making decisions. The alternative is that the healthcare system will be transformed out from beneath them.

I have no idea whether leaders are made or born. I'm sure circumstances may awaken latent leadership qualities. We all know physicians who seem to have been born with natural gifts that enable them to get beyond the daily grind and focus on solutions rather than complaining about the problems. I believe a critical characteristic to look for is unbridled optimism and the ability to never feel like a victim. Leadership is all about having a clear vision and the certainty that one step at a time, that vision can be obtained.

What makes physician leaders effective? Many of the same attributes that drive people to become physicians in the first place. Caring about the healthcare system and what happens to it; caring about and advocating for patients; an insider's knowledge of what is wrong with healthcare and what could work to transform it.

I'm encouraged by the trend of more physicians going back to school to learn business and management skills. When physicians pair their clinical training and natural leadership aptitudes with business education, they can be a powerful force for change. However, getting a business degree doesn't necessary guarantee that a physician will be a good leader. If nothing else, it can help open doors for clinicians switching from clinical care to management. However, healthcare needs fresh new thinking. Anything that inculcates physicians in 'traditional' business-think could be counterproductive.

I'm a fan of **Clayton Christensen's** ideas about disruptive innovation. I highly recommend both of his books – *The Innovator's Dilemma* and *The Innovator's Solution*. A professor at the Harvard School of Business, his theory describes how large, successful enterprises often are unable to successfully keep up with innovation, because most of their effort is on incremental changes requested by their demanding customer base. As a result, their products become ever more complex and expensive. This leaves room for tiny companies to do an end run around the larger business by producing products which are simpler, cheaper, and more in line with what the market as a whole, who can't afford the sophisticated products of the large company, wants. I'm greatly oversimplifying an elegant business theory – but the bottom line in my opinion is that healthcare needs disruptive innovation to transform itself quickly. This requires that physician leaders learn how to think out-of-the-box, getting beyond the delivery paradigms we have been living with over the past 30 years.

There are so many books that are relevant for physicians who aspire to become leaders. I would recommend **Regina Herzlinger's** *Market-Driven Healthcare*. Although somewhat dated, it's a wonderful example of re-thinking the whole system from the customer point of view. A perspective on the history of medicine is critical. A book by **Paul Starr,** MD, called *The Social Transformation of American Medicine* shows how far we've come in the science of medicine, and how far we must go in healthcare delivery.

Physician leaders should ideally have been in practice for at least 8–10 years. There is no substitute for the perspective that can be gained only through practicing medicine – perspective both on what is fundamentally wrong from the physician's perspective, but also on the incremental changes which would be acceptable by physicians with limited emotional room for change."

J. Peter Geerlofs, MD
Family Physician
Chief Medical Officer, Allscripts Healthcare Solutions, Inc.

Physician leaders whose abilities and interests draw them to serve as pioneers of innovation often devote their attention toward the development and use of information technology in healthcare. According to Atul Gawande, MD, a physician named William Baxt, MD, was one of the first to champion the notion that computers – specifically artificial neural networks – can make better sophisticated clinical decisions than can humans (Gawande 2002: 37–39). Dr. Baxt did so by demonstrating that computers readily outperformed physicians in diagnosing heart attacks among patients with chest pain. That research was further extended by Lars Edenbrandt, MD, whose expertise in artificial intelligence enabled him to show that computers read EKGs 20 percent more accurately than physicians. Gawande points out that the keys to perfection in such procedures are routinization and repetition – rigid adherence to standardized protocols. He cites a Swedish study that indicates the individualized, intuitive approach we cherish in modern medicine actually causes more mistakes than it prevents; that algorithmic approaches usually trump human judgment in making predictions and diagnoses. Why? Gawande and the social scientists whose work he reports, find that, "Human beings are inconsistent: we are easily influenced by suggestion, the order in which we see things, recent experience, distractions, and the way information is framed" (Gawande 2002: 40–44).

Lest we misconstrue that Dr. Gawande is naive about the resistance of many physicians toward reliance upon technology, he goes on to assure his readers that " . . . as systems take on more and more of the technical work of medicine, individual physicians may be in a position to embrace the dimensions of care that mattered long before technology came – like talking to their patients . . . In the increasingly tangled web of experts and expert systems, a doctor has an even greater obligation to serve as a knowledgeable guide and confidant. Maybe machines can decide, but we still need doctors to heal" (Gawande 2002: 45–6).

Even if physicians are willing to embrace new technologies and procedures, the challenges of innovation persist. With the ever-increasing pace of medical innovation, all practicing physicians remain embedded in unceasing and sometimes very steep learning curves. The "see one, do one, teach one" philosophy of learning and leading is nowhere more applicable than the practice of medicine. Thus with the experimentation and learning that are inextricably enmeshed in the adoption of new innovations, we find the axiom "trial and error" to be disturbingly true. The fact is, "Patients do eventually benefit – often enormously – but the first few patients may not and may even be harmed" (Gawande 2002: 27). We hate to admit that any patients will suffer as a result of our quest for continued progress, but the fact remains that they can and some will.

> "There are two ways of spreading light: to be the candle, or the mirror that reflects it."
>
> Edith Wharton

It can be quite challenging to work in a newly emerging field. By definition, emerging fields preclude evidence-based medicine because the medicine that is being developed is quite literally on the leading-edge. Senator Frist, MD, describes what that experience can feel like for the physicians involved:

> "On dreary October nights, I found myself sitting at my desk flipping through stacks of phone messages, thinking about Jim Hayes [a transplant patient]. This field is just too young, I'd say to myself. We don't know enough. It's all word of mouth, or something picked up at a conference, maybe, or a clue hidden away in an inconclusive research report published in some obscure medical journal. There was no textbook to consult, no rules to follow . . . It [total lymphoid

radiation therapy] seemed to work, though there was no scientific evidence, no clinical proofs, that it would and no prospective clinical trial to demonstrate its efficacy. But when you are working in a new field, one full of unknowns and the unexpected, you don't always have the luxury of having well-accepted recipes to choose from."

> Senator William H. Frist, MD
> Cardiothoracic and General Surgeon
> Senate Majority Leader, U.S. Congress
> in his book *Transplant* (1989)

Dr. Frist summarizes the tongue-in-cheek description of seven stages that happen with the development of any new idea according to his colleague Norman Shumway, MD:

> "In the first stage, doubters all around you say 'It won't work; it's never been tried before.' After several successful experiences with animals, you enter the second stage, and the same doubters say, 'But it won't work in man.' One successful clinical patient later, they turn around, shake their heads, and mumble, 'Very lucky. But the patient really did not need the operation in the first place. Too bad the tragedy occurred; they'll probably try it again.' ... After four or five clinical experiences, critics call it 'highly experimental. Too risky. Probably immoral. Certainly unethical.' And someone in the back adds in a whisper, 'I understand that they probably had a number of deaths that they have not reported.' The fifth stage is characterized by critics saying, after 10 or 15 successful patients, 'May proceed cautiously in carefully selected cases, but most patients with this defect don't need the operation anyway.' In the sixth stage, after a large series of success, some critics, say, 'I hear that a number of their patients are now dying late deaths,' while other critics are saying, 'So-and-so elsewhere cannot get the same results.' Finally, in the seventh stage, the critics now say, 'I know this is a very fine contribution. A straightforward solution to a difficult problem. I predicted this. In fact, I had the same idea long before they even started. Of course, we didn't publish.'"

> Senator William H. Frist, MD
> Cardiothoracic and General Surgeon
> Senate Majority Leader, U.S. Congress
> in his book *Transplant* (1989)

Physician leaders serving as pioneers and champions of change are determined to find ways to minimize such sacrifices. They collaborate with organizational executives where such innovations are adopted to institute policies and procedures that safeguard patients and professionals from medical mishaps. These physician leaders are not just brilliant visionaries – "idea people" – some may call them. They're also catalysts for change, systems-thinkers, masters of influence who understand the human psyche and how to motivate risk-averse professionals to think outside the box and move beyond their comfort zone.

Another physician who is dedicated to leadership of clinical innovation is Charles Jaffe, MD, PhD. Working to "raise the bar" for all physicians – Dr. Jaffe leads several initiatives designed to further diffuse the use of information technology through adoption of standards:

"I have a terrific job. Who knows how that happened? The time, I suppose, was right. A confluence of increasing demand in healthcare technology and surprising opportunity, I suppose. The work is extraordinarily demanding, both in time commitment and devotion, but the rewards are commensurate. The emphasis placed on healthcare information technology is expected to reduce medical errors, improve patient privacy, and enhance cost-effective delivery. It's quite a challenge.

Why did I choose to earn an MD and a PhD? Because I wanted to be an academician and thought the combination of an MD and PhD would serve me well. At the NIH [**National Institutes for Health**] I met extraordinary talents who couldn't play within the system, and marginally competent scientists who were very politically agile. The rest of us just did our jobs. I had some wonderful allies who stuck up for me so I didn't have to play the game. To be really successful, you either must be a good politician or fabulously talented.

In pharmaceutical companies, the political environment is very challenging. The individual who first recruited me explained that the corporate world was not a meritocracy. In the more structured environment of academia, the tenure system is fairly clearly defined. In the business workplace, advancement is based on many subjective attributes, not the least of which is political allegiance.

In many large structured businesses or even some academic communities, it is very possible to be widely successful in the external environment and unrecognized within your own. Sometimes, it's hard to be a hero in your own backyard. On numerous occasions, I was invited to travel to Europe or Asia to speak or to consult, but not included in a local committee of experts.

I was very motivated to join 'big pharma' (the pharmaceutical industry) because I believed that I would have impact on a broader and much deeper plane. The sphere is influence is greater but the pace of change is sometimes excruciatingly slow.

Healthcare information standards, like CDISC and HL7, are being developed by people who are conscientious and innovative thinkers. It's rewarding to have a sense of accomplishment about my role. Within the pharmaceutical industry there are many activities and functions that rely upon decades old processes and are not eager to change.

When I was in medical school, my heroes were a couple of general internists. They seemed to have a credible grasp of almost everything. It was remarkable to listen to them expound on medical knowledge. It was also an accomplishment that I could never hope to duplicate. For me, I was more comfortable choosing a subspecialty for which I might have a command. In 1970 we were told that medical knowledge doubles every 18 months. I can barely calculate the immense body of knowledge that today's graduates must confront. To be successful, we need technologies to help physicians do things that the human brain cannot even appreciate. It enables us to broaden our perspective so our interventions don't have to begin and end with our own experience.

Many years ago I hoped to see the widespread acceptance of electronic medical records before I retired. It has taken a lot longer than I had envisioned. To quote **Shakespeare**, 'The fault, dear Brutus, is not in our stars but in ourselves.' As physicians, we could have taken a leadership role in getting the technology and processes we needed, but, by and large, we abrogated that leadership role until it was far too late. Now, we are committed to follow the dictates of a bureaucracy before that vision can be realized."

Charles Jaffe, MD, PhD
Director, Medical Informatics
Astra-Zeneca Pharmaceuticals

Another physician leader who has been actively involved in clinical informatics as well, but from a completely different vantage point is Daniel Z. Sands, MD, MPH. He still practices medicine, though he has had to cut back a bit in order to invest time in his other endeavors. Somehow, he juggles care for his own patients with his faculty appointment, his frequent speaking and consulting engagements that take him literally all over the world, and his executive role. Why would anyone juggle so much? Passion. Dr. Sands is passionate about accelerating the adoption of electronically-enabled physician–patient communications. Though he would likely be too humble to admit it, through his leadership of the task group that generated the seminal guideline for physicians' use of electronic messaging with patients, Dr. Sands quite literally "wrote the book" on electronic physician–patient communications.

Insights from Daniel Z. Sands, MD, MPH

"You've asked me to share my story. I'll do so in order to help other physicians, but talking about myself kind of offends my modesty. I'd been involved in patient care and clinical information technology a long time. During the early 1990s I began communicating with a lot of patients via email and noticed that I was evolving methods of incorporating email into my practice. Those methods became a best practice, and I wanted to share the ideas, so I began lecturing and speaking with others about it.

In the late 1990s I led a group of AMIA (American Medical Informatics Association) members to produce the first ever guidelines for use of email in patient care. I was able to infuse a lot of my ideas into the group and the document. It was published in January 1998. I kept speaking, lecturing, and writing about it and started a web site on this subject. Nine months later, I began spreading my ideas further through use of the popular press in order to get the ideas out there. I gained confidence and communication skills.

Continued

Many physicians have good ideas but can't express them in ways that are helpful to others. By age five I was performing magic shows, so I found it easy to communicate with groups. In college, while working in a lab at **The Cleveland Clinic** with a lot of PhDs and surgeons, I learned the importance of speaking up. My mentor at the time told me to admit it whenever I didn't understand something, and to ask for clarification. I took that lesson to heart.

I've chosen to be more involved at a national level but within a specific field – clinical informatics. I work through national medical informatics associations to get the word out. The fact that I'm at a university that has prestige associated with it doesn't hurt. People listen to what I have to say.

People who aspire to lead should choose the level and field they want to impact. Many people who make medical discoveries are not leaders, or agents of change. It takes a certain type of person to create new innovations, but these skills are different from the skills required to bring about the dissemination and adoption of innovation. For example, I didn't invent email, nor was I the first to use it in clinical care. I did spread the idea – at policy levels, and through speaking and writing."

Daniel Z. Sands, MD, MPH
Internist
Faculty, Harvard Medical School
Chief Medical Officer and Vice President, Clinical Strategies,
Zix Corporation

In a presentation he gave (Jessee 2004), Dr. William Jessee explained why the traditional approach to healthcare service delivery does not and can not foster the environment we need if we are to bring about innovative and substantially improved means of assuring care quality and patient safety. Dr. Jessee said:

"Neither issue is purely clinical. Both involve systems – which are primarily administrative. In the traditional view, physicians are responsible for clinical work, while administrators handle the scheduling, billing, personnel problems and clerical support functions. Each stays out of the other's domain of expertise, or else!

The problem? Cost-effectiveness in chronic disease management, for example, or patient access to care, are not purely administrative matters. Business-savvy clinicians can help make better decisions that will contribute to improvements in operational efficiency and overall effectiveness in healthcare service delivery.

Only by working together in physician–administrator teams can we bring patients the needed diversity of skills and perspectives. Only by working as teams can we respond quickly to changing demands, reduce over-dependence on individuals, be willing to take risks, and enhance results.

But we must beware of the frequent challenges faced by teams. Namely, lack of accountability for performance, using the team for all issues rather than being selective, placing too high a value on individual autonomy, stereotyping team leaders or members, or simply going through the motions with 'pseudo teams.'

Gone is the old compact in which physicians see patients and administrators provide autonomy, protection and entitlement. The new imperatives are all about improving care quality and patient safety, delivering accessible services, reducing costs. Doing these things requires that we attract and retain competent, committed staff who have high morale, and who trust one another. The new compact still allows physicians to focus on patients, and accept accountability for outcomes, perhaps now more than ever. However, the new compact also requires physicians to collaborate on care delivery, to listen and communicate, to lead and participate in change. The healthcare compact of today requires that we all work better – together."

William F. Jessee, MD, FACMPE
Pediatric, Preventive and Emergency Medicine Physician
President,
Medical Group Management Association

Points to Ponder

1 What do you believe to be the driving forces behind the chaos and complexity of healthcare today?
2 In what ways do significant improvements in healthcare delivery seem impossible, naïve, idealistic?
3 What role do you believe physicians should take in improving overall healthcare delivery?
4 If that doesn't happen, how will healthcare evolve – from the perspective of physicians, other clinicians, administrators, patients, and society at large?
5 Why, do you believe, it is often difficult for physicians to identify and address the warning signs that imply threats to the profession?

References and Further Reading

Berwick D.M. (2003) Disseminating innovations in health care. *The Journal of the American Medical Association* **289**: 1969–75.

Berwick D.M., Godfrey B., and Roessner J. (2004) *Curing Health Care: New strategies for quality improvement.* San Francisco, CA: Jossey-Bass Publishers.

Berwick D.M. and Nolan T.W. (1998) Physicians as leaders in improving health care: A new series in Annals of Internal Medicine. *Annals of Internal Medicine* **128**(4): 289–92.

Christensen C.M. (1997) *The Innovator's Dilemma.* Boston: Harvard Business School Press.

Christensen C.M. (2003) *The Innovator's Solution.* Boston: Harvard Business School Press.

Crooks G. (2000) *Creating Covenants: healing health care in the new millennium.* Old Lyme, CT: Medical Vision Press.

Ferlie E., Fitzgerald L., Wood M. and Hawkins C. (2001) *The diffusion of innovation in health care: the impact of professionals.* Paper presented at the Academy of Management Annual Congress. August 2001.

Frist W.H. (1989) *Transplant: a heart surgeon's account of the life-and-death dramas of the new medicine*. New York: The Atlantic Monthly Press.

Gawande A. (2002) *Complications: a surgeon's note on an imperfect science*. New York: Picador, Henry Holt and Company.

Goldratt E. and Cox J. (1992) *The Goal: A Process of Ongoing Improvement*. 2nd rev ed. New York: North River Press.

Gruen R.L., Pearson S.D., and Brennan T.A. (2004) Physician-citizens: Public roles and professional obligations. *Journal of the American Medical Association* **291**(1): 94–8.

Healy B. (2004) Keynote presentation at the Medical Group Management Association annual convention.

Herzlinger R. (1997) *Market Driven Health Care: Who Wins, Who Loses in the Transformation of America's Largest Service Industry*. Reading, MA: Perseus Books.

Jessee W.F. (2004) *The Physician–Administrator Team: fostering a partnership*. Presented at the Southern Medical Association in Charleston, South Carolina on July 31, 2004.

Mullan F. (2002) *Big Doctoring in America: profiles in primary care*. Berkley, CA: University of California Press.

Reinertsen J.L. (1998) Physicians as leaders in the improvement of health care systems. *Annals of Internal Medicine* **128**: 833–8.

Starfield B. (1998) *Primary care: balancing health needs, services and technology*. New York: Oxford University Press.

Starr P. (1984) *The Social Transformation of American Medicine*. New York: Basic Books.

Chapter 8

Physician Leadership in the United States Senate: Lessons From the Past, a Vision for the Future

William H. Frist, MD

Thoracic and General Surgeon and Senate Majority Leader (since 2003), the United States Congress

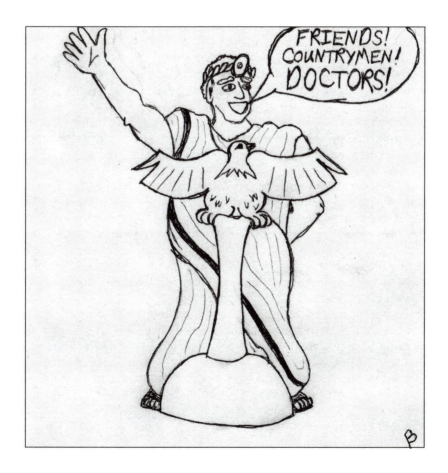

Introduction

Doctors have consistently been among the most trusted members of our society. In the Hippocratic Oath we as physicians swear to do our best to benefit the sick, do no intentional harm, and ensure our actions are never dictated by external motives. Even now in modern twenty-first century medicine, this ancient code governs the approach to our most important and sacred vocation.

However, I think it is vitally important we explore the possibility that the values outlined in Hippocrates' writings describe our obligations not just as doctors, but civic leaders. As caretakers for people of all backgrounds and social classes, we have been imbued with implicit trust from our patients. Suitable to this most intimate responsibility, we are regarded as trustworthy, independent, and fundamentally moral and ethical professionals. These traits are not only crucial to effective medical practice; they provide the foundation for effective leadership in virtually all arenas of human interaction.

In light of the similarities between successful medical practice and public leadership, it is unfortunate that there are so few doctors currently serving as legislators in our nation's government – and specifically the United States Senate. A historical survey of physicians who have served in the Senate demonstrates the unique contributions made by physician-lawmakers. They have rendered tremendous influence in the lawmaking process with their specific medical knowledge and their scientific training.

Yet sadly, over the course of America's history the story of physician-senators has been one of decline rather than growth. In the Senate's history, a total of 49 members trained as physicians and only 38 ever actively practiced medicine. While the numbers might seem impressive, the majority of physician-senators practiced in the Senate's earliest decades – they have nearly vanished in modern times. Within the United States Senate, I am the first medical doctor to have served since 1938 and the only doctor trained as a medical scientist.

In an era where important and controversial medical issues are center-stage in public discourse, the absence of physician leaders is conspicuous. Imagine the contributions trusted physician leaders could make in legislating major healthcare issues like medical insurance, AIDS education, and bioterrorism to name a few. It is ironic that as public policy and medical practice have become increasingly complex and interconnected, that the number of physician-senators has dwindled. Perhaps even more tragically, the very virtues of goodwill and trust embodied by the medical profession are the ones commonly cited as lacking in America's public leaders.

In these next pages, I would like to explore the history of physician leadership in the Senate. Unfortunately, there are few records that expound upon their accomplishments as America's earliest medical practitioners and lawmakers (of the 49 medically trained senators, 31 have no existing memoirs or scholarly biographies). Regardless, by examining those records that do exist, I have found common themes that have united all of these great doctors and public servants. Specifically, I have highlighted three physician-legislators who have demonstrated the profound and unique influence that physician-senators can have on public health policy.

In exploring our profession's past successes in civic leadership, I hope to foster a renewed commitment to expanding the values and ethics of our profession outside of traditional private practices, and allow them to inspire us to fulfill Hippocrates' oath on a larger scale.

Early National Period

The first physician-senator in America's history was Jonathan Elmer of New Jersey. A graduate of the first medical class at the University of Pennsylvania in 1763, his motivation for serving in public office accurately represents the reasons many of the first physician-senators became involved in early national politics. In the late eighteenth century, medicine was still in its early stages of development in the United States. Unlike today when being a physician is an around-the-clock occupation, early American medicine was not a lucrative source of income for practitioners. Doctors had fewer vocational obligations and felt less pressure to choose between a political career and practicing medicine. As a result, physicians often sought alternative sources of revenue and professional satisfaction.

For two of the earliest physician-senators, the transition to public service stemmed from their experiences as surgeons in the Revolutionary War. Doctors such as Senator Henry Latimer of Delaware and Senator John Condit of New Jersey served as surgeons in battle, and as a result of their experiences, took an interest in the welfare of the young republic. Their endeavors as both doctors and lawmakers served an important public service to the growing nation. Dr. Joshua Clayton, a U.S. Senator in 1798 from Delaware, was able to continue practicing medicine throughout his political career. During the Revolutionary War, Senator Clayton was responsible for discovering a substitute for Peruvian Bark, a vital medicine for treating gangrene and mortifications that was in short supply. In 1798, while serving in the Senate, then meeting in Philadelphia, Clayton united his roles as a physician and public servant by advising the city's medical community during an epidemic of yellow fever. In his valiant efforts to serve as a civic leader and medical caretaker, Dr. Clayton contracted the fever and died before completing his Senate term.

Finally, it was Samuel Latham Mitchill who best personified the scientist-turned-statesman of the early national period. While his short period of service – from 1804 to 1809 – is brief by today's standards, Dr. Mitchill served as the model for the several other physician-senators who would follow him over the course of the nineteenth century.

Samuel Latham Mitchill

Samuel Latham Mitchill is one of the finest examples of a physician successfully marrying the practice of medicine with the opportunity to shape public policy. A true polymath, Mitchill was known to his contemporaries as the "Nestor of Science" because of his interest in a wide variety of disciplines. There were seemingly no limits to his interests and few bounds to his knowledge; attributes that would later become an invaluable resource for him and his Senate colleagues in creating informed and successful public policy.

Mitchill was born in 1764 and received a classical education at Kings College in New York, followed by a three year apprenticeship with Dr. Samuel Bard.

Mitchill's earliest medical education came while serving under Dr. Bard during the American Revolution. This early training helped Mitchill appreciate the connection between medicine and its potential impact on the broader social context. "There I went to college," Mitchill later reflected, "observing fevers and witnessing amputations before I had been made to read the fables of Aesop." (Mitchell 2003) Lacking opportunities to advance his medical education in America, in 1783 Mitchill sought further training at the University of Edinburgh in Scotland. Awarded the MD in 1786, he returned to America and began practicing medicine.

Yet it would be grossly insufficient to describe Mitchill as strictly a physician. Dr. Mitchill's extensive interests demanded that he be an excellent physician while still inspiring him to continue nurturing what he called, "the mighty march of the mind." A true renaissance man, Mitchill was one of the finest intellectuals of the early republic; a statesman and teacher, philosopher and poet, and a true pioneer in the natural and physical sciences.

Upon his return from England, Samuel Mitchill was soon drawn to the ongoing debate over the new federal Constitution. This newfound interest prompted him to study law under Robert Yates, Chief Justice of the New York Supreme Court. Thereafter, he was appointed to a chair at Columbia University (formerly Kings College) in natural history, chemistry, and agriculture.

Exposure to academia allowed Mitchill to begin demonstrating how scientific discoveries could directly impact public regulations and policies. As a medical researcher, his experiments with toxins and what he referred to as "septons" led to investigations into public sanitation and hygiene. His concern for society and his concomitant interest in science would foreshadow the modern public health crusade. Already a respected author, in 1797 Mitchill co-founded the *Medical Repository*, the first medical journal published in the United States. As editor for 23 years, he shared scientific news from around the world and educated the American public about the world's greatest scientific advancements.

Samuel Mitchill's zeal for knowledge and its practical social applications primed him for an effective career as a public servant. Consistent with his broad base of academic pursuits, his interest in the American democratic experiment soon drew him into politics. Mitchill's savvy for understanding and practicing law caught the attention of New York Governor George Clinton, who appointed Mitchill to negotiate the purchase of land from the Iroquois Nation in 1788. This accomplishment propelled him to being elected to the New York State legislature in 1790 and later to the United States House of Representatives in 1800. The ability to integrate sophisticated elements of divergent thought helped create Mitchill's reputation in Washington as the "Congressional Dictionary." His scientific training, commitment to learning and vast experience uniquely enabled him to shape congressional debates. His contributions in the House of Representatives would not go unnoticed, and in 1804 Samuel Mitchill was elected to the United States Senate.

Samuel Mitchill sought office in the Senate because he deemed his vote would be "greatly more ponderous" in the United States' upper-legislative body. Indeed, his efforts to pass legislation had an incalculable effect on the social well-being of the young country. His medical experience inspired him to fight for better quarantine regulations, improved naval sanitation, and hospital relief for sailors. A champion of public hygiene, Mitchill also believed in the importance of other social programs, as evidenced by his promotion for better transportation infrastructure, improved educational programs and increased opportunities for the deaf. According to one observer, Mitchill "brought to these legislative halls an understanding of scientific problems which was as rare as it was beneficial."

As a physician-turned-statesman, Samuel Mitchill furthered the debate over public health, while fostering a deep respect for the contributions of physicians, in government and society. His life was a prime example of the limitless contributions that a doctor can make to a society. Mitchill's medical background offered a substantive base for formulating thoughtful public health policy, and his honest, objective, scientific approach was beneficial to the young republic on a range of non-medical issues. "Whether in the capacity of legislator, of medical savant or of a devotee of pathological history, of sanitary chemist or of surgeon-general of militia, of hospital surgeon or of private practitioner," wrote one biographer, "he was always the physician, laboring to find the truth which might save the lives of human beings."

The Nineteenth Century

The mid-to-late nineteenth century brought profound changes to medicine in America. Pervasive medical challenges like cholera epidemics, casualties from the Civil War, and the need for veterans' healthcare taxed medical knowledge and pressed the scientific community to research and develop more sophisticated means of treatment. These growing threats to social health in turn provided additional opportunities for men of science to shape public policy. In the United States Senate, Dr. Simon Conover introduced legislation that called for procedures designed to help stem the tide of yellow fever. For Missourian Lewis Linn, his Senate career developed as the direct result of his medical experience. His extraordinary efforts during an outbreak of yellow fever led to his election to the Senate.

However, as the nineteenth century progressed and the scope of public health broadened, there was a marked decline in the role of physician-legislators in the Senate. Medical issues became increasingly complex, and physicians spent more time developing and improving community health treatment and preventive medicine. This rapid development inspired doctors to become better educated, more specialized, and increasingly professionalized. In turn, there was less available time to legislate as public officials. Ironically, as the field had become more complex and integrated into society, medical practitioners had less time available to complete the important connection between public health practice and public health policy.

Transition Era (1891–1938)

Over the course of the nineteenth century, the number of medically trained senators continued to steadily decline. Yet, those physician-legislators that remained in office provided impressive snapshots of the potential influence that medical-legislators can wield.

Jacob Gallinger

Dr. Jacob Gallinger's 27-year career, spanning from 1891 to 1918, is the longest of any physician-senator. Moreover, this Senator from New Hampshire was the only other physician-senator, aside from me, to serve as a leader of his party in the Senate.

A model of diligence and hard work, Gallinger distinguished himself at a young age. Born to a family of modest means, he financed his medical schooling by simultaneously working as a printer. Upon graduation, he settled in New Hampshire and began a surgical practice.

Jacob Gallinger's political career began with involvement in municipal politics. His meticulousness served him well both in surgical practice and in the state legislature. Inexhaustible, Gallinger managed to attend legislative sessions while still attending to patients. Even after abandoning his practice for a political career, he remained connected to his medical roots by reading medical journals and remaining associated with his physician colleagues. Indeed, after his election to the United States Senate, he was well-known to his colleagues not as Senator, but 'Doctor Gallinger.'

Gallinger's legacy in the Senate centers on his unique ability to apply medical knowledge to public health policy. His bills addressed a wide array of public health issues, ranging from hospital improvements to sanitation and healthcare provisions for the poor. As Chairman of the Committee on the District of Columbia, he had a profound impact on improving the practice of medicine in the federal district. Recognizing critical shortcomings and gaps in the public health system, he pushed for heightened regulation of medical practices and called for standardized qualifications for physicians. His expertise inspired the confidence of his colleagues and enabled him to mold broad consensus for his legislation. As a result, in his final five years in the Senate, Doctor Gallinger chaired the Senate Republican caucus and served as his party's floor leader.

Jacob Gallinger's tenure in the Senate serves as an impressive model for future physician-legislators. His ability to synthesize his medical training with public leadership demonstrates the unique contributions that physicians can make in the policy arena, by improving individual, communal, and national healthcare.

Modern Era

The twentieth century saw the advent of tremendous public health programs like Social Security and Medicare. Yet these landmark federal achievements were accomplished with a conspicuous absence of physician-legislators serving in the United States Senate. Before I was elected to the Senate in 1994, only two such men had served in the body during the previous 60 years. And while both Dr. Royal Copeland and Dr. Ernest Gruening served in the Senate, only Dr. Copeland practiced as a physician. Significantly, however, while he may have been the only true physician-legislator for the majority of the twentieth century, his Senate career is a shining example of what a physician-statesman can accomplish in the field of public health.

Royal Copeland

Even before becoming an elected official, Royal Copeland was interested in improving public health. An 1889 graduate of the University of Michigan Medical School, Copeland initially practiced as an ophthalmologist. Despite his optic specialty, he clearly viewed his role as a physician within a wider social context and saw the potential benefits of communicating with the public on health issues.

Royal Copeland used his talents as writer to publish a number of medical books geared towards promoting safe and hygienic practices for the general population. In addition to his books *Healthbook* and *Dr. Copeland's Home Medical Book*, he also wrote a widely syndicated newspaper column to provide health education and warnings about epidemics to the broader population. A genial, practical, and astute practitioner, Royal Copeland was soon recognized as a strong advocate for public health reform.

In 1908, Copeland was drawn from Michigan to New York City where he assumed the position of dean of the Flower Hospital Medical College. Soon thereafter, he was appointed the City's Commissioner of Public Health. This influential position enabled him to make dramatic improvements to the city's public health systems. By all accounts a natural leader, he masterfully utilized the media to publicize health warnings and rules of healthy living. Additionally, his medical savvy guided him to make numerous proactive civic health advancements that improved the quality of life for all of his citizens. As commissioner, he helped double the city's milk consumption, which drastically reduced the infant mortality rate, and he helped contain the 1918 influenza epidemic.

In 1922, fueled by his state-wide popularity and particular credibility with the New York City public, Royal Copeland defeated incumbent William M. Calder for a seat in the United States Senate. Serving from 1923 until his death in 1938, Copeland continued to champion health issues at the federal level. Copeland was particularly committed to food and drug legislation, which eventually became the hallmark of his public service. Using his unique role as a physician-legislator, he established a federally funded public health program to control venereal disease and more stringent regulation of potentially harmful cosmetics and drugs.

Ultimately Royal Copeland's legacy would stem from his work to pass the Copeland-Lea Act of 1938. After laboring for over five years to establish this meaningful health reform, the passage of the bill signified a landmark event in the regulation of food, drug, and cosmetic products. Though undergoing later amendments, the law remained the centerpiece of drug regulation policy for almost 50 years, and is a tremendous example of the enduring policy that can result from physician involvement in national politics.

Physician Leadership: A Call to Public Action

By all measures, it is clear that in the past physician-senators were, as a group, tremendously qualified and educated individuals. They were largely men of vision, creativity, and imagination, with an interest in addressing complex social problems. As legislators, they all seemed to recognize the close connections between health problems and social policy. Indeed, by reviewing the careers of physician-leaders in the Senate, it is possible to highlight a number of key traits shared by doctors and politicians. The ability to rapidly assimilate information, listen carefully to recognize intricacies of complex problems, and formulate clear and accurate solutions are all vital attributes shared by both professions.

Given these profound similarities between vocations, it is curious that the number of physician-legislators drastically declined over the course of the twentieth century. While the reasons for the decline are fairly obvious (the development of clinical science, more advanced and specialized medical training, increased professional demands on physicians' time and energy), it is paradoxical that as health issues have become increasingly complex and central to public debate, that there are fewer and fewer physicians involved in shaping public policy.

We – as physicians – have a long and proud history of public service to our nation, and particularly in the Senate. But in more recent times we have not been as involved. Our participation has diminished drastically. In the Senate, 25 physicians served in the first 50 years; 14 served in the second 50 years; eight served in the third 50 years; and now only two physicians have served in the last 50 years.

I am not making the case for more physician-legislators based on a facile comparison of vocational traits. Physicians should not pursue public leadership positions strictly because of the similarities between the jobs. Rather, we need physicians in positions of public leadership because our expertise in the medical field could dramatically alter and improve the course of the world's medical care in the twenty-first century. We are experts not only on medicine, not only in our specialties, but on healthcare in general.

Recall the vision and beliefs espoused in Hippocrates' ancient oath. As physicians it is our obligation to do our best for our patients – to ensure that we never do them intentional harm. While we may be meeting this goal on an interpersonal level, I believe we are grossly underachieving on a social scale. Whether we realize it or not, physicians have the capacity to be trusted civic leaders. Indeed, I would contend that one of the single greatest impediments to a rebirth of public physician leadership in the last century has been our inability and unwillingness to acknowledge our potential.

That does not mean every doctor should run for the U.S. Senate. However, we must examine ways we can influence public policy at every level. For some of us, that may mean spending a few hours each week writing our legislators, participating on community boards, supporting candidates, and educating ourselves on policy issues. For others, it may mean running for public office. Regardless of the methods, we must acknowledge the legacy of previous physician-legislators and act on our profound obligation to do no harm to patients in every way possible – both through conducting appropriate medical practice and actively crafting responsible health policy. In the words of President Theodore Roosevelt: "It is not the critic who counts; not the man who points out how the strong man stumbles, or where the doer of deeds could have done them better. The credit belongs to the man who is actually in the arena ... who spends himself in a worthy cause; who at the best knows in the end the triumph of high achievement, and who at the worst, if he fails, at least fails while daring greatly, so that his place shall never be with those cold and timid souls who neither know victory nor defeat."

Our medical training is the prism through which we see humanity and the world in ways no one else can. Equipped with this unique perspective, we must actively and aggressively shape our profession, or it will be shaped by others who might not put the patient first. We must once again recognize our place in the larger world. We can lead medicine and healthcare with vision. It is both our privilege and our obligation.

"Senator Frist's comments are instructive for physicians who wish to become directly involved in Congress. It is important for physicians to realize they can influence health policy and legislation in other ways as well. For example, Donald J. Palmisano, MD, JD, the immediate past President of the American Medical Association, was a driving force behind the passage of tort reform legislation in the U.S. House of Representatives through his impassioned pleas which were credibly substantiated by evidence in support of his recommendations. He helped non-clinical decision makers understand the impact of capping damages for economic recovery by arming himself with facts from our experiences in California and Colorado.

To be a persuasive advocate for any cause or constituency, physicians must not only be articulate and insightful, we must do our homework and have a thorough knowledge of the issues at hand. This is vital. Otherwise, we will be discounted, or worse, discredited. Our country needs evidence-based health policy, evidence-based medicine, and evidence-based management of health services delivery. Physicians are ideally positioned and equipped to gather and share the evidence – if we're willing to invest the time and effort required."

William F. Jessee, MD, FACMPE
Pediatric, Preventive and Emergency Medicine Physician
President, Medical Group Management Association

References and Further Reading

Mitchill S.L. (2003) *Letter from Dr. Samuel L. Mitchill of New York to Samuel M. Burnside.* Temecula, CA: Reprint Services Corp.

Saultz J.W. (1995) Effective leadership in a reformed health care system: New skills for family physicians. *Family Medicine* **27**(6): 393–6.

Chapter 9

Leading Physicians in Unique Settings

"Encouragement means holding others to high standards, recognizing their potential and not underestimating them. It can mean encouraging them, not just to become self-reliant and capable of achieving their goals, but to develop integrity and the character traits that accompany it. We not only can, but must, encourage others to be honest, fair, and reliable. Further, we must encourage them to exhibit self-discipline and to work hard, to be accountable, and to persevere at what they do in order to achieve their fullest potential."

Dick DeVos

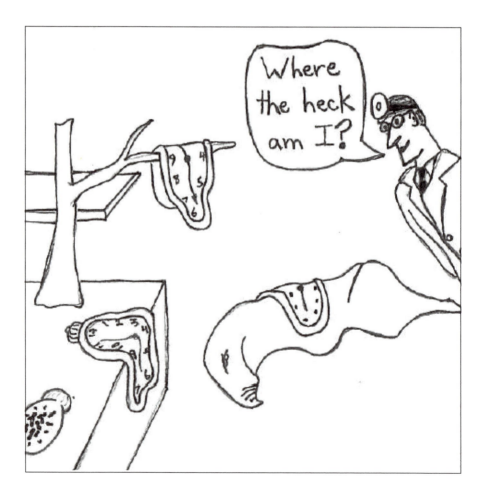

Physician leaders often encounter challenges from multiple directions, some of which are situation-specific. In recent years the medical profession in general and physicians in particular have been challenged to be more involved in leadership to improve the state of healthcare in this nation, including public health domains. Some conceptual shifts need to occur for physicians to assume the work of leadership in any healthcare setting, let alone the public domain.

Leading in the Public Health Domain

There are many compelling reasons why physicians need to increase their involvement as leaders in the public domain. First of all, among the most serious challenges faced by the people of this nation is that of access to healthcare. Physicians possess unique knowledge that would be valuable in addressing access, quality of care, public health and even policy concerns. As Gruen *et al.* (2004) point out, public trust in members of the medical profession has declined in recent decades; greater visibility by physicians as leaders and advocates for public interest may help regain that public trust.

In the public setting, physicians can find innumerable opportunities to make functional contributions to the communities in which they live and work, and these provide an opportunity for leadership. Opportunities exist within school boards, local public offices, advisory committees to large employers, charities, and advocacy roles for groups of all types. In any of these settings, physicians can function like ambassadors, representing the healthcare professions to those groups. Like ambassadors, physician leaders must acculturate to their environment, developing an intimate understanding of its sphere of influence, target constituencies, and, yes, even biases. Yet practicing physicians must never forget their "citizenship" as professionals. Practitioners' foremost responsibility is always to address the needs of their patients.

Physicians' leadership in their communities may be mediated by several variables. One, for example, is that of career stage. Young physicians who are just beginning to establish their professional reputation will have a role and impact quite different from that of physicians who have been working in the community for an extended period of time (Rosof and Felch 1992). Why? Experienced physicians will have had multiple opportunities, throughout the evolution of their careers, to establish personal as well as professional credibility.

Another variable is that of context. Physicians' involvement with a school board, for example, will entail different and broader challenges than involvement in a community advocacy group, which is likely to focus more specifically on a narrower range of issues.

Physicians' personal background, training and chosen discipline will substantively impact their capacity to provide leadership in the public domain. Physicians who are trained in pediatrics, for example, will enjoy greater natural credibility when advocating on behalf of children's health issues than might those physicians from other specialties, even though their interests might be equally heartfelt.

Leading in Not-for-Profit Clinics

Not-for-profit health clinics represent another environment in which physicians are often called to demonstrate leadership. Leadership of vision – the ability to see the possibilities rather than just the challenges; leadership of collaboration – the ability to enlist tireless dedication from others, often without the enticement of lucrative rewards or stature; leadership of resource allocation and utilization – to ensure scarce resources are leveraged for maximum patient benefit.

As Medical Director of the Jackson County Free Health Clinic, Bridget McCandless, MD, deals with challenges such as these each and every day. She describes for us what it means to be a physician leader in the not-for-profit environment, and challenges any physician interested in supporting the delivery of care through not-for-profit health clinics to consider these ways to make an impact:

"From the beginning, healers have cared for patients based on need and not on the ability to pay. Medicine has changed substantially in the last 50 years but that same commitment to care still exits. In addition to the long hours spent in regular practice, physicians continue to provide countless volunteer hours in their communities. We serve on boards, conduct school physicals, and volunteer time in countless other situations.

Some physicians are having an increasingly difficult time adapting patient care to fit a 'business model.' It is becoming more challenging to provide pro bono care in private offices so many providers have chosen to offer services at non-profit health clinics. There are approximately 1,000 formal free health clinics currently operating in the United States providing $3 billion in free or reduced cost healthcare. More than 375,000 clinician volunteers make this happen. Freed from the constraints of time pressure and the bottom line, physicians can do what we enjoy most – care for and connect with people. Patients are grateful for the care they receive and we are able to make some contribution to ease the problem of the burgeoning uninsured.

Healthcare professionals are increasingly asked to weigh in on the issues of medical structure, straining public safety nets, and limited resources. To date, the public debate has been shaped by those other than direct care providers. For years, most doctors believed that even the mere discussion of money in the setting of patient care was a betrayal of the tenets of medicine. By keeping the practice of medicine pure, clinicians have neglected the disparity between scarce resources and an increasing menu of diagnostic and therapeutic options. There is no right answer or one right way to solve the problem. What is clear is that the system now in place is not working. The costs of delaying care and prevention cut to the core of our economy, standard of living, and life expectancy.

To bring the issue of medical finance to a less abstract level, it is worthwhile thinking about medicine at the individual level.

Physicians are in the unique position of being intermediary consumers. We order tests and medications on patients' behalf without the ability to see their budgets, bank accounts, and financial reserves. Consider the cost of medical tests in terms of hourly wage rates – for example, a Chemistry panel at a regional Mid-West hospital costs $194.50 or nearly 38 hours of work at minimum wage ($5.15/hour). Physicians need to be cognizant of the financial position in which patients may end up due to our 'leave no stone unturned' approach. Doctors cannot fix all of the financial issues facing medicine, but we need to be especially conscious of the fiscal management of resources that are not our own.

In the area of philanthropic medicine, it is necessary lead with our hearts but essential to strategize and plan with our heads. Basic business acumen is needed to be able to discuss matters of public policy. For too long, the business aspects of medicine have been relegated to the accountants. Physicians are losing our ability to shape the future of this precious charge with which we have been entrusted.

To identify how best to proceed, consider the following:

- Who provides free care in your area?
- Who helps patients with the cost of medications?
- Do you understand the basics of the Medicaid and CHIP (Children's Health Initiative Program)?
- Do you know that most pharmaceutical companies provide medication for compassionate use at no cost to patients who qualify?
- Are you aware of the costs of tests that you order every day?
- Who are your local government representatives and do they know what challenges you face everyday in your practice?

Every day you are a leader. You get up and go into an office or a hospital and face unknowns. You solve problems. You hold hands. You give guidance in difficult decision making. You travel the journey of life with patients. In some simple way, look at your surroundings and find one thing that you can fix or improve. Our jobs can be exhausting and overwhelming. It is too easy to be passive in the face of the enormity of the issues. The most important thing we can do is to have an opinion and care enough for what is happening to make our opinions known. Together, we will shape the future of medicine."

Bridget M. McCandless, MD
Internist
Medical Director
Jackson County Free Health Clinic

Leading in the U.S. Military

Within the U.S. Military, physicians are often called upon for leadership through a variety of roles, ranging from administrative roles in military medical institutions to managing the health and well-being of both soldiers and noncombatants in the theater of warfare. These physician leaders face pressures of personal danger, uncertain resources, and unpredictable conditions of monotonous boredom and frantic chaos. Nevertheless, physician leaders in the military must balance the priorities of the well-being of their troops, the safety of their coworkers and the ethical obligations to provide the greatest good for the greatest number.

> "As a physician in the **U.S. Army Reserves**, I'll soon receive orders to report either to Iraq or to Fort Hood in Texas. If sent to Iraq, I'll care for soldiers. If sent to Texas, I'll care for soldiers' families. It doesn't really matter to me, because either way I'll be using my gifts to help people. I consider it an honor to do my duty and to serve my country. I go where I'm called."
>
> Gary Morsch, MD
> Family and Emergency Medicine Physician,
> U.S. Army Reserves
> Founder, Heart to Heart International

Another physician who exemplifies leadership in the military is John Bucholtz, DO. Here is how Dr. Bucholtz describes the challenges associated with leading others to practice medicine in the United States Army.

Insights from John Bucholtz, DO

"I sometimes find it ironic that I have been so influenced by an infantry specialty whose primary objective is to kill people and break things. Yet they are all volunteers as we are in medicine. As they go out in a world that has become a more dangerous place, I have come to appreciate them more. They are and have been my friends, neighbors, Godparents to my children, and recently the recipients of more of my prayers.

Like my colleagues, I am the product of my upbringing. My professional upbringing occurred while completing 20-plus years of active and reserve time with the United States Army. I spent the entire time affiliated with Martin Army Hospital located at Fort Benning, Georgia. For those not well versed in the military, Fort Benning is home of the Infantry School, Airborne School, and the Ranger Course. It is a place where a culture of leadership is the norm and schooled to all those who serve there. Soldiers are trained here who do the grunt work of military operations – infantry men who carry their equipment into harm's way to occupy and defend. Rangers deploy around the world on very short notice, their whereabouts unknown to their spouses and loved ones who might watch CNN to figure out where daddy may be. I soon came to the realization as a resident working every third night that there were a lot of soldiers I cared for working a lot more than I was. I have a particular fondness for drill sergeants, who reported for work at 4 am and brought the last of their charges to the ER at 10 pm on their way home. No one told them about an 80-hour workweek. I had it almost easy then in hindsight. The experience surgically removed whatever part of my brain had been conditioned to whine and complain as I watched and learned how responsible infantry officers and noncommissioned officers cared for their charges. I learned that the guy in charge has to care for those under him to allow the subordinates to reach their potential. I learned how to be resourceful with ever dwindling resources."

John R. Bucholtz, DO
Family Physician
U.S. Army Medicine

Leading in Academia

In academia, leadership opportunities for physicians are often presented by the inevitable internal politics, long boring meetings of unclear purpose and scarce resources. In the academic setting, personal ego, and discipline-driven prejudices are not uncommon. These can provide unique challenges for physician leaders who strive to help communities of academic physicians achieve positive working relationships, consensus positions, and functional progress toward the academic medical center's goals.

"Through my IHS work I learned the importance of recognizing there are two sides to every story. For example, academic medical center physicians may not respect local medical doctors and vice versa. Be humble, realize you don't know it all, and you're not the only one with 'the right answer.'"

David G. Fairchild, MD, MPH
Internist
Chief of General Medicine, Tufts – New England Medical Center

Leading in Rural Areas

In rural settings, physician leaders face unique challenges as well. The local community will have an "opinion" of the physician's status, commitment and integration into that geographically limited constituency. Physicians considered to be "outsiders" will carry with them substantially less credibility and potential for influence than those who have long exhibited a vested personal interest in the good of the town.

Leading in Policy Setting Bodies

Policy setting bodies such as advisory committees, boards of directors, and other elected and appointed positions can also present unique challenges for physician leaders. Often physicians in such settings are expected to carry out an ambassadorial role on behalf of various healthcare causes and constituencies. Many physicians have found, however, that in order to influence policy beyond that of healthcare, they must shed their mantle of "physician" to have a broader impact. Why? Doing so offers physicians the opportunity to build alliances with constituencies that will further goals that range well beyond the limits of healthcare.

> "More so than most other professions, a physician's sense of self-identity is very closely tied to his day-to-day role as a clinician. This can make the transition from active practice to a full-time leadership or management role difficult. Those who can continue to practice while playing a leadership role in healthcare are fortunate. Academic physicians, for example, may have more opportunities to do so.
>
> Also, for many physicians the financial rewards of leadership may not be as great as their earning potential in full-time practice. Ideally, leadership and the opportunity to impact a wider spectrum of healthcare needs to be a calling, much like one's calling to medicine in the first place. It helps to view leadership in healthcare as a way to extend to even more patients the benefits of one's accumulated skills and wisdom."

> J. Peter Geerlofs, MD
> Family Physician
> Chief Medical Officer
> Allscripts Healthcare Solutions, Inc.

Leading in Your Community

The question must be addressed: "Why don't we see more physician leaders in active roles within their own communities?" Are increasing pressures in the healthcare provider environment preventing physicians from extending themselves into the community? Perhaps a different conclusion may be drawn. In many cases, physicians are actually leading within their communities but doing so as "quiet" leaders. Many physicians volunteer their time and expertise without seeking recognition for doing so. History has demonstrated repeatedly that the impact and magnitude of many physicians' contributions were poorly understood or not even recognized at the time those contributions were made. We believe that many physicians are unsung heroes – quietly working in their communities to advocate for various causes and constituencies. Visible? Mostly not. Challenging? Indeed. Valuable to society? Undoubtedly.

Points to Ponder

1 In what ways does your own work setting influence your goals as a leader?
2 Which aspects of your situation support your effectiveness?
3 Which aspects hinder you from achieving your full potential?
4 Why is it important to adapt your leadership goals and approach to the specific context in which you're working?

5 To what extent have you consciously done so?
6 How could the "best practices" of physician leaders in one setting be more readily transferred and adapted to other settings?
7 To what extent are you involved in helping make that happen?
8 If you find yourself in a situation that's not ideally aligned to your work style – the pace or amount of interaction, for example – how can you adapt your behavior to better fit the setting, or how can you alter the setting to better fit your style?

References and Further Reading

Gruen R.L., Pearson S.D., and Brennan T.A. (2004) Physician-citizens: Public roles and professional obligations. *Journal of the American Medical Association* **291**(1): 94–8.

Masaoka J. (2004) *The Best of the Board Café: hands-on solutions for non-profit boards.* St. Paul, MN: The Wilder Foundation and CompassPoint.

Masaoka J. (2000) *All Hands On Board: a handbook for boards of all-volunteer organizations.* St. Paul, MN: National Center for Nonprofit Boards.

Masaoka J. and Allison M. (2004) *Why Boards Don't Govern.* St. Paul, MN: National Center for Nonprofit Boards and CompassPoint.

Rosof A.B. and Felch W.C. (1992) *Continuing Medical Education: a primer.* 2nd edn. Westport, CT: Praeger Publishers.

Section III

Stepping Stones for Successful Physician Leadership

"A leader achieves success when creativity, motivation, and the relentless pursuit of excellence coalesce."

Elissa J. Palmer, MD, FAAFP
Family Physician
Director, Altoona Family Physicians Residency, Pregnancy Care
Center and Women's Health and Wellness of Altoona Regional
Health System

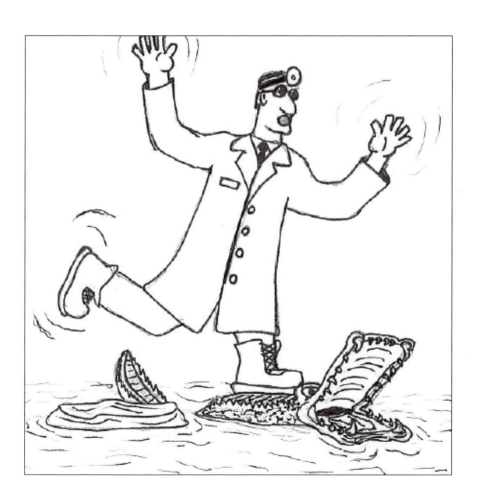

What are the hallmarks of an effective leader? Several characteristics are worthy of our consideration. Effective leaders exhibit self-awareness, they conduct ongoing self-assessment. Effective leaders are self-regulated, comfortable with ambiguity, and open to change. Effective leaders are highly motivated to achieve results; they remain optimistic and determined to persevere despite encounters with inevitable obstacles. Effective leaders establish strong relationships; they're able to do so because they exhibit empathy and sensitivity, they find common ground with others whose backgrounds, work styles, and interests may be quite diverse from their own. Effective leaders are persuasive; they create an atmosphere in which people are highly loyal – toward the vision, and toward each other.

How do we define, measure, and reward effective leadership? One indicator of great leadership is the number of "followers" – or colleagues. "Don't look at the decisions and actions of the leader, but of those the leader has led" we often hear. Leaders have followers who buy into the ideas they envision and the changes they champion. Effective leadership is also indicated by the attainment of the group's vision, mission, and goals. Successful leaders produce remarkable results, enabling their organizations or colleagues to achieve excellence as well.

Organizational effectiveness is measured in the "business world" in a wide variety of ways, including quality of products and services, market share (volume), growth rate, customer satisfaction and loyalty, capacity utilization, adaptability and innovation, stability and flexibility. Financial metrics of organizational results are also quite varied – profitability, liquidity, and stability measures encompass a range of factors including revenue, profits, earnings per share, earnings before interest and taxes, return on investment, return on equity, return on assets, and so on.

Organizational ineffectiveness is also measurable. Astute leaders can spot signs and symptoms of organizational malaise as readily as astute physicians can spot signs of physical disease. And just as physicians realize that patients' headaches are usually more appropriately addressed by having them swallow a tablet than by performing brain surgery, so too can good leaders discern which course of action is advisable for addressing various organizational dysfunctions.

When people show signs of confusion ("I don't understand") or conflict ("I don't agree") effective leaders have insights and skills to make a differential diagnosis and seek data to confirm whether their hypothesis regarding the root cause holds true. Perhaps the vision isn't clear or compelling, the staffing levels and job structures don't equip people to competently perform their responsibilities, the communication systems are inadequate to coordinate tasks, people lack the information needed to complete the tasks, or the organization's resource allocations are misaligned with its values (its deeply held beliefs and priorities that guide all major decisions, investments, and actions).

Dr. McKenna uses a metaphor of "Stepping Stones" when coaching leaders and consulting with organizations in order to help them enhance their effectiveness. The "Stepping Stones" metaphor provides a mental model for envisioning and practicing essential leadership attitudes and behaviors. What are those stepping stones to successful leadership?

> ## Stepping Stones to Successful Leadership™
>
> ### Credibility
> Successful leaders exhibit *competence* (skills, knowledge, ability) and *character* (values, beliefs, and behaviors). Credibility is the starting point for anyone who desires to earn others' trust and respect.
>
> ### Clarity
> Successful leaders provide clear *direction*; they clearly *communicate* a compelling vision that attracts others to contribute toward the achievement of that vision.
>
> ### Collaboration
> Successful leaders create *cohesive teams* of *diverse individuals* who respect one another, and are deeply committed to the purpose they share.
>
> ### Coordination
> Successful leaders ensure decisions and actions, resources and processes are aligned with key goals and priorities; they manage and measure the achievement of results.
>
> ### Change
> Successful leaders equip themselves and others with the resilience and the capacity for renewal that are necessary to withstand the pressures of continuous change and the ongoing quest for further innovation and improvement.

These "Stepping Stones for Successful Leadership" are built on the premise that anyone who aspires to lead well must live well, that we must first *be* leaders before we demonstrate strong leadership. Leading involves being, not just doing. We must be leaders – earning credibility through our competence (knowledge, skills, experiences, and expertise) and our character (values, beliefs, attitudes, and trustworthiness). To lead well, we must bring clarity of direction (vision, mission, purpose, and goals); we must communicate the vision in clear and compelling ways to those whose involvement and insights we seek.

> "There is no necessary connection between the desire to lead and the ability to lead and even less the ability to lead somewhere that will lead to the advantage of the led."
>
> Bergen Evans

Leaders are, by nature or necessity, great collaborators. To lead successfully, we must inspire others' commitment toward a shared vision. To the extent we're able to build shared commitment, we build highly cohesive and yet richly diverse teams of people who work well together in order to achieve what none could accomplish individually.

Virtually all successful leaders recognize that vision and inspiration alone are insufficient to achieve remarkable results. Leading well requires the alignment of decisions and activity for the achievement of goals; the coordination of resource utilization for optimal impact.

> "Everyone knows that on any given day there are energies slumbering in him which the incitements of that day do not call forth. Compared with what we ought to be, we are only half awake. It is evident that our organism has stored-up reserves of energy that are ordinarily not called upon – deeper and deeper strata of explosible material, ready for use by anyone who probes so deep. The human individual usually lives far within his limits."
>
> William James

Successful leaders equip those they lead to flourish in the midst of change – to cultivate resilience and renewal that are necessary for continuous change and improvement. Strong leaders are adaptable and they persevere, and more importantly, they enable others to do so as well. Without resilience and renewal, people experience burnout – the stress and fatigue that result from an environment brimming with chaos and complexity.

We have good news for you. All of us can develop these attitudes and practice these behaviors. All of us can enhance our credibility, clarity, collaboration, coordination, and capacity for change. Read on to find out how.

Points to Ponder

1 What practical steps do you believe physicians (or people in general) must take to become successful leaders?
2 Think of someone whom you consider a strong leader. In what ways has that person inspired, challenged, or enabled you to be more effective or fulfilled in your work?
3 What is the value of using a "mental model" of leadership?
4 How can such a "mental model" help you stay focused on the attitudes and behaviors that lead to successful leadership?
5 What specific steps could you take to become more effective or fulfilled in your work?

Chapter 10

Credibility Through Competence and Character

"What do people want to know about someone whose lead they're being asked to follow? Are you competent? Can I trust you? Do you care about me?"

Lou Holtz

Do you share our belief that anyone who aspires to successfully lead others must first and foremost *be* a good leader? Do you recognize that without *being* a successful leader, it is virtually impossible to successfully *do* the work of leadership? The reasons for this are intuitive if we pause to ponder them. For we

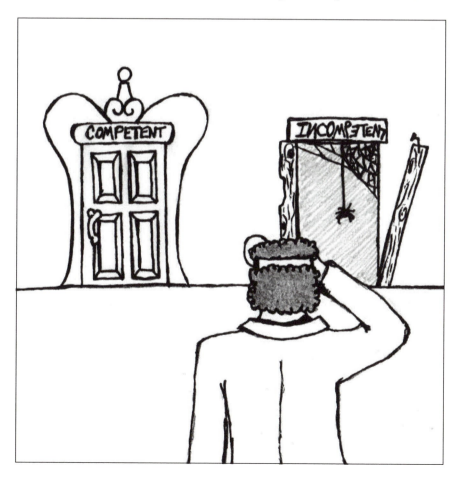

know that successful leaders come in all types – of personality, and passion, of capability and credentials. And we also know the one thing that all successful leaders have in common. All true leaders have followers! People who trust and respect the leader thoroughly enough to follow their lead.

And who do people trust and respect? We trust and respect those who are credible. That leads, does it not, to the next question: Where does credibility come from? Credibility is earned through the demonstration of competence (skills, knowledge, abilities, experiences, and expertise) and character (values, beliefs, attitudes, behaviors, and general trustworthiness). Credibility is the starting point for anyone who aspires to lead well – whether in the practice of medicine or in life overall.

> "A competent leader can get efficient service from poor troops, while on the contrary an incapable leader can demoralize the best of troops."
>
> John J. "Black Josh" Pershing

Physician Leader Attributes and Values

What are the attributes and values of successful physician leaders? They vary widely, of course, depending on the physician and the leadership being provided. In general, however, we can suggest several common traits, based on our collective decades' of experience working with physician leaders in a variety of roles and settings. We've found that effective physician leaders, regardless of specialty, are likely to:

- value patient care and the healing mission of medicine
- be driven by the need for excellence in all that they do
- understand the importance of shared vision and goals
- be drawn to the possibility of helping many people, not just one patient at a time.

> "Docs want someone who understands our world and sets an example. We're turned off by platitudes – like business management fads. For example – 'promoting excellence' is receiving a lot of attention. Most docs feel excellence is core to their profession, so for an outsider to push it as a 'new initiative' seems silly to us. Physicians are pretty hard on themselves and our leaders. We expect a very high level of integrity."
>
> Randall Oates, MD
> Family Physician
> President of Docs, Inc.

In fact, most of the effective physician leaders we've known exhibit several attributes or values that seem to be integral to their success. Those include integrity, life balance, external focus, and humor. Perhaps you like to follow general management and leadership literature. If so, you may already have some familiarity with these notions.

Twenty-six Characteristics of a True Leader

1 A leader is trustworthy.	14 A leader knows when to change his mind.
2 A leader takes the initiative.	15 A leader does not abuse his authority.
3 A leader uses good judgment.	16 A leader doesn't abdicate his role in the face of opposition.
4 A leader speaks with authority.	
5 A leader strengthens others.	17 A leader is sure of his calling.
6 A leader is optimistic and enthusiastic.	18 A leader knows his own limitations.
7 A leader never compromises the absolutes.	19 A leader is resilient.
	20 A leader is passionate.
8 A leader focuses on objectives, not obstacles.	21 A leader is courageous.
	22 A leader is discerning.
9 A leader empowers by example.	23 A leader is disciplined.
10 A leader cultivates loyalty.	24 A leader is energetic.
11 A leader has empathy for others.	25 A leader knows how to delegate.
12 A leader keeps a clear conscience.	26 A leader is Christlike.
13 A leader is definite and decisive.	

Excerpted from *The Book on Leadership: the power of a godly influence* (MacArthur 2004).

Do you believe these characteristics are important for physicians? In your experience, is their importance obvious to most physicians? We believe, and perhaps you do too, that physician leaders, by virtue of their role in society as healthcare professionals, bear unique obligations and characteristics. Physicians have traditionally been perceived by the general public as carrying the moral imperative of "life and death decisions." Such decisions are complex and not fully understood by the lay person, yet their gravity is generally well appreciated. Physicians and the public both recognize that physicians must, as a matter of course, make decisions that affect others in uniquely intimate ways. Consequently, trustworthiness is an absolutely essential characteristic for physicians.

At the same time, physicians can be particularly vulnerable to the negative consequences of success. The demands of professional life can be seductive. Many successful physicians have found that clinical practice and other professional activities can easily overwhelm any semblance of a personal life. Yet, physicians all need personal lives that provide emotional rest, support, and reality perspective. Rejuvenation, relaxation, renewal, re-invigoration are necessary to contextualize the burdens of complex professional decisions and priorities. Success in the professional environment can generate substantial positive reinforcement. Praise for success, however welcome, if excessively embraced, can delude leaders into an inflated sense of self-importance. Excessive internal focus can support the stereotypical behaviors of paternalism and arrogance that are too often justifiably associated with physicians.

> "I believe every person has a heart, and if you can reach it, you can make a difference."
>
> Uli Derickson

Thus those aspiring to be effective and fulfilled physician leaders invariably cultivate these attributes and values in their lives, and in the attitudes and behaviors of those they lead. Successful physician leaders recognize that integrity, life balance, external focus, and humor are essential stepping stones to living well and leading well.

Integrity

Integrity is essential for success as a physician leader. Other words, such as "trustworthiness" or "high moral values" may be substituted, but the point is that integrity is consistently identified as the number one reason why an individual is considered capable of leadership. Integrity is the number one reason why others will follow someone. It is the key to "trust" during periods of change and as leaders move into new and uncharted areas. Leaders with integrity enjoy sustained support over the long term. Leaders with integrity can tolerate disagreement and even draw from disagreement the alternative perspectives that expand their context of understanding. Those who follow leaders with integrity recognize that no one is perfect, so they tend to forgive minor shortcomings and errors, confident that leaders with integrity learn from their mistakes, are open to alternative viewpoints, and thus have a broader context for avoiding a repeat of their mistakes.

> "In **Dr. Stephen Covey's** book *The Seven Habits of Highly Effective People*, **Cecil B. DeMille** observed that 'It is impossible for us to break the law. We can only break ourselves against the law.' Of course he is referring to laws or basic principles of personal character that have governed social behavior forever. Covey goes on to mention basic characteristics such as fairness, integrity, honesty, human dignity. Certainly leaders of the health insurance companies of the early twenty-first century seem to be losing sight of these basic principles as they strive to increase their short-term 'bottom line' quarter after quarter. Their behaviors may be interpreted as driven by 'greed' in some quarters. I think we (physicians) must work hard to remain aware of these powerful, enduring principles as we negotiate with powerful partners in the healthcare arena."
>
> John M. Pascoe, MD
> Pediatrician
> Professor and Chair, Wright State University

Life Balance

Life balance is the thing that sustains leaders and permits them to be successful over an extended period of time. The capacity to balance personal and professional life is required for leaders to maintain a reality-based perspective. It guides their decision making by taking into account a diversity of viewpoints and the evolving environment. Life balance also adds an element of "freshness" to a leader's capacity to evaluate environment changes and predict their direction. Finally, life balance allows leaders, and especially physician leaders, toward more appropriate prioritization for themselves and the constituencies they support.

Paul Tsongas, a former U.S. representative, is credited as having said: "No one on his deathbed ever said, I wish I had spent more time at the office." Physician leaders are more than just physicians and leaders. They are also spouses, parents, children, and citizens, members of their society and of their communities. Just as social diversity is a well-recognized strength in communities, life balance is a strength in individuals.

Vision

Another essential attribute for success as a physician leader is a vision of the future and the capacity to communicate it. Good communication skills without vision produce a speaker whose listeners say, "That was beautiful but he really didn't say anything." Vision without the capacity to communicate it is equivalent to having a world-changing idea that is never shared. Vision to be successful must be for a future that most listeners would agree is "better" than the present. The capacity to communicate it means more, however, than simply painting a picture of how things "might be," but to articulate in clear, concise, and understandable terms what must be done to achieve that vision and to convince at least the majority of listeners that it is within their grasp. Physician leaders must not only develop a vision of the future. They must be able to communicate the vision in ways that inspire others to similarly integrate it into their own values and visions, and be willing to work together to make that enhanced future a reality.

External Focus

External focus reins in the tendency toward arrogance that can be particularly seductive for some physician leaders. Leaders with external focus are capable of directing sustainable behavior change. For example, such leaders can build self-directed teams. Effective leaders direct their focus toward succession planning so that the benefits of what they have built will be sustained by others for the future. Strong leaders commonly note that they begin succession planning on the first day of each new job – looking for, developing, growing, and empowering successors who will build upon their contributions.

Humor

Humor is essential for successful physician leadership. Although a good sense of humor does not typically rate much attention in traditional business literature, it is of particular importance for physician leaders. Humor helps physicians avoid the trap of arrogance. Humor is helpful in connecting leaders and followers. Humor conveys that you, the leader, "don't take yourself too seriously." Humor is the ultimate tension breaker; it opens communication and gives "permission" for a candid exchange of ideas. This is not to say that physician leaders need to be accomplished comedians. But it doesn't take more than a little dry or self-deprecating humor to convince others that a physician leader is a regular person they can talk with and potentially come to trust. In many ways, humor facilitates communication by breaking down barriers of prejudice and preconceived notions that might otherwise hinder clarity of direction and purpose.

> "Humor is one of God's most marvelous gifts. Humor gives us smiles, laughter, and gaiety. Humor reveals the roses and hides the thorns. Humor makes our heavy burdens light and smoothes down the rough spots in our pathways. Humor endows us with the capacity to clarify the obscure, to simplify the complex, to deflate the pompous, to chastise the arrogant, to point a moral, and to adorn a tale."
>
> Sam J. Erwin, Jr.

Points to Ponder

1 What attributes and values do you believe are characteristic of effective physician leaders? Why do you believe that? How might your view differ from the views of your colleagues?
2 What do you suppose your colleagues would say are your key values? Would their perceptions be consistent with what you'd hope them to be?
3 Are you aware of any attributes or values that you should alter in order to enhance the effectiveness and fulfillment you experience in your work?
4 How do you convey your values to those you lead – specifically, how do your values guide the decisions you make and actions you take on a day-to-day basis?
5 How do you deal with ethically complex or ambiguous situations? What factors do you take into consideration? What approach do you use to resolve or at least address such concerns?

Monte Anderson, MD, is a firm believer in the importance of credibility for any physician who aspires to make an impact inside or outside of healthcare. Dr. Anderson asserts that patients and colleagues deserve to be able to trust physicians to be truly "rock solid."

Insights from Monte L. Anderson, MD

"How do I define physician leadership? Any good executive has to be a leader. Some special prerequisites are involved in being a physician leader. Before doctors will respect others as leaders, they must respect them as 'rock solid' physicians. After that, it becomes more similar.

How does one physician know whether another is 'rock solid?' We see patients who've been referred by other doctors, and those patients let us know. So we can tell from the consults we do. Also, we hear it from the nurses. For example, over 40 nurses help with endoscopies here at the **Mayo Clinic – Scottsdale**. They work with physicians every day; and it is clear to see which ones they hold in high esteem.

People expect doctors to be leaders, and they want to think their doctor excels in his field. Many doctors reveal leadership skills while they are in college – heading committees and project teams of various sorts – so many of them expect leadership of themselves. Most doctors who are effective leaders focus far beyond passing their clinical boards. More and more, there is a realization within medicine (it came later to us than to most people in business) that we can accomplish far more through teamwork than we could ever accomplish alone. This concept is well established in the Mayo Clinic practice. In my opinion, those who do not understand the value of teamwork are short-changing themselves but, sadly, some of us still continue to strive only to outdo one another.

Leaders must be smart and knowledgeable. But most doctors are. Effective physician leaders have rock solid competency in medicine. Once you know this about a colleague, you never need to doubt it again. When I have a question in another field I contact a doctor who specializes in that field. During our brief interaction I can tell who is reliable because they're obviously well-versed in their own field; they're medical dictionaries with experience.

Effective physician leaders realize the importance of being trustworthy. They're consistent, understanding, and compassionate.

I have been shocked to observe a senior doctor, residents and students in tow, walk into a patient's room and barely acknowledge that person's presence. That patient is what we are all about! People learn by watching what others do. There is a science to teaching. All doctors have the opportunity to teach and nurture other doctors. Being good at that requires genuine respect for patients and trainees. The compliment that has always meant the most to me is being called a good role model by the residents.

I've always been interested in science and medicine – even as a kid. Any money I had while growing up was money I had earned myself. I started with a paper route, then I got a job with a veterinarian taking care of dogs and cats. They trusted me to the point that they allowed me to assist in surgery. I liked seeing sick animals get better.

I met **Pat** (my wife) while in college, fell in love with her, and was married soon after. No one in my family had even gone to college. Pat was a huge influence on me. She was a stellar student and I wanted to be as well. I took a huge number of classes; earned a high grade point average. We had children right away, while still in school. So after graduating, I got a job in the pharmaceutical industry. I was reasonably successful at it; but it wasn't a substitute for actually working as a physician. Then one day, Pat said to me 'If you really want to go to medical school, this is the time to do it.' So I quit my job, took a couple of prerequisite courses, and passed the MCAT exam with very high scores. I hadn't been in college in over 10 years at that point, but was thrilled to begin.

Continued

The first year I applied, I received a letter from the **University of Nebraska Medical Center (UNMC)** stating that I was too old for medical school. I was so upset about it, I threw the letter away. A few days later, after reflecting on the situation, I made an appointment with the Dean. I told her how serious I was about wanting to be a physician, and said I couldn't understand how someone with my credentials would not be admitted. After that conversation, I was appointed to the **University of Nebraska – Omaha** for a year, working as a graduate teaching assistant.

I reapplied to UNMC the following year. The Dean called me and asked if I thought I could go through medical school in three years (rather than four) without taking any vacation time. I knew I could do it, and told her so! UNMC was starting an experimental program and I was to be a part of it. So I began medical school at age 33 – the oldest student in my class. I was elected to leadership of the Senate and served on search committees for various Department Chairs. I placed very well in my graduating class, and because of the academic scholarships I'd earned, only owed $5,000 when finished.

Despite my surgical inclinations, I chose to go into Internal Medicine, believing it would be important to keep my options open for the future. All of that time, my family didn't have much money but we had fun. My teachers and peers elected me to the **Alpha Omega Alpha (AOA)** honor medical society. I later became Chief Resident in my internal medicine program. Gastroenterology really appealed to me, particularly GI endoscopy, which was still very new and seemed about as close as an Internist could come to being a surgeon.

Some faculty members at the University invited me to join their practice, but at the same time, the **United States Army** offered me an opportunity to do a GI fellowship, paying back one year for each year of training. So I recruited another resident to take my place with the physician group and went into the GI fellowship. On completing my Army obligation, my children were in high school, and our family decided we wanted to stay awhile in the same city. I joined some great colleagues at **Scott and White Clinic** in Temple, Texas.

I went to work for a month with **Dick Fleming**, MD, at the **Mayo Clinic – Rochester**. A wonderful friendship was born. A couple of years later we discussed my coming to Rochester, but I had learned by then that I could get depressed in places where there is a paucity of sunshine so the discussions went no further.

A couple of years later, I was again contacted on behalf of Mayo Clinic. They were starting a new clinic in Scottsdale. A good friend and medical school classmate, **Gretchen McCoy**, MD, and I started the GI program together. The planning of what we'd need to get the GI department up and running, and the goals that we hoped to attain were very exciting projects. I was later appointed the Department Chair, Gastroenterology. Over the next several years I recruited some terrific colleagues and our department flourished.

A few years later, I was appointed Chairman of the International Committee and Director of International Affairs for **Mayo Clinic – Scottsdale**. With the help of some great administrators, we started the program and opened an office in Mexico City. We wanted to make it easy for patients to come to Mayo Clinic. We ran the program in Mexico like a business – with a business plan, budget, and annual goals. After about seven years of being on gastroenterology call and traveling internationally, the absences from home began to take a toll. So I stepped out of the role. In October 2003 I was asked to step back in, and I did.

At this point, I'm semi-retired, working two weeks each month at **Mayo Clinic – Scottsdale**. On Mondays I see International patients – especially those who don't speak English. I really enjoy seeing these patients who have come all the way to Scottsdale to have an appointment at Mayo. Out of sensitivity to the cost those patients incur, we've found ways to streamline the episode of care so their visits begin on Monday and are completed by the end of the week.

I've done a lot of speaking at Medical Schools and Congresses in Mexico. A few years ago, I was invited to give a keynote speech at one of the Medical Schools in Mexico City. The auditorium was huge, and completely full. Afterward, a young man approached me and said that he wanted to carry on his studies at the **Mayo Clinic**. I helped him get a surgical residency in Rochester, where he was recognized as the outstanding member of his class. **Keith Kelly, MD,** Chair of Surgery here in Scottsdale, brought the young man to our Clinic for the remaining four years of his residency. He continues to excel and is now a Fellow in transplant surgery. My involvement in such relationships has been one of the most rewarding parts of my career.

Several years ago, I developed a heart arrhythmia and experienced rapid heart beats that caused me to pass out. My career was seriously threatened. I became one of the first patients to undergo radio frequency ablation. It restored my life to normal. Our youngest son Chris [Chris Anderson, MD] was living at home at the time and knew of my condition. Chris decided on his own that he wanted to become a physician. He was an outstanding first year surgical trainee, but chose to drop out of Surgery and go into Pediatrics instead. Chris spent a year in Emergency Medicine. Then he trained in the Pediatric Residency Program at **Baylor University** in Houston. He went on to complete a Fellowship in Pediatric Cardiology at **UCLA**. At graduation, the cardiac surgeons invited Chris to attend their award ceremony where they asked him to come forward to be recognized for his outstanding cooperation with the surgical program. Chris later left academic medicine. He is now in a private practice of Pediatric Cardiology in Spokane, Washington. He works long days, but he loves what he does. And that's what counts.

Our daughter, Elizabeth, is also in healthcare. Our other son, Mark, majored in English at the University of Texas and works in high tech computer operations in New York City."

Monte L. Anderson, MD
Gastroenterologist and Hepatologist, Mayo Clinic Scottsdale

Dr. Anderson has chosen to apply his leadership abilities toward the advancement of clinical excellence in the specialized field of gastroenterology. Not only does he provide the highest quality care for his own patients, he is mentoring and guiding the "next generation" of physicians to ensure the standard of excellence is as high as possible. Dr. Anderson represents one way that leading physicians can make a difference – in the health status of their own patients and in healthcare overall. He is a clinical standard bearer whose credibility stems from both his "rock solid" technical competence and his "rock solid" character.

Points to Ponder

1 What, in your opinion, does it mean to be credible, competent, and of trustworthy character? Specifically, what attributes, values, behaviors, or other factors do you look for when seeking to determine whether someone is credible and competent, someone whose character you can trust and respect?

2 Some people would describe "integrity" as the integration of our decisions, actions, attitudes, and behaviors – with the values we claim to cherish. Using "integration" of values and behaviors as the metric, do you exhibit as much integrity as you'd like to? What challenges do you face in that regard?

Another physician who believes strongly in the importance of credibility is Richard Birrer, MD, MPH, MMM, CPE. Having been Chief Executive Officer of St. Joseph's Regional Medical Center in New Jersey, Dr. Birrer understands the importance of maintaining credibility with his clinical colleagues, even while earning credibility with administrative colleagues.

Insights from Richard Birrer, MD, MPH, MMM, CPE

"The mark of a good leader is followership – being credible and having followers. Leaders attract people who follow, not because they fear job loss or oppression, and not because they are forced to comply. Real leadership is about commitment, not compliance. Real leaders instill in others a sense of ownership and motivation. Servant leadership is an important concept.

Many doctors (and people in general) are recidivistic; that may explain the popularity of that old saying: 'Change is good, as long as it doesn't involve me.'

Effective physician leaders recognize the importance of focusing on the needs and interests of their constituencies. They make the time to get out there and listen to all their key stakeholders. And they let people know they've listened. They take a stand and act on the insights gained from the interaction.

Savvy physician leaders understand the pitfalls to avoid. For example, they don't waste time trying to gain consensus. It is futile to expect consensus all the time. Physicians respect the outlier, sometimes to the detriment of progress.

Physician leaders listen to others' input, in order to increase the likelihood of making optimal decisions and taking appropriate actions. Then they exercise the self-discipline to say: 'Thanks! We're going to move forward now!'

Effective physician leaders understand the importance of having credibility with other physicians. They need to be credible in order to gain physicians' commitment, involvement, and loyalty to the cause at hand. Effective physician leaders offer other doctors plenty of opportunity to participate, to partner, to 'hold a stake' in the outcome of the matters at hand.

To develop physicians' leadership abilities, give them the money, the time, and the opportunity to be involved. They will make the right decisions – *if* – you've been mentoring, coaching, and leading them appropriately.

Effective physician leaders make the effort to remain clinically credible. They do so by going on rounds, asking questions that show they still understand and appreciate the practice of medicine.

I recommend aspiring physician leaders identify their developmental needs, create a list of options to pursue, and then prioritize which of those options to focus on.

I use my 'kitchen cabinet' – a team of colleagues that happens to include a surgeon, an internist, and a cardiologist – to kick around issues. I can count on them to give me suggestions of where to go, what to do, and how to do it. Their collaboration and our forum for interaction has really helped me succeed."

Richard R. Birrer, MD, MPH, MMM, CPE
Family, Emergency, Sports and Geriatric Medicine Physician

Dr. Birrer has become a very effective organizational leader through a combination of natural aptitude, formal education, and progressively broad job responsibilities. He isn't content to rely upon his current capabilities, though, but continuously seeks out additional experiences, relationships, and resources to even further enhance his ability to contribute to the advancement of excellence in healthcare delivery.

> "A man too busy to take care of his health is like a mechanic too busy to take care of his tools."
>
> Spanish proverb

Points to Ponder

1 To what extent are you responsible for the credibility, competency, and character of those you aspire to lead?
2 Think about your own abilities and the abilities of those you aspire to lead. How exactly can you help others enhance their credibility by strengthening their competence or character?

Another physician who is passionate about the importance of character and credibility is Gary Morsch, MD. In fact, Dr. Morsch believes strongly that no one should concern themselves with what types of leadership work they will *do* until they've become clear about who they are called to *be*. Dr. Morsch is a board certified Family Physician who has served as an Emergency Physician in the U.S. Army Reserves in Kosovo, Iraq, and elsewhere. However, he is perhaps better known for his numerous and varied entrepreneurial endeavors. In particular, Dr. Morsch is respected by Ministers of Health in countries all over the world for having founded Heart to Heart International, a philanthropic organization that delivers medical supplies and medical education to people in underdeveloped countries and places that have been devastated by natural or man-made disasters.

Insights from Gary Morsch, MD

"Anyone can be a leader. Leaders care about and help others. They do the right thing. Some people mistakenly think I work all the time. I don't. I give the world eight or ten or twelve hours, but then I 'turn work off' in the evenings when I'm with my family. I don't knock myself out 48 weeks per year so I can take a break four weeks per year. That doesn't make sense to me. I've known too many people who are materially wealthy but unhappy. Maybe some would call them successful; I wouldn't. Society sometimes pressures us to view ourselves in light of what we 'do.' But first, we must be clear about who we are called to 'be.' The notion that 'if you can, you should' isn't necessarily true. For instance, a student might be able to earn all 'A's in school, but prefers to invest more time and energy in other things and so earns some 'B's. We all need to be clear about who we are called to be, what we are called to do. Then we may choose to set goals for how much income we want to generate, or how many projects we want to complete.

I learned a great deal from Mother Teresa about values, priorities, and time commitments. I've also learned a lot from Protestants, Hindus, Buddhists, and people of all faiths and cultures. What works for me is a matter of personal preference as well as theology. I'm often asked to speak with others – to motivate groups, get them fired up, get them to donate money to charity. Do you recall that saying from the seventies: 'I'm OK, you're OK?' Well, my theme is 'It's OK, you're OK,' meaning that it is important to relax and trust things to work out. When we know ourselves, and who God has designed us to be, then we can begin to glimpse what we're called to do. The world has it backwards. Too often, we're encouraged to focus on 'doing' and then tack on 'being' as an extra. This applies to people in healthcare, business, and churches – to people in all walks of life.

Leadership, we're often told, is about setting goals and getting people to get work done. I disagree. I'm not saying my view is right and that view is wrong; or my view is good and that view is bad. But the perspective that fits my abilities, experiences, and dysfunctions (said with a smile) is different. My personal view of leadership – my calling – is to help people find their place in the world – to help them gain a sense of purpose and mission.

As a Christian, physician, businessman and entrepreneur, founder, and owner of several organizations, I've learned that helping others is the right thing to do. For me, first! And then if I can do it for others – that's great! I have to resist viewing things the way the world portrays them – judging what's good or bad, valuable or worthwhile based upon money, or visible success. Taking a plate of cookies to a neighbor may be just as meaningful as developing a software operating system that ends up being used worldwide. The important thing for all of us is to know who we are and serve others through our gifts and abilities.

My message isn't always received well by everyone. I learned that when I ran for Congress in 2002 and was not elected. My level of transparency about my beliefs wasn't what 'won' in the voting polls. I don't view that as a failure or setback. To do so would imply the world's view of success. I truly believe success is 'doing the right thing' – it's how you respond or act in any given situation. I did 'the right thing' by running for Congress. It doesn't matter that I wasn't elected.

I like the character Don Quixote in the musical '**Man of La Mancha.**' He succeeded even though the world laughed at him and thought he was nuts. He knew his purpose and lived it out every day of his life. He was happy. He didn't focus on what others thought of him.

My goal isn't to accumulate material wealth (assets) or accolades (degrees or other credentials). People who express regrets when on their deathbed are very consistent in what they say they wish they'd done differently. They always say they wish they had spent more time with their families and loved ones; that they had treated others better. We (physicians) definitely know that. We hear it consistently from dying patients. So why don't we live that way?

I don't have any goals to start anything (i.e., new businesses). I never did. My goal is to know myself. Every day. That's why I believe in prayer, meditation, reflection. It is important to invest time pondering 'Who am I?' 'Where am I going?' 'What does this day hold for me?' 'Who will I see today?' 'What am I irritated about right now, and why?' 'What is that telling me about myself?'

Continued

I have this tendency to bring people together, help create a vision, and find the resources to bring it about. 'Risk everything!' I tell them. 'If we lose it all, so what?' Because I believe that what's 'right' is not about making money. What's 'right' is about 'doing the right thing.'

In fact, having more money can distract us from happiness because the presence and the pursuit of money can pull us away from focusing on the real meaning of life. It can create barriers, cause people to treat you differently, put pressure on you to take it to the next level and make even more money.

I launched **Docs Who Care** (a temporary physician staffing company) because I saw a need – there was, and still is, a shortage of doctors in rural areas. I later launched **Priority Physician Placement** (a physician recruiting service) because I saw a need – traditional recruiters weren't serving doctors very well because they didn't know the communities or the docs they were placing into them; they were putting the wrong people in the wrong places, so attrition was high. I launched **Heart to Heart International** (a humanitarian organization) because I believe in serving others we find our meaning in life. Those who serve others are more likely to know themselves and to accomplish their purpose. So Heart to Heart 'helps' the recipients of the medicines, yes, but it also helps those who donate products, or money, or time. It gives people the opportunity to become aware of needs and to address those needs – hopefully by personally getting involved in serving others. Some people go [on one of our international delegations] because they view it as an interesting adventure. But some go and are transformed – their lives are changed forever, for the better! It isn't about the quantity of product we deliver. It's about the people we impact by getting them involved.

In 1989, I challenged my local **Rotary Club** to identify a meaningful project that would serve people's needs. So they asked me to take a dozen people to remodel a **YWCA** in Belize. We did. The next year we went to St. Croix. The third year I suggested we serve our 'enemies' in Viet Nam or Russia. So we did an airlift of medicines to Moscow. That's how **Heart to Heart International** began. Now, after 11 years of operation, some see **Heart to Heart** as a professionally run organization and lose the heart-based passion on which it has always been based.

I was recently in Belize again (this time on a family vacation) and went to see **Mrs. Harris**, the woman who ran the **YWCA** back in 1989. She is still in Belize; still running that **YWCA**. She told me what we did for them back in 1989 went far beyond wiring and plumbing. What we did gave them hope, and a means to convey their vision to others, so that more people could be served. She, of course, was thinking of people in their local community. So I told her our side of the story – how that project inspired us to do another project the following year, and another, and another. I told her that Heart to Heart International has supplied over $300 million worth of medicines to people in over 100 countries around the world. And most importantly, I told her, it has mobilized literally thousands of volunteers. People who decided to share their time and their resources to see others' needs and respond.

My initial book, *Heart and Soul* written with co-author **Dean Nelson**, was created to help people understand the importance of finding their purpose and helping those in need. I'm currently working on a book that will challenge people to ask themselves what life is really all about; to help people live and die feeling good about themselves and their lives.

I still work in the emergency room, and whenever I begin my shift, I always say to myself (and others) 'Whatever happens, it's going to be great!' That's my attitude. Whether we see 100 patients and get no sleep, or whether we don't see any patients that shift. It doesn't matter.

Did this journey I've found myself on begin after I'd already completed medical school? Yes, I suppose so. But the seeds of it were there from the beginning. I grew up in a family that was always generous – we give of ourselves, serve others' needs, do the right thing. That's true of many physicians.

My son Graham **[Graham Morsch]** is named after **Ms. Mattie Graham** – a patient of mine back during my residency days. Ms. Graham was confined to her wheelchair, so she spent her days recycling birthday and anniversary cards to send to others. Then Ms. Graham lost her eyesight, and arthritis crippled her hands. So I asked her 'What will you do now?' and she replied 'I can still pray for people!' Ms. Graham was 'Don Quixote crazy' – and she was an inspiration to me.

I'm blessed because I get to leverage my gifts and my work to mobilize others. Some people are impressed that I personally know so many Ministers of Health in countries all over the world. But I'm not any more important than anyone else. I, just like everyone else, must focus on 'being' before I focus on 'doing.' My skills and abilities, time and interests, can only be appropriately directed when I'm clear about who I am and why I'm here."

Gary Morsch, MD
Family and Emergency Medicine Physician,
U.S. Army Reserves
Founder, Heart to Heart International, Physicians Who Care, and Priority Physician Placement

Through his entrepreneurial endeavors, his many books, and his gripping presentations, Dr. Morsch has inspired thousands of people – physicians and others – to rethink our place in the world. Few of us are blessed with such exceptional gifts of innovation, or the ability to mobilize such vast coalitions of collaboration toward service to those in need. And yet all of us can learn a great deal about leading well and living well from Dr. Morsch's words and more importantly, the example he sets for us.

Points to Ponder

1 Is your commitment to those you lead readily apparent in the way you allocate your time, energy and attention?
2 Suppose someone were to look through your calendar to see how you spend your time, and your checkbook to see how you spend your money. Would they see the person you claim to be?
3 Are you as credible, competent, and trustworthy as those you lead deserve you to be?
4 If so, congratulate yourself. If not, what are you willing and able to do about it?

"A person who is fundamentally honest doesn't need a code of ethics."

Harry S. Truman

Another physician servant-leader is the Reverend Pamela Harris, MD. Deeply devoted to the health of all people, Dr. Harris believes that a return to the traditional community-centered, faith-based medical model is essential for the provision of holistic care and thus the full healing of people – on physical, spiritual and social levels. She explains:

"I knew I was 'supposed' to be a doctor when I was 10 years old. My fourth grade class in school had been asked to consider various career options. When I told my mom that I was thinking of becoming a nurse, florist, or forest ranger, my mom said 'You know, Pam, nowadays, women can become doctors too.' And it clicked.

I grew up in Madison, Kansas in a town of 1200 people. During high school, I worked in a pharmacy and as a nurse's aid at the local nursing home. I even helped start an ambulance program at age 15. You see, our town had one volunteer EMT (emergency medical technician) but federal legislation required EMTs to have ambulances. We were 20 miles from Emporia, the next largest town. My dad, who worked for **Kansas Power and Light**, and another man, who did telephone repairs, knew where everyone lived, so they drove the ambulance.

I've always had a strong commitment to justice and a strong drive to reduce suffering. In our town, if someone was really sick, they would call the doc off his ranch to come help. We would wake up the pharmacist in the middle of the night if someone needed medicine right away. I saw community care at its finest. We all helped each other.

So that was the perspective I brought with me to medical school at the **University of Kansas**. While there, I took a job handling questionnaires in physical medicine and rehabilitation. I observed a huge contrast between that field versus the subspecialties, where docs get patients to baseline, discharge them, and move on. I liked rehabilitation medicine because it is holistic – the focus is on the whole person, who they are, not just what medical condition they're experiencing.

But the business of medicine kept interfering, and that caused me to consider other paths. I reflected on the way religious organizations had traditionally founded hospitals and schools as well as churches. My dad was Roman Catholic, and my mom was anything but, so my family wasn't encouraging me in that direction or anything. But I was fascinated by a book called *Primitive Physick*, written by the **Reverend John Wesley** back in 1791. In that small book of less than 200 pages, **Reverend Wesley** gave 289 tips for healing and wholeness. I had a conversion experience at age 20. Having only been in a Protestant church once – for a wedding – I found the variety of denominations interesting, and visited quite a few churches in Lawrence, where I was attending college. Mostly I attended **First Presbyterian Church** in Lawrence – I liked the pastor there. Later, living in Kansas City to attend medical school, a friend took me to **Old Mission United Methodist Church**. The United Methodists' framework of 'head, heart and hands' really fit. My husband and two daughters are still active in that church, even though I came to the **United Methodist Church of the Resurrection** in 1997. So we're a 'two-church family.' I need to be in a large church (COR has over 12,000 members) for the work I do as Minister of Health.

I envision myself as a consultant for the entire Kansas City district of Methodist churches – initiating programs that can be replicated, going into other churches as a speaker. I founded a 'Health and Wellness Speakers Bureau' here at COR to equip doctors, nurses, and various para-professionals to provide health education in the community. I want to reduce the incidence of insensitive remarks made to patients by people who mean well, but who make comments that are more hurtful than helpful. When, for example, people tell a patient 'Have faith and you will be healed' or 'God let this happen for a reason,' they often aren't considering the systematic theology of their comments, or what they're conveying about God or their beliefs of how the world works. They're simply repeating the socially acculturated traditions passed on to them by others. I've helped form a new group for bereaved parents – they need to believe God shares their agony and is welcoming their loved one with open arms.

I was in private practice for $8\frac{1}{2}$ years, including responsibility as Associate Director of the Rehabilitation Department at **Bethany Medical Center** in Kansas City, Kansas and **Rehabilitation Medical Director for Providence Hospital** in Kansas City, Kansas and **St. John's Hospital** in Leavenworth. It wasn't the most lucrative of practices, because a lot of the patients were uninsured, but I saw it as my mission as well as my practice.

Someone told me a job was opening at the **Veteran's Administration (VA) Hospital**. It wasn't immediately clear to me that the job was for me, but I was very confused by the changes that had been happening in my medical practice. I usually don't make demands for answers from God, but on this occasion I 'laid down a fleece' as Gideon had in the story found in Judges Chapter 6 in the **Bible**. I told God that I could not see what I was supposed to do, so if God wanted me to take the job at the VA, God should have them offer me the job; if it was not supposed to be, God should have them offer the job to the other candidate. So when offered the position I saw that as God's will and I accepted the role (in the year 2000).

I considered seminary for quite some time before applying. Usually my decision making is logical and rational; and rational physicians don't head off to seminary. But my VA job was only 25 hours per week and **St. Paul School of Theology** was only 10 minutes away, so it all fit. My first seminary class included a mixture of theology and pastoral care. The pastoral care resonated for me. I've come to realize that my call is to be a healer, not just a doctor. The education and experience I've gained through seminary has fleshed out that other side of my calling.

I yearn to help bring medicine back to its roots. That's why I wanted to become the Minister of Health at **Church of the Resurrection**. The fact that they'd never considered such a position, or that no other church in town has such a position wasn't going to stop me! I sent **COR** a 25-page proposal, outlining why they needed a physician with seminary training – essentially describing a role for which I knew I'd be the only candidate qualified to fill. It worked! I joined the staff in July 2002, having gradually increased my volunteer involvement the prior two years.

In my role as Minister of Health at COR, I've put together resources for people dealing with serious grief. I've been with people while they are dying. I don't second guess their own doctors' decisions, but I can offer translation of medical terminology. Plus, while doctoring, if spiritual questions come up, I don't have to refer them to others.

One time prior to claiming my 'religion,' I found myself with the wife of a patient who was 'coding' (dying). The chaplain wasn't available. Was that ever nerve-wracking! I grabbed some Kleenex for the woman, and patted her hand furiously, wondering what else to do. So I called a nurse, who sat with the woman until the chaplain arrived.

It seemed to me the chaplains got to deal with the really important questions. I mean, patients and their loved ones aren't usually as interested in the scientific mechanics as they are in the meaning behind the science. Chaplains have the societal permission to ask 'Are you scared?' Most doctors wouldn't see that as appropriate to their own role. Things are changing, but the traditional medical model hasn't positioned doctors to address patients' needs on all levels. Community care and holistic care models do – they take medicine back to its roots.

I want the way we provide care to return to the pre-enlightenment time when body, mind and spirit were recognized as being inseparable. Ancient practices across two thirds of the world saw the spiritual component as much a part of healing or wholeness as the medical science component. They acknowledged the emotional, spiritual, and relational ramifications of a person's physical disabilities.

I want doctors to incorporate this awareness into the treatment plans and care they offer. I want the church to be one of the best sources of legitimate information for people seeking health and wholeness. In church, we not only minister to the soul, we honor the body as well. As a Deacon, I'll be ordained to serve, to bring the concerns of the world to the church, and to empower people in the church to use their gifts in service to the world. This is the bridge from head to heart to hands. A pitcher, basin, and towel (reminiscent of Christ's washing the feet of his disciples) are the symbols of Deacons – they remind us that whoever would be great must be a servant."

Reverend Pamela S. Harris, MD

"Great ideas reflect ancient wisdom and have the power to bind people together while creating unity and making good things happen. But no great idea exists alone. Without the innovators and servant leaders with heart and soul, no system can live for very long."

Nikitas J. Zervanos, MD
Retired Residency Program Director
in his presentation "The Family Physician as Servant Leader"
for the Ohio Academy of Family Physicians, April 3, 2004

Reverend Harris, MD, continues:

"I've never taken any business courses. My first boss at the VA Hospital mentored me in the mechanics of the hospital. Mostly I just jump in and swim. I follow my internal compass by considering whether something is fair, just, and reasonable. Although I was a resident at the VA many of the new employees don't know me, so I have to walk the talk, and demonstrate consistently over time that I am who I say I am, that I really do care about them.

The past four years my path has been illogical, but it has also brought me balance. My primary appointment under the United Methodist connectional system is ministry at the **VA Hospital**. My church recognizes this. I set boundaries and am clear about what I need in order to do what I'm called to do. My internal compass is my guide – not just in moral/ethical matters, but also time/energy boundaries. If I were to work in traditional medicine, I could make four times more money. But not being paid for my work as Minister of Health at the **Church of the Resurrection** is freeing – it allows me to express who and what I am, and it prepares me to do my paid job."

Reverend Harris, MD, offers us an example of a physician leader who is both innovator and executive, practitioner and healer. Using her clinical training, spiritual beliefs, and administrative abilities, Dr. Harris coordinates the application of resources toward the holistic well-being of patients and citizens – in her community and beyond.

Another physician leader who champions the explicit focus on ethics in leadership is Dr. Erich H. Loewy. A renowned medical ethicist, he has made a significant contribution to our understanding of this complex subject. Here are his insights:

Insights from Erich H. Loewy, MD

"For many topics, we turn to textbooks as reliable sources of authority. When it comes to questions of ethics, no such handy authority is available. To mediate between distinctly different senses of morality we must settle it by:

1 using power – but that does not alter a sense of right or wrong
2 turning to the law – but there are numerous laws many would consider unethical
3 turning to our particular religion or belief system – but that will convince no one who does not adhere to the same beliefs
4 following our 'conscience' or 'gut feeling' – but the conscience of some will be deemed unconscionable to others
5 accepting anything in the spirit of complete cultural relativism
6 voting to accept as 'right' the views of the majority – but because most people believe something does not make it 'right'
7 settling on a framework of inevitable human capabilities and experiences within which we develop laws and guidelines.

In using such a framework, I believe we must make a few assumptions:

1 Force – either tacit or explicit – will not be used.
2 Everyone's voice will be equal.
3 The weak – children, mentally deficient, the senile, etc. – will be represented by an Ombudsman of some type.

In looking at other cultures, religions, or at ethical theories, we find similarity in their basic rules. All prohibit murder, theft, and lying. Almost all recommend being helpful toward others. Tolerance for other customs, so long as they fall within this framework, must emerge. Such systems have at least six components:

1 the desire to be – all normal creatures under normal circumstances want to live
2 access to resources that support biological needs – food, water, shelter, etc.
3 equal access to the social needs of the society
4 prevention of useless suffering
5 a common sense of logic, sufficient to acknowledge that we cannot be in two places at once
6 opportunity to pursue our interests and optimize our talents.

Thus, in such an ethical system, we would not murder, steal, lie, let others go hungry when resources exist, deprive people of education, or cause (or fail to alleviate when possible) needless suffering. We would have universal access to healthcare.

Leadership in general denotes showing the way to others. It implies a common goal, and knowledge and skill in working toward the agreed upon goal. There is more to leadership than being knowledgeable and motivated. Leaders must have wisdom, be trustworthy, competent, and experienced. Physicians can assume several leadership roles:

1 leadership to their patients
2 leadership to their students if they are in an academic position
3 leadership in their institution
4 leadership in their professional associations
5 leadership in their community
6 leadership in international health.

In each of these, physicians themselves can be therapeutic agents, bringing about good, in part, by being role models for others. The ethics of leadership, then, is to have well thought out goals developed in dialogue among the public with the advice and consent of the profession."

Erich H. Loewy, MD
Professor of Medicine (emeritus)
Founding Alumni Association Chair of Bioethics
Associate, Department of Philosophy
University of California, Davis

Spirituality in Healthcare

While physicians' religious backgrounds are, of course, as diverse as those of the patients they treat, most physicians share a deep regard for the sacredness of life. And for many, that includes a respect for patients' spiritual condition, as well as their physical and emotional health status. The impact of prayer on wellness or recuperation has been the subject of more published research in the past 10 years than in the previous 100 years. The data regarding statistically significant association between faith and healing are debatable. And yet, few physicians practicing medicine today would debate the fact that we are complex, integrated beings, whose spiritual, emotional, mental, and even socio-economic status often impacts – directly or indirectly – our physical health status.

Physicians who aspire to lead significant progress in the delivery of healthcare may find themselves drawn to make a contribution in this relatively underdeveloped aspect of medicine. Though resources are not yet plentiful, some do exist, and are being used with success. Steven Jeffers, PhD, Director of the Institute for Spirituality in Health describes some of the resources the Institute offers physicians.

"Spirituality, often expressed in a cultural or religious tradition, provides a personal framework for the understanding of life's purpose and meaning, the sense of well-being and the relationship with humanity and the divine. It is a determining factor in how individuals explain and react to life events. Spirituality is an important element in patients', families', and healthcare providers' ability to cope with illness, dying, and death. Thus spirituality is an indispensable component of quality holistic healthcare.

This definition of spirituality is the guiding principle of the Institute for Spirituality in Health. An overarching goal of the Institute is to help physicians remember the real reason for choosing the medical profession – to serve humanity. We rely upon four strategies to achieve this goal – education, publication, research, and a national prayer ministry. Our educational offerings include conferences, CME programs, and physician/clergy dialogue groups. We publish books, booklets, and other print or electronic resources for physicians who wish to understand, or help their patients and families understand and address the spiritual aspects of their medical conditions. We regularly gather and disseminate research on spirituality and health.

For example, the Institute generated a 'CARE Spirituality History' framework to help physicians and patients address spiritual concerns at end-of-life. We saw this as important because 84.5 percent of physicians who participated in one of our surveys cited the importance of religion or spirituality and 80 percent indicated belief that 'a patient's involvement in religion or spirituality reduces morbidity and mortality,' yet over 70 percent of those physicians never or rarely initiate a spiritual history with patients, often because they lack training to do so.

The Institute developed a CARE Spiritual History model for provision of **C**omfort, **A**ssessment of needs, mobilization of **R**esources, and **E**mpowerment of patients and families to grow through the difficult experience. That model has reportedly benefited patients, patients' families, and physicians, both in our local medical center and through its publication in the online journal of the American College of Physician Executives.

Spirituality shapes who physicians are as individuals. When physicians incorporate spiritual convictions into their professional roles, they connect with patients at a deeper level and with more sensitivity. In that sense, spirituality enhances the well-being of physicians and those they serve."

Steven Jeffers, PhD
Director
The Institute for Spirituality in Health
Shawnee Mission Medical Center

References and Further Reading

Covey S.R. (2004) *The Eighth Habit: from effectiveness to greatness.* New York: Free Press, a division of Simon & Schuster.

Covey S.R. (1992) *Principle-centered Leadership.* New York: Simon & Schuster.

Covey S.R. (1989) *The Seven Habits of Highly Effective People.* New York: Simon & Schuster.

Estes M.L. (1997) Core competencies for physician practice success. *Physician Executive* **23**(1): 9–14.

Ferrell O.C., Fraedrich J., and Ferrell, L. (2002) *Business Ethics: ethical decision making and cases*. Boston: Houghton Mifflin Company.

Jeffers S.J., Hightower D.P., Kelley G.R., McKenna M.K., Nelson M.E., and Schwartz A.M. (2005) The CARE spiritual history. *The American College of Physician Executives The Leading Edge Online Journal for Medical Management* **2**(1). Posted online 1/01/05 at www.acpenet.org/MembersOnly/leadingedge/jan_2005_vol2_no1/spirit.htm.

Kouzes J.M. and Posner B.Z. (2003) *Credibility: how leaders gain it and lose it, why people demand it*. San Francisco: Jossey-Bass.

Lane D.S. and Ross V. (1998) Defining competencies and performance indicators for physicians in medical management. *American Journal of Preventative Medicine* **14**(3): 229–36.

MacArthur J. (2004) *The Book on Leadership: the power of a godly influence*. Nashville, TN: Thomas Nelson Publishing.

Maxwell J.C. (2001) *The Right to Lead: a study in character and courage*. Nashville, TN: Thomas Nelson Publishing.

McKenna M.K., Gartland M.P., and Pugno P.A. (2004) Development of Physician Leadership Competencies: Perceptions of Physician Leaders, Physician Educators and Medical Students. *The Journal of Healthcare Administration Education* **21**(3)(Summer): 343–54.

Nash D.B., Markson L.E., Howell S., and Hildreth E.A. (1993) Evaluating the competence of physicians in practice: From peer review to performance assessment. *Academic Medicine* **68** (2 Suppl.): 19S-22S.

Schneerson M.M. (2001) *The Unbreakable Soul: a chasidic discourse by Lubavitcher Rebbe Rabbi Menacham M. Schneerson of Chabad-Lubavitch*. New York: Kehot Publication Society.

Strack G. and Fottler M.D. (2002) Spirituality and effective leadership in healthcare: Is there a connection? *Frontiers of Health Services Management* **18**(4): 3–18.

Wesley J. (1791) *Primitive Physick, or An Easy and Natural Method of Curing Most Diseases*. Accessed 8/21/05 at: http://195.12.26.123/404.asp?404;http://195.12.26.123/encyclopedia/wesley.htm

Chapter 11

Clarity of Vision and Communication

"To be an effective leader requires skills in listening, speaking, and writing. Physician leaders need to be good communicators as well as idea people. Thinking outside the box is not natural for many physicians, who spend years functioning within a fairly narrow confine. I believe many physicians have the innate ability to lead, but haven't nurtured or developed their ability to do so."

J. Peter Geerlofs, MD
Family Physician
Chief Medical Officer
Allscripts Healthcare Solutions, Inc.

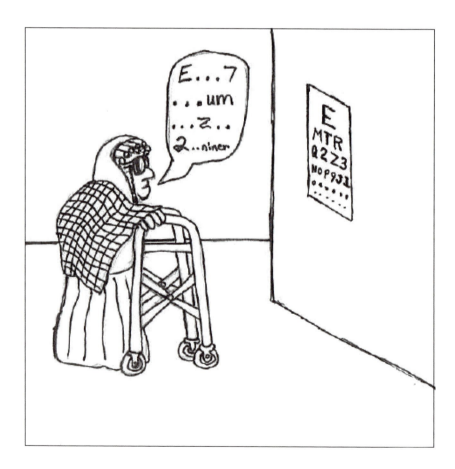

Clarity of Direction

To lead well we must bring others a clear sense of direction. This occurs at several levels. Leaders offer a clear vision of the future that is desired for all involved; a clear mission, or reason (purpose) for the expenditure of effort and sacrifice; and clear goals that serve to guide our activity while helping us measure the extent of our progress. Often, the ability to provide such clarity of direction involves a keen power of observation, and a frame of mind that is conducive to contemplating complex situations – both familiar and unfamiliar – in fresh new ways.

> "Discovery consists of seeing what everybody has seen and thinking what nobody has thought."
>
> Albert von Nagyrapolt Swent-Gyorgyi

> "The 'elephant in the room' is looming larger than ever. Healthcare delivery simply doesn't work the way its consumers and payors need and want, but many physicians are too overwhelmed to do anything about it. That's a large part of why I'm so passionate about the potential for a new breed of physician leaders. Even with managed care and the advent of large practices and IDNs, healthcare remains largely a cottage industry – with each organization or clinic operating as though it were an island. Physician leaders must help physicians grasp how infinitely better healthcare could be if we changed our minds and decided to operate as regional and national teams on behalf of our mutual customer – patients!"
>
> J. Peter Geerlofs, MD
> Family Physician
> Chief Medical Officer
> Allscripts Healthcare Solutions, Inc.

Catalysts for Shared Vision

Not only are successful leaders visionary. They're able to *communicate* that direction in a clear and compelling manner. They "paint a mental picture" that is so powerful – relevant, engaging, credible, and inspiring – that others are naturally and irresistibly drawn to contribute to its achievement. We do not mean to imply that leaders must be the font of all brilliance. Just the opposite, in fact. The most effective leaders are those who're able to trigger otherwise untapped creativity and insight of those they lead, much as enzymes are catalysts for biochemical reactions and processes.

> "Some doctors think they're the smartest person in the world. Good leaders realize they're not smart enough to know everything. They seek insight from others."
>
> Monte L. Anderson, MD
> Gastroenterologist and Hepatologist
> Mayo Clinic Scottsdale

Vision and Optimism – Synergistic Leadership Attributes

We know that a typical attribute of successful leaders is their unwavering optimism. What isn't clear is whether those leaders are optimistic because they can envision a better future that many of us don't yet see, or they're able to envision a better future because they view the world through a positive lens. Either way, the fact remains, successful leaders anticipate positive outcomes, and then bring them about!

> "Leadership requires time, patience, confidence and the belief that things can be better. With those commitments a great deal can be accomplished."

> Edward T. Bope, MD
> Family Physician
> Residency Program Director

Clarity of Direction Exemplified

One physician leader who understands the importance of clear vision and direction is Ronald Riner, MD. Trained as a cardiologist, Dr. Riner now consults with leaders in healthcare organizations of all types and sizes, helping them develop strategies and set goals that improve the quality and cost-effectiveness of the services they deliver.

Insights from Ronald Riner, MD

"How do I define leadership? Leadership is something we all recognize when we see it, but find difficult to define. Most bona fide leaders have a very strong value structure that doesn't get compromised; their values permeate their interactions with others. Most effective leaders share several common denominators. They are typically ethical, and communicate well. They're flexible. They focus on others (versus themselves) and focus on accomplishing results. Leaders are not necessarily charismatic, though some certainly are. Good leaders can be counted on – in adverse and in favorable conditions. Leaders are, to a certain extent, dilettantes. They aren't focused exclusively on their own organization. They bounce multiple balls, they see multiple agendas, they are intrigued by multiple opportunities. Good leaders can focus, but typically have a broad horizon.

I view healthcare leadership (of which physician leadership is a component) as very important. Money should be invested in the education and development of healthcare leaders – both clinical and non-clinical professionals. Everyone talks about leadership, but few plan for it and even fewer are blessed to experience or exhibit leadership. I view it primarily as an organizational issue in clinical practices and healthcare systems. The presence or absence of leadership is what makes or breaks organizations. People and organizations consistently seek leaders; but leaders aren't readily available.

Healthcare organizations are far more complex than they were in previous eras; as a consequence, leaders must understand and interface with many facets of business. Effective leaders are effective communicators and relationship builders. To become an effective leader, one must first have an interest in it. Some have innate leadership qualities. Even so, they must expose themselves to multiple avenues of education and experience in order to become truly effective as leaders.

Effective leaders are capable of crafting a 'big picture' that others buy into. Why do we lack leadership in healthcare? Perhaps because most of us were trained to focus on our particular clinical specialty, not the big picture. Also, the complexity of medical advances and healthcare delivery systems cause all of us to experience great demands on our time, simply to 'keep up with' advances in our own specialty.

I was born in South Dakota, but grew up on the East Coast – White Plains New York for high school, then Princeton for undergrad, Cornell for residency, etc. I joined a cardiovascular surgical program at the **Mayo Clinic – Rochester**. I was Program Director of Internal Medicine for a 600 bed university-affiliated hospital and Department Director of Cardiology. I've worked with **St. Louis University** and **Washington University** in St. Louis. For a while, I continued my private practice while growing my consulting business. My consulting focused on practice management and cardiovascular data acquisition for clinical trials.

In the early 1980s, the quality movement led by **Deming** and **Duran** permeated healthcare. I worked with the management team of one of the largest Integrated Healthcare Systems in the country. I was Chairman of the Board of the **Alleghany Health System** in Florida – one of the largest healthcare systems on the East coast some time ago. That's where I gained much of my current understanding of governance.

Finally, I stopped practicing medicine around 1992 or 1993 because I couldn't honor my travel commitments and provide continuity of care. Now I focus entirely on the business side of healthcare, by helping healthcare organizations with strategy, new business development, and performance improvement.

Much of my medical training has applicability to my consulting work. I miss patient care sometimes. When that happens, I remind myself that I'm practicing 'vicariously' by helping my clients understand and improve their own provision of care for their patients.

What have been the keys to my success as a physician leader? I've been blessed with good health, a supportive family, a strong educational foundation and a curious mind.

I've been fortunate to work with many strong healthcare leaders, such as **Dr. Hugh Smith**, Chairman of the **Mayo Clinic Board of Governors**, for example, and **Bill George**, former CEO of **Medtronic, Inc**. I've also known

Continued

> many hospital CEOs and clinical department chairs/managing partners of medical groups who are superb leaders. Those individuals exhibit compassion and influence others in positive ways."
>
> Ronald N. Riner, MD
> Cardiologist
> President, The Riner Group

Dr. Riner certainly exemplifies the way in which physician leaders can bring clarity of direction to healthcare organizations. In his work as a consultant, he is helping physicians and others become visionary, effective leaders.

Points to Ponder

1 Do you believe it is appropriate to challenge the status quo before having a clear vision of a better approach?
2 In what circumstances do you believe challenging the status quo is appropriate? When is it not a good idea to challenge the current situation? Why?
3 How clear and compelling is your vision? By that we mean, how clear are you about who you want to be, what you intend to accomplish, what will be different if that vision is realized, and who (besides yourself) will benefit from its realization?
4 What exactly are you doing to provide clear, compelling direction and communication to those you lead? What else can you do to help those you lead gain greater clarity of vision and direction?

Clear and Compelling Communication

Successful leadership doesn't stop with the creation of a vision. It also involves the communication of insight – through various methods, with various constituencies, in various settings. **Dr. Daniel Sands** emphasizes the importance of communication and optimism. Both, he says, are essential characteristics for anyone who aspires to lead – in healthcare or in general.

> "Physicians aren't necessarily good leaders. Some physicians are good leaders. It is not a sure thing. Physicians don't usually get that kind of training. Some are, and some learn to be. My favorite quote on leadership was stated by **President Eisenhower**."

"Leadership is the art of getting someone else to do something you want done, because he wants to do it."

President Dwight D. Eisenhower

"An important part of leading involves communications. Leaders need to be able to convey ideas effectively in ways that won't offend people. Some physicians have contrarian's notions, and air them in public settings and in negative ways. Good leaders are good communicators. They use appropriate settings and the appropriate tone. Leaders need to be able to communicate, not just to others one-on-one, but also to groups. And they must be able to communicate through speaking, through writing, through email. Email communication is really important in a group setting. Doctors can make asses of themselves in a medical staff meeting by speaking without thinking or sending ill-conceived emails.

People look up to leaders and respect them. Leaders need to be positive, not negative; constructive, not destructive. Leaders don't say 'They're trying to screw us again, isn't it terrible.' They think of constructive ways to challenge and improve the status quo.

Leadership is not the same thing as management. Anyone in a management role with responsibility for other staff should show leadership. But people don't have to be in management positions to be leaders: individuals can be good leaders without being good managers.

Leaders inspire confidence. They're constructive; and good communicators. Some are respected by clinical colleagues who look to them for clinical guidance. Others are administrative leaders – they may head departments and committees.

Many physician leaders who are making a difference in healthcare are heads of medical societies at state and national levels. They're working on healthcare, not working in healthcare. **Tom Sullivan** is a physician leader in Massachusetts. **Jack Sloan** is a physician leader in California.

You can sense who the leaders are by seeing who people naturally seek out and go to. In informatics, I can name the leaders because that's my domain. Your area of focus depends on what specialty, institution, or practice type you're working in and who or what you choose to lead.

In a book I read many years ago called *Fine Art of Flirting*, the author, **Joyce Jillson**, advocated being friendly, open-minded, and personable as a commendable way of being. I think these are traits that leaders should exhibit. Effective leaders generally aren't shrinking violets, but they should not be outspoken in an obnoxious way. If you don't have anything nice to say, don't say it. Bringing it up isn't the best idea sometimes. People can learn to be more positive, to see the glass half full."

Daniel Z. Sands, MD, MPH
Internist, Faculty, Harvard Medical School
Chief Medical Officer and Vice President, Clinical Strategies
Zix Corporation

"To listen well is as powerful a means of communication and influence as to talk well."

John Marshall
Chief Justice, U.S. Supreme Court

Dr. Sands stresses the importance of listening actively and accepting responsibility to seek clarity if the message isn't understood.

"Many years ago I had a mentor, who, following each presentation we heard, would ask me whether I had understood everything. If I hadn't, he'd then ask me why I hadn't asked the speaker to answer my questions. I learned a great deal from that. People can be leaders in many different spheres of influence with their families, practices, hospitals, communities, medical societies, or politics at large. All are important. Decide which you want yours to be and chart your course accordingly. If you aspire to a national position, volunteer to serve on a national committee. Great physician leaders are extraordinarily gifted at herding cats and making good things happen."

Daniel Z. Sands, MD, MPH
Internist, Faculty, Harvard Medical School
Chief Medical Officer and Vice President, Clinical Strategies
Zix Corporation

As you no doubt would agree, Dr. Sands is an excellent role model for physicians who aspire to see best practice innovations diffuse throughout medicine to become mainstream approaches that are used by the typical physician. His perspective – especially his advice about learning to communicate well – is echoed by Doug Henley, MD, FAAFP who emphasizes, in particular, the importance of listening.

"Successful leaders listen. They use a lot of common sense in their decision making ... and they listen. Leaders use their intuition along with moral and spiritual values ... and they listen. Leaders communicate clearly and directly ... and they listen."

Douglas E. Henley, MD, FAAFP
Executive Vice President
American Academy of Family Physicians

"The phrase 'I didn't learn that in medical school' has been exclaimed countless times, by nearly every physician who has ever gone into practice – or assumed a leadership role of some sort."

Perry A. Pugno, MD, MPH, CPE

Points to Ponder

---

1 Considering that effective communication involves understanding on the part of the recipient, as well as articulation on the part of the speaker/writer, how effective is your typical communication with those you seek to lead?
2 In what ways could you more clearly convey your vision, or convey it in a way that is more compelling to those you seek to lead?
3 What are you doing to help others become clearer and more compelling in their own vision and communication?

"It is vital to align your core values, strategic goals and outcomes with those of the greater organization to be seen as a value to top leadership. Keep your goals, vision and mission in mind when planning and evaluating opportunities. Preparation, perseverance and hard work are often requirements on the road to success; intelligence is also helpful but often less valuable – when doing the right thing – don't give up too soon or allow nay-sayers to talk you out of a good idea."

Tim Munzing, MD
Family Physician
Kaiser Permanente – Orange County

Authentic Conversations with Colleagues

Another physician leader who understands the importance of clear, candid conversation is Dr. Francine Gaillour. As a certified Executive Coach who decided to forego clinical practice in order to help other physicians become more effective and fulfilled in their practices, Dr. Gaillour draws from a deep reservoir of training and experience when advising physicians on the nuances of clear communication. Here are a few communication tips from Dr. Gaillour:

"Authentic leaders communicate candidly and constructively with others, and help others become respectful, honest, effective communicators. Using effective dialogue skills, leaders help others solve problems and move forward. The Greek roots of the word 'dialogue' could be loosely translated as 'meaning flowing through.' Dialogue is the respectful, two-way, open-ended flow of communication that balances listening and speaking for the purpose of learning. Other forms of communication – debate, directing, discussing – may influence or control people, but are unlikely to maximize productivity or effectiveness to the extent possible through meaningful dialogue.

Authentic leaders create dialogue by asking effective questions that lead to enlighten and engage others. Effective questions are often open-ended; for example: 'What do you think about this idea?'

'How would you solve this?' 'What other factors should we be considering?' 'What do you see as the obstacles we face?'

To respond, others are required to share their thoughts and ideas. The discussion should flow naturally. You may begin, for example, by inquiring about the person's hopes or intentions: 'What do you want to accomplish?' This leads to problem identification: 'What problems are you encountering?' which can be followed by assistance in exploring solutions: 'What do you see as your options?' The leader can then encourage action, by asking, for example: 'How do you plan to proceed?' and offer support: 'What can I do to support you?'

Many physician leaders squirm at the thought of 'confronting' colleagues about inappropriate behavior. Focus on the behavior, not the person. Be aware of any bias you may harbor because of behavior style differences between you and the other person. Speak frankly, without anger or judgment. Don't settle for simply 'defusing' such situations – seize them as opportunities to help others achieve their full potential. Here is a seven-step discussion format I often suggest to the clients I coach:

1 Describe the observed or reported behavior and the effect it had on others.
2 Probe for additional information.
3 Probe for acknowledgment of the event and the effect.
4 Suggest or request a new behavior.
5 Ask for agreement.
6 Encourage the person to develop skills to address the behavior in the future.
7 Agree on next steps for follow-up.

Authentic leaders are respectful, honest communicators, and help others communicate effectively as well. By communicating and collaborating, leaders help others overcome challenges and achieve results."

Francine R. Gaillour, MD, MBA, FACPE
Internist
Founder and Director of Creative Strategies in Physician
Leadership™

Points to Ponder

1 How comfortable are you when communicating with colleagues on matters of sensitivity that could lead to defensiveness or confrontation?
2 What steps can you take, in advance of such conversations, to reduce your discomfort and increase the likelihood that your colleague will be able to hear and respond to you appropriately?
3 What specific options are you willing to consider, in order to help others enhance their clarity of direction and communication?

Authentic Patient Communication Involves Matters of Spirituality

Some physicians maintain a strictly "'professional" relationship with patients in the sense that they converse only about physical diagnoses and interventions. This often falls far short of the conversation patients need to have with their physicians, as Andy Schwartz, MD, has discovered over the years. He describes in candid detail how his view of his responsibility to patients has evolved beyond that of "care provider" to that of "healer."

Insights from Andrew M. Schwartz, MD

"Physician leadership is one facet of who I am. My role as a physician, my expectations and goals in healthcare enhance my participation in medical staff leadership, and help to fulfill my global responsibility of service to myself, my patients, my peers in the hospital and its administrative leadership. For me, there is no clear demarcation between the person, the doctor and the medical staff leader.

The person I am today and the way I practice medicine had its conception around 1967. Until that time, I was your regular young teenager with a daily agenda of just getting through the school day and getting home to enjoy simple boyhood pleasures. We had no computer, little television, no Nintendo games. My greatest resource for amusement was my imagination, which frankly, often led to mischief. Neither of my parents completed college. I was a 'B' student, nothing spectacular from an academic standpoint. I was raised in a Jewish home where little Judaism was practiced. I became Bar Mitzvah, but it was a chore getting there. I was quick to laugh and quicker to smile. At age 13, I had no goals, no aspirations with regard to the future. I have three sisters and no brothers. My father was simple, hot tempered and not demonstrative with his emotion. My mother was chronically depressed. They offered the best they could. I captained my own ship, and chartered waters with little guidance.

In 1967, **Dr. Christian Barnard** performed the first human heart transplantation in Cape Town, South Africa on a dentist. The patient lived, but briefly, following surgery. I was smitten by this event.

I fell in love with the medical book section at Barnes & Noble on 5th Avenue, just outside of Greenwich Village in New York City. The shelves containing medical texts were canyons of vast medical knowledge, which allowed the 'want-to-be-doctor' in me to run wild. Not long thereafter, I began collecting all sorts of animal hearts, putting them in glass jars with preservatives and adorning my shelves with them. Those preserved hearts were almost sacred to me. I was awed by these unassuming engines of human existence and their roles as the epicenter of our physiology. Honestly, I felt no connection to wanting to serve or save others as physician; I was just purely immersed in the fascination of this incredible beating organ. Using a reel-to-reel tape recorder, window caulking, a

---

Continued

microphone, a kitchen funnel, the diaphragm and tubing from a stethoscope, I fashioned my own echocardiogram recorder. My future was starting to take shape. In high school I volunteered at two hospitals. Proximity to the healthcare environment was numbing for me. Everything was new. I felt a step closer to joining the fraternity of healthcare practitioners. I envied those wearing long white coats with stethoscopes hanging from their necks. I was attracted to the dynamic nature of medicine in which no two minutes were ever the same.

Medicine seemed like a life 'on the go.' I suspect the probably-undiagnosed adult attention deficit disorder in me relished the constant surges of adrenalin. At age 16 or so, I attended an evening education program sponsored by the American Heart Association. The featured speaker was chief of cardiology at a local hospital. I sat next to his wife. She recommended that I call her husband at work, which I did, and subsequently spent a summer in his department, working alongside third and fourth year medical students. I had arrived. That summer I observed heart surgery and co-authored a published article on coronary artery collateral circulation. My career goal became clear as I realized the allure of operating room drama. As a heart surgeon, I would live and breathe the basic elements of human existence, witness first hand the fragility of life, use my hands and mind in synchrony. The fact that people would benefit from the healthcare I rendered was still elusive. I had not yet imagined the eventual impact of spirituality in my practice of medicine.

College education's primary role was to provide me the opportunity to gain entrance into medical school. My devotion to cardiac surgery remained unwavering throughout medical school. I was one of a few in my 200-student medical school class who knew the very first week what discipline of medicine I wanted to practice. Through medical school, general surgery training, and cardiothoracic surgical fellowship, the patient was never defined as a person with emotions, expectations, or spiritual uniqueness. For that matter, neither was the healthcare provider. I did not recognize the responsibility of connecting patients' physical illnesses to their spiritual, emotional and intellectual selves. Nor did I recognize those fundamental needs in myself until I'd been practicing medicine for 14 years. Throughout my evolution to medical doctor and surgeon I never entertained the impact on patients and their loved ones of a worrisome diagnosis or declaration of a terminal illness. I didn't appreciate the fear and anxiety that discussion of a planned operative procedure might generate. Nor was I ever engaged in dialogue addressing the impact of the practice of medicine on my being, my emotional and spiritual framework. Surgical training involved endless hours of rigorous rituals of patient care, preparations for surgical procedures, and the potential for crucifixion of our self-worth at medical grand rounds or mortality and morbidity conferences. Patients were educational exercises – appropriateness of their healthcare algorithm failed to include quality of life. Healthcare was provided by physicians out of touch with the process of delivering healthcare information; physicians who bordered on becoming emotional eunuchs, unable to synchronize the mind-body connection in their patients and in themselves.

Clearly, my own upbringing did not adequately provide the needed tools to abort my own disengagement. As a physician in training and eventually newly in practice, I was focused on efficiency, accuracy, and growing my fund of knowledge. I enjoyed what I was doing and felt no sense of a lack of fulfillment. I felt blessed, for I was living my dream.

A failed marriage should have notified me of my underdeveloped human skills, but instead I interpreted it as a matter of wrong timing. Years later, I married a woman who loved and nurtured me, opening my eyes, my heart, my ears, and my mind to a life outside of medicine. The subsequent birth of my two children was pivotal in helping me define myself. Marriage and parenting changed my priorities – almost undermining what I had thought was my primary life role. That conflict required establishing a balance. The innate emotional and spiritual parts of me jockeyed for position in defining myself as a person, a father, a husband, and a physician. Not surprisingly, my religious roots had floundered and my Judaic connection extended little beyond my birthright. I slowly began re-establishing observance of religious tradition; acknowledging and desiring inclusion of prayer and God in my life.

By 2002, I had been involved in the care of thousands of patients. I had improved and prolonged life. I remained awed by the same poetic unity of anatomy and physiology that had captured my attention in 1967, but I felt something was lacking. How could I operate daily on hearts and lungs, yet feel unfulfilled? My wife would often comment that I had 'not yet found my niche.' She was right.

The establishment of the **Institute of Spirituality in Health Care** at **Shawnee Mission Medical Center** and the vision of its director, **Dr. Steven Jeffers**, would profoundly affect my life in ways that I could not have envisioned. I came to realize the pure joy in patient care; the fulfillment in treating the whole patient. The **Institute** provided a lattice for my emotional and spiritual components to evolve and to thrive.

Interestingly, at the same time I was not only returning to my Judaic roots; I was enthusiastically embracing them. I have come to realize that my gift as a physician is a responsibility and obligation bestowed upon me by God. I am thankful to God. I often seek counsel and find guidance in caring for my patients through prayer. I am seldom disappointed or left unfulfilled. I appreciate that I am blessed with skill, and that the final determination of outcome is in the hands of God.

Teachings by **Rabbi Schneerson** include the belief that 'life and health of every man is in God's hands. God guides the destinies of every man and whatever happens to him, in all places and at all times, is predestined by God ... no man should lose heart under any circumstances. He should pray to God and trust God to save his life and protect his health' (Schneerson 2001).

I recall visiting an elderly patient a day before her scheduled heart

Continued

surgery. She was frightened. She asked my religion. I told her I was Jewish. She told me she was Catholic. The woman then asked if she could anoint me with holy water on my hands and my forehead. I said yes. As she smiled, I readily identified a new sense of calm in this patient. Her request did not violate my own religious identification, and I fully appreciated the importance of this event towards her spiritual welfare. While visiting her four days after surgery, I could see she was in trouble, so I asked if she wanted to pray. She said yes and we did. Catholic and Jew, patient and physician, both in need of spiritual fulfillment – found fulfillment at the bedside.

Understanding the importance of words not spoken, of emotions that are not visible; encouraging patients to share their thoughts and concerns; these have become essential in my climb to a spiritual peak where I can achieve a sense of wholeness in my relationships with my patients. When talking to patients about newly identified lung nodules, I outline the clinical diagnostic work-up and subsequent treatment options. But my obligation in caring for the whole patient falls short unless I also acknowledge the fear and sense of doom generated by the word 'cancer.' For patients, this diagnosis often implies dying. Once the word 'cancer' is used, patients invariably can no longer focus on any other element of the physician-patient dialogue. I frequently encourage patients and their loved ones to tell me what the illness means to them, and how their view of their lives has changed with the illness. By doing this, my patients can know that the physician caring for them also cares about them.

I recall being a medical student on an internal medicine rotation and noting that an elderly physician had an extraordinarily large patient population. He was clearly not a pedigreed university physician, yet his patients loved and trusted him. The reason his patients were so loyal eventually became obvious. This physician was dedicated to the person with the illness. He listened intently and caressed their emotions with warmth and gentleness. He had mastered the art in the practice of medicine.

As technology continues to advance and new therapies are developed, the emphasis seems to be on preservation or prolongation of life, without sharing in the life of the patient. Mr. Abramowitz (name changed) was an elderly Jewish patient who required dialysis due to renal failure. Jewish patients in our institution are infrequent. The holiday of Passover had begun. Unable to attend the celebration meal of this holiday, the Seder, I shared with Mr. Abramowitz the symbols of the holiday, the Matzah and wine. This brought much satisfaction to the patient, to his family, and to me. Too often, hospitalized patients are stripped of their uniqueness, their self-identity. Too often, patients are referred to by their illnesses, such as 'the myocardial infarct in room 424,' or 'the stroke in the intensive care unit.' Helping this patient observe his religious holiday returned to him some of the defining parts of his life. Too often physicians fail to relate to the emotional and spiritual needs of their patients.

Too often physicians fail to talk with our patients in language that is plain and simple enough for them to understand. I suspect some physicians use 'Medspeak' to maintain the distinction between patients and physicians, thus creating self-imposed boundaries to protect the physicians from spiritual vulnerability. By having an emotional safe harbor, physicians are shielded from their own ineptness in dealing with the humanistic elements of patient care.

About a year ago I evaluated a patient with abnormal changes in his chest and neck. I believed his x-ray suggested an aggressive malignancy that had already spread. Even with aggressive treatment, I believed the odds for long-term meaningful survival were not in this patient's favor. With the patient's encouragement, I was honest and forthright as I shared my assessment of his illness and probable limited prognosis. With his head half cocked to one side, the patient looked at me and asked 'what do I do now?' I had not anticipated his question, and at first felt ill-prepared to give him the answer he deserved. After pausing, I responded:

1 Allow your family, friends and neighbors to help you, to support you and your family.
2 Make every day, every hour, and every moment count.
3 Do the things you always wanted to do.
4 You will be most remembered during this time of illness in your life, ensure as many good memories as you can.
5 Be sure your questions and those of your family are clearly answered by your healthcare providers.
6 Get your affairs in order: financial, end-of-life care decision and funeral arrangements.

As the patient and his family left my office, his daughter-in-law, who is an operating room nurse, said to me 'you did good.' I realized then that the ideals of spirituality in healthcare had successfully taken root in me, and were being harnessed to help me better care for my patients.

I believe the elements of spiritual care are collectively nebulous but individually specific. Our spirituality, I believe, is innate. Through our lives and through our interactions with others and with the world around us, we are helped to express and define more clearly our spiritual needs. For many, including myself, recognizing how to address the spiritual needs of patients and their families is not always obvious. There are no texts, edicts, or treatises on spirituality – particularly on its role in wellness and healthcare. Our own needs are sometimes better recognized when we become the patient instead of the healthcare provider. Walking in the shoes of patients provides us an opportunity to better understand patients' emotional and spiritual needs. Such experiences cannot be smoothly translated into a written text on 'how to give spiritual care to your patient.'

Spiritual care is really an eclectic phenomenon. Spiritual care draws on our own interpretation of our spirituality and that of our patients. It requires a clear understanding that the patient and healthcare provider's spiritual needs and expectations can be very different, and the ability to bridge that gap.

Spirituality in healthcare is not the same necessarily as religion but can

Continued

include it. Spirituality in healthcare should not be perceived primarily as end-of-life experiences. Spirituality should be an everyday part of our patients' lives and our own – when designing care plans and discussing intervention options, risks and expected outcomes. Spiritual care should not be limited to our patients, but should include patients' families and loved ones. An article I recall having read in my local newspaper years ago quoted a trauma surgeon saying something to the effect that 'families do not remember that you have the most modern monitor or loveliest waiting room; they do remember what time you spent with them to help them.' That notion really stayed with me.

Exploring spirituality in healthcare has led me to conclude that the science of medicine looks for the cure, while the art of medicine seeks to heal when there might not be a cure.

Appreciating how I have defined myself as a practitioner may help you understand my expectations of physicians as leaders in the healthcare arena.

It has become clear to me that physicians communicate better to physicians about their dissatisfaction than they do to administrative leadership. Most 'visits to the front office' by physicians are too late for all involved. 'Griping physicians' often express distrust and have low expectations of administration leadership. Understanding this is vital.

Great leadership flourishes because the surrounding support is as good, or even better than the leadership itself. Leadership looks for an environment in which there will be unification among physicians, administrators, and hospital staff. Creating an atmosphere where honesty and open communication are encouraged, where leadership is kept equally informed, will nurture camaraderie and results.

Good physician leaders understand the spiritual and emotional uniqueness and needs of our peers and the community in and outside of the hospital. This is necessary to create a hospital environment where people will want to come to receive their care. 'State-of-the-art care' should include just that – the 'art of caring.' This mentality must flow from the top."

Andrew M. Schwartz, MD
Cardiac Surgeon
Vice President, Medical Staff
Shawnee Mission Medical Center

Tips for Communicating Clearly

"Having the intellectual knowledge needed to help a patient does little good if the physician cannot communicate this in a way that a particular patient can understand it. As a medical reporter on television for over 20 years, I've had the opportunity to interview numerous physicians and observe their communication skills. All the doctors had the book knowledge, but many lacked the ability to transform this into simple language.

Before all interviews, I suggest that physicians follow some simple rules in communicating both on television and with patients. I ask them to first think about the 'One most important message they want to convey.' After that, I ask them to practice the following:

1 Follow the KISS principal (Keep it Simple Stupid).
2 Your #1 job ... 'Tell a Story.' We all learn best and relate to stories.
3 Realize that even when you are not talking, you are communicating. The non-verbal messages you send are powerful.
4 Talk in sound bites. If you can't say it in 20 seconds, you are not communicating well or sending too much information at one time.
5 Remember that eye contact is essential for understanding.
6 Use visual tools or aids to help with understanding. Some people learn best visually.
7 Check for understanding and ask if there are any questions.

If you follow these simple rules, your communication with anyone will be enhanced greatly."

Kevin J. Soden, MD, MPH
Emergency Medicine Physician
Medical Correspondent for NBC News
Soden Consulting Services

Points to Ponder

1 Do you encourage physicians to listen intently to their patients – for words not spoken as well as those expressed? Do you encourage physicians to use plain language with patients, and to ask questions in order to ensure the patients understand what is being explained?
2 What do you believe is the role of spirituality in medicine?
3 How do your religious belies and spiritual values influence – directly or indirectly – your work as a physician and as a leader?
4 Do you believe spirituality in medicine is being addressed sufficiently to fully meet patients' needs? If not, what are you willing and able to do about that?

Confrontation: A Particularly Challenging Aspect of Communication

"Nearly all physicians feel that we are good communicators – it's what we do all day. Very few of us are good at confrontation. We are used to an unbalanced power structure that does not leave much room for confrontation. We have learned to avoid troublesome patients, staff, colleagues, or dissention on committees. Of course, that doesn't mean we don't complain about it. We need to learn how to deal with confrontation, and how to assert ourselves in inherently asymmetric power structures – say, when dealing with a Chief of

Staff, or health plan insurers, the head of the medical group practice, or the senior partner."

Bridget McCandless, MD
Internist
Medical Director
Jackson County Free Clinic

References and Further Reading

Berwick D.M. (2004) *Escape Fire*. San Francisco: Jossey-Bass Publishers.

Berwick D.M. and Nolan T.W. (1998) Physicians as leaders in improving health care: A new series in Annals of Internal Medicine. *Annals of Internal Medicine* **128**(4): 289–92.

Clarke-Epstein C. (2002) *78 Important Questions Every Leader Should Ask and Answer*. New York: AMACOM, division of the AMA.

Deming W.E. (2000) *Out of the Crisis*. Boston, MA: MIT Press.

Gaillour F.R. (2004) Want to be CEO? Focus on finesse. *The Physician Executive* **30**(2): 14–16.

Jillson J. (1986) *Fine Art of Flirting*. New York: Fireside Publishing.

Kirschman D. (1996) Physician leadership: Physician executives share insights. *Physician Executive* **22**(9): 27–30.

Linney G.E., Jr. (1995) Communication skills: A prerequisite for leadership. *Physician Executive* **21**(7): 48–9.

Peters T. (1991) *Thriving on Chaos: Handbook for a management revolution*. New York: HarperCollins.

Reinertsen J.L. (1998) Physicians as leaders in the improvement of health care systems. *Annals of Internal Medicine*. **128**: 833–8.

Royer T. (1995) Physician executives of the future moving from management to leadership. *MGM Journal* **10**: 12.

Royer T.C. (2003) Good doctor/good leader: It's not an oxymoron. *MGMA Connexion* **September**: 26–7.

Schneerson M.M. (2001) *The Unbreakable Soul: a chasidic discourse by Lubavitcher Rebbe Rabbi Menacham M. Schneerson of Chabad-Lubavitch*. New York: Kehot Publication Society.

Soden K.J. and Dumas C. (2003) *Special Treatment: How to get the same high quality health care your doctor gets*. Berkley, CA: Berkley Press.

Chapter 12

Collaboration Through Commitment and Teamwork

"No one can really 'lead' doctors. To motivate doctors, one must understand the world they live in. Real leaders understand perfection isn't possible. Physician leaders understand that doctors are just as wounded and flawed as anyone else, but are sensitive of their need to protect the mindset that they lack flaws and wounds. Docs typically have a strong need for achievement and independence. How do you herd cats? You get out the tuna fish. Anyone who aspires to lead physicians must figure out what will motivate physicians at a gut level."

Randall Oates, MD
Family Physician
Founder and President, Docs, Inc.

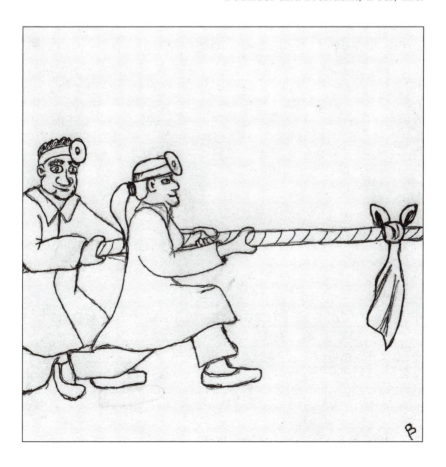

The Importance of Interpersonal Skills

As pointed out by Kagarise and Meyer (2004), "... interpersonal skills are an increasingly important factor in determining the physician's ability to practice medicine successfully." Why? In part, because medicine has become sufficiently specialized and complex as to require a team of diversely trained professionals collaborating together on behalf of the patients they serve. Another reason stems from the societal changes that have occurred in the past two decades. No longer do patients automatically comply with physician "orders." Instead, patients determine the extent to which they'll heed physicians' advice based on the trust and respect they hold for the physicians – and patients, like all humans – tend to trust and respect those with whom they have some sort of relationship. No longer are medical knowledge and clinical competence sufficient for the practice of medicine, let alone the leadership of positive changes in healthcare.

In fact, the Accreditation Council on Graduate Medical Education (ACGME) now considers "Interpersonal and Communication Skills" to be one of six core competencies required for successful practice of medicine. Specifically, the ACGME holds that "Residents are expected to demonstrate interpersonal and communication skills that enable them to establish and maintain professional relationships with patients, families, and other members of healthcare teams."

Physician Leaders' Roles in Committees and Meetings

If you peruse the shelves of the business and management of any bookstore, you will undoubtedly find a number of publications with titles that relate to meetings and how to manage them. The purpose of this chapter is to not reiterate the information in those books but to highlight a few key issues of pertinence to physician leaders and their role within the relatively generic experience of attending committees and meetings.

For the purposes of this discussion, we'll examine the role of the physician leader from three perspectives:

1 meeting participant
2 meeting chair and
3 providing staff support to committees and meetings.

Each role demands somewhat different behaviors and responsibilities, so each will be dealt with separately.

Physician Leaders as Meeting or Committee Participant

For any physician aspiring to be a leader, meetings provide an opportunity to demonstrate the unique knowledge, skills, and attitudes that qualify one for being a leader. Although many feel that entirely too much time is spent in such settings, the reality is that they are special opportunities to either help or hinder your efforts toward leadership. Along that line, there are a few basic principles:

1 **Preparation:** It is safe to say that the meeting participant who has clearly

prepared for the meeting, read the agenda and any accompanying materials, has thought about the issues to be discussed, and is well prepared to offer observations and recommendations will be immediately identified as a unique individual at the table. While recognizing that physicians' lives are busy and time for meeting preparation is limited, those who demonstrate sufficient interest and commitment to fully prepare for a meeting distinguish themselves as possessing the qualities of a leader.

2 **Active participation:** Notwithstanding different personality types, to passively sit in a meeting, listen to the discussion, and offer no comments, reflections, or contributions will not support your aspirations toward leadership. Appropriately active participation and contribution during a meeting provides others the opportunities to learn your viewpoints, hear your vision and at least have the opportunity to decide whether your contributions exhibit leadership in the directions they want to go. Notice, however, that I use the word "appropriate." Active participation in a meeting is to be distinguished from monopolizing the conversation, being argumentative, or constantly attempting to steer the conversation toward your unique viewpoint. However, actively participating in decision making and facilitating the achievement of consensus are additional distinguishing characteristics of those with leadership potential.

3 **Seek first to understand:** Meeting participants who actively engage in conversation directed toward understanding the issues involved and, from that understanding, offer observations and recommendations that support and build on the experiences and priorities of others will again distinguish an individual with the qualities of leadership. If your priority is seen as understanding what others feel is important and helping to achieve that, you will be viewed in a much more favorable light than making your first priority to be that of everyone else understanding what *you* think is important.

4 **Keep your promises:** Most meetings and committees are conducted in order to make decisions and follow up on them. It is only too common, however, that in the heat of the moment, many individuals at a meeting will promise to provide a piece of information, create a product, contact another individual, or in some way do something ... that never actually occurs. For those aspiring to be physician leaders, it is also very easy to become overcommitted. Caution is recommended to avoid overextending what it is you are willing to do as you volunteer to contribute to future meetings. It is most important, however, that if you make a commitment to do something, you will honor that commitment. I suppose it goes back to the primary quality of a leader being that of integrity. If your word is seen as consistently trustworthy, you will have taken the first giant step toward a future role as a leader.

"Spending the time and effort in recruiting and developing the right team is vital to success. Most major successes are the result of team efforts, not individual efforts. Find mentors and learn from them."

Tim Munzing, MD
Family Physician
Kaiser Permanente – Orange County

Physician Leader's Role as Meeting or Committee Chair

Among the roles of a committee chair is one which occurs only periodically. That is the role in identifying appropriate representatives or members to participate in a given meeting or committee. For the physician leader, this can be among the more challenging demands of that role. Although a great deal has been written on this subject, including the identification of a diversity of expertise and perspectives, committee composition really boils down to two central principles.

The first principle is to have the appropriate people at the table. Meetings and committees are designed to make decisions. Those decisions affect many more people than the ones sitting at the table. It is important the composition of a committee be designed such that relevant constituencies and their viewpoints are adequately represented, that the meeting participants are capable of accurately reflecting the priorities of their constituencies, and that once a decision has been made, the representative can engage their constituencies in acceptance of the decision.

A second key principle is to structure meetings or committee to include the optimal number of members necessary to achieve the goals. Generally, that means involving the smallest number of individuals that can provide adequate representation on behalf of the majority of interested parties. Various authors have suggested optimal committee sizes from five to ten individuals, but if a smaller group can achieve the same ends, what purpose is served by consuming more people's time? Similarly, in settings with a wide array of interested and potentially affected parties, meeting groups and committees must sometimes of necessity grow a bit larger.

Another matter of concern to physician leaders involves the creation and use of meeting agendas. Although this may seem somewhat like an oversimplification, the guiding principles should be:

1	have an agenda
2	stick to it and
3	provide and ensure appropriate follow-up.

Meeting agendas should be designed so that the work of the group is achieved. If a meeting agenda is constructed but the discussion varies substantially from it, the goals for which it was designed may not be addressed and its core purpose therefore subverted. Similarly, even though an agenda may be present and the meeting discussion adhere to it, if the leader of the meeting does not ensure follow-up of the decisions made and commitments addressed, again its purpose will have been compromised.

Along the same lines, one of the most important roles of a committee chair or meeting leader is to ensure not only the presence of interested parties but their active participation as well. For physician leaders, it is vitally important to understand that some people speak early in meetings while others prefer to listen awhile before speaking. Perhaps the most effective technique employed to assure that meeting participants are actively engaged in the discussions being held is periodically to directly address individual members who have yet to comment on the subject at hand and invite their observations.

A final point involves the sometimes controversial subject of seating. Much has been written describing the "power of positions" of various seating arrangements and places at the table. In the vast majority of situations, however, only two principles need be considered. First, the chair or leader of the meeting should sit somewhere conducive to seeing and being seen by every member of the committee. This permits the chair to address individuals directly and to monitor their engagement with the discussion at hand. Second, the chair should be able to see the entrance to the meeting room, thus monitoring the incoming and outgoing flow of individuals with minimal effort.

Effective leadership of meetings or committees is likely if these simple principles are followed. Nothing is gained by making the straightforward more complicated than it needs to be.

Leadership involves working well with others

"I came out of **Stanford** knowing how to care for the sick, how to assess difficult clinical situations, how to move quickly and efficiently, how to work with all support people, including – and especially – the nurses. I learned how to make the people around me trust me and have faith in me, to feel good about the work they did, to open up, to give me the right information unhesitatingly when I needed it. In short, I think, I hope, I learned how to be a leader."

William H. Frist, MD
Cardiothoracic and General Surgeon and
Senate Majority Leader, U.S. Congress
in his book *Transplant* (1989)

Physician Leaders as Staff Support for Meetings and Committees

Emerging physician leaders often encounter opportunities to function as a support staff or staff executive to an existing and functioning committee. This role, although superficially a subservient one, provides ample opportunity for a demonstration of leadership skills. A few examples will illustrate my point.

One of the more common responsibilities of a staff executive role is to prepare and distribute summaries of meeting activities. This is an exceptionally important and potentially influential role since the individual responsible for the meeting summary has the opportunity to identify and emphasize aspects of the meeting event and decisions made in ways that ultimately support their own vision for what the group they are supporting should be accomplishing. In addition, a well prepared meeting summary, which clearly identifies not only the decisions made but who will be responsible for what and when, can serve as one of the most effective drivers of that meeting's effectiveness. An important principle is to get a meeting summary prepared and redistributed to the meeting participants as soon following the meeting as is reasonably possible. While memories are still fresh and commitments are still closely held, the meeting summary with clearly identified task commitments will serve to reinforce those commitments and result in more of them eventually being honored.

From the meeting summary eventually flows the agenda for the next meeting. A well prepared agenda with clearly identified areas of discussion, decisions to be made, and support information with appropriate background materials can serve to substantially enhance the effectiveness of the meeting itself. Agenda placement of controversial items in congruence with the attendance behaviors of influential members of a committee, for example, can also serve to influence and facilitate decisions to the ultimate benefit of the constituencies served by them.

In addition to preparing the agenda itself, an important staff role is to assure that the individual actually chairing or leading the meeting is well prepared to do so. Reviewing a meeting agenda with its chair, clarifying the decisions to be made (including the alternatives available), and ensuring that appropriate background material is available again serves to facilitate the overall effectiveness of the meeting and ultimately the effectiveness of its decisions. Helping a committee chair to be well prepared for the meeting and having anticipated additional information available during the meeting may seem like somewhat "invisible" support for the aspiring physician leader, but it is nevertheless an opportunity to substantially influence the direction of decisions and the carrying out of plans in ways that ultimately will support the aspiring physician leader's objectives.

> "A leader will share what they have learned. For it is in sharing knowledge that we can gain from the points of view and insights of others and thereby see the world through different eyes per se, as well as exponentially expand our knowledge bases. A leader realizes that it is through others that true leadership thrives and survives. The utmost example of this is in their ability to develop, mentor, and encourage leadership in others. A true attestation to leadership is when their protégée has become perhaps a 'better' leader than themselves, that the physician leader has achieved success. (Socrates-Plato). Leaders develop other leaders."
>
> Penny Tenzer, MD
> Vice Chair, Department of Family Medicine and Community Health
> Director, Family Medicine Residency Program
> University of Miami School of Medicine

Avoid Pitfalls to Achieve Remarkable Results

Some "traps" exist in leadership – traps to which physician leaders are particularly prone. Being aware of the traps is the first step leaders take to minimize their negative impact, or better yet, avoid them altogether.

The "Ego Trap"

The first pitfall we advise physician leaders to avoid is something we call the "ego trap." The nature of the physician's role in clinical settings often involves leadership of the healthcare team, decision making in a "high-stakes environment," and being someone upon whom patients depend when they are most vulnerable. That is why the "ego trap" can ensnare ineffective or inexperienced physician leaders. How does it happen? Physician leaders come to believe, or convince themselves that they must "always know best." As this attitude becomes internalized, it is easy to begin believing that if others would just listen and do as they are told, everything would be okay. When our peers begin to express admiration, gratitude, and appreciation for what we are providing or accomplishing, it is all too easy to fall into the seductive trap of believing that we are always right, and that other's opinions have little merit. Is there an easy defense against the "ego trap?" Unfortunately, the answer is no. Effective leaders, especially seasoned ones, are aware of the risk, and rely on a combination of discipline and intellectual honesty to guard against this counterproductive mindset. By assessing ourselves on a regular basis, seeking candid feedback from trusted friends and family, and mustering up enough humility to accept that feedback as being in our best interest, we can more quickly notice if our ego begins to swell disproportionately.

> "The trouble with most of us is that we would rather be ruined by praise than saved by criticism."
>
> Norman Vincent Peale

In fact, the times when we are most in need of a little constructive criticism are often the times when we are least ready to receive it. Sometimes our unwillingness to admit the need for improvement indicates a lack of self-awareness. Often, when we hold inflated opinions of our skills and abilities we are least able to recognize tell-tale signs of incompetence. When this happens, we need someone with strong leadership skills to help us become aware of the gap between our perceptions and reality, and to help us close that gap. Sometimes we are unwilling to accept criticism from others – not in spite of, but actually because of, our awareness of our shortcomings. We may find our deficiencies too painful or embarrassing to admit. In these situations, we don't need help realizing the issues, but may very well need help in addressing them.

Self-Promotion

Another trap that leaders often face is the trap of *self-promotion*. Physician leaders may be particularly prone to experience this. In all communities and organizations there exist high-profile leaders who enjoy honors, accolades, and high visibility from those they lead. Unfortunately, most of us have known leaders who direct large amounts of energy toward the promotion of their own perceived importance. Of course, a certain amount of visibility is necessary in order to gain opportunities to utilize our leadership capabilities. But when we focus excessively on making ourselves seem more important than we are, our potential contributions become diluted and our effectiveness is curtailed.

Inattentive Listening

Listening is important for several reasons – it serves as a source of information, an opportunity to consider situations from an alternative perspective, and a way of connecting with those to whom we are listening. Think about times you've wanted to talk about something – because you were excited about it, you wanted to "talk out loud" in order to gain insight into your own understanding of a situation, or you simply needed to feel "heard." The very best thing others could do for you at that moment was simply to listen, right? *Not* merely to refrain from talking, but to actually listen. Actively. With interest. We've all experienced just how disheartening, annoying, or hurtful it can be when someone nods their head and periodically says "mmm hmm," but one glance at their face reveals that their mind is a million miles away.

Listening – active, purposeful, high energy listening – is altogether different from merely keeping quiet. True listening requires concentration, empathy, engagement of both intellect and emotion. Effective listeners hear not only what is said. Effective listeners also hear what is left unsaid. Effective listeners absorb the words and the body language, the pitch and the pace of our voice inflections. Effective listeners absorb a host of signals that include words, yes, and much more than words.

How can we further develop our listening skills to become truly effective listeners? Here are a few suggestions:

- Concentrate only on the person to whom you're listening – don't multi-task by reading, typing, watching someone or something else in your peripheral vision.
- Mentally ask yourself questions that will help you more fully experience and understand what the person is conveying – why are they telling me this and what response are they likely to be wanting.
- Interact with the person who is speaking by asking questions to clarify or confirm what they're seeking to convey, rather than simply replying with facts or opinions of your own.

> "Professionally, family physicians were just starting to make senior colonel and general officer level where they could influence impor-tant medical issues. As I was more involved in the politics of the departments of the hospital, my chief reminded me that family doctors would rise to positions of authority and responsibility if for no other reason that hospital departments are like dysfunctional family members and who better than a family doctor to cut through the crap and get things done. That concept – cut through the crap and get things done – has served me well."
>
> John R. Bucholtz, DO
> Family Physician
> U.S. Army

Insufficient Personal Interaction

Effective leaders make a point of spending time face to face with people. One reason is because face-to-face interaction often allows deeper connections than any other form of communication. Sure, email and telephone conversations offer certain advantages of expediency when time is short or distance is great. But just try to imagine your only daughter's wedding. Would you be willing to listen to a tape recording of the event, or would you make every effort to be there in person? A dramatic example, perhaps, but one we believe makes the point.

"When dealing with people, remember you are not dealing with creatures of logic, but with creatures of emotion."

Dale Carnegie

Just as photographs are often less revealing and engaging than videotapes, so too are email messages and printed memos often less powerful than live interactions. The deep, transformative relationships that effective leaders build with others require personal involvement that is typically best mediated through shared experience and physical presence, not just static communications or phone conversations.

"Learning techniques of negotiation are invaluable to physician leaders. Many physicians instinctively negotiate like they are selling a used car. They sell for as high a price as possible no matter the setting and do not expect to ever see the buyer (or the car) again. In healthcare management this is risky. Although the nineties seemed to promote a business process that was a 'take all that you can' model, the 2000s are not the same. In all likelihood you *will* see whoever you negotiate with again, and it will likely be in another negotiation process. The best advice is to 'not burn bridges' with any negotiating party because you may need their consideration or help in the future."

Roland A. Goertz, MD, MBA
Family Physician
President, McClennan County Medical Education and Research
Foundation

Insufficient Teamwork

"Great achievements involve the cooperation of many minds. Nowhere is it truer than in healthcare because no one person is ever personally responsible for the care of a person. Quality healthcare requires effective communication between various health professionals. Unfortunately, there is often a lack of understanding of the roles, responsibilities, and skills of other team members. This is highlighted by the all-too-frequent turf battles between specialists and primary care physicians. Whether we like it or not, doctors' egos often get in the way of working with other healthcare professionals.

Can you imagine going in for cardiac bypass surgery without the pump technician, the scrub nurse, the recovery room nurses, or the respiratory care team members? I can't. The cardiac surgeon wouldn't be as successful without the team, nor would any physician. Isn't it time to think about how we communicate with and relate to the other members of our team? Respectful communication between team members can only enhance the quality of care we deliver."

Kevin J. Soden, MD, MPH
Emergency Medicine Physician
Medical Correspondent, NBC News
Soden Consulting Services

> "Leadership involves surrounding yourself with individuals smarter than you and after observing them, putting them into positions where their talents will shine ... when they all shine together, the whole organization will take on a tremendous glow."
>
> Mark H. Belfer, DO, FAAFP
> Family Physician
> Residency Director
> Akron General Medical Center/NEOUCOM

Leaders are – whether by nature or by necessity – great collaborators. Why? Because leading successfully requires that we inspire others' commitment toward a shared vision. To the extent we're able to do this, to build an atmosphere of mutual respect and cooperation, we're able to build highly cohesive and yet richly diverse teams of people. Such teams work well together, and by doing so, achieve remarkable results – results none of them could have ever hoped to accomplish individually.

> "Teamwork is the ability to work together toward a common vision, the ability to direct individual accomplishment toward organizational objectives. It is the fuel that allows common people to attain uncommon results."
>
> Successories

Successful leaders create cohesive teams of diverse individuals who respect one another; teams who are highly motivated and deeply committed to the purpose they all share.

> "Never doubt that a small group of thoughtful citizens can change the world. Indeed, it is the only thing that ever has."
>
> Margaret Mead

The Power of Collaboration

A physician who demonstrates the power of collaboration in order to enhance the delivery of quality healthcare is David Fairchild, MD, MPH. As Chief of General Medicine at Tufts – New England Medical Center, Dr. Fairchild is a champion of teamwork. Read on to learn from his example of one way leading physicians can make a positive impact on healthcare through their attention to organizational excellence.

Insights from David G. Fairchild, MD, MPH

"I attended **Hershey Medical School at Penn State**; then did my residency in Internal Medicine at Yale having become involved in Internal Medicine in part due to an advisor's influence. After residency I became a Chief Resident and left my residency program thinking I would eventually go into pulmonary medicine. However, I went into the Indian Health Service directly after my Chief residency (on a Navajo reservation) because my wife and I were interested in international health (I had been to Haiti and Zimbabwe while in residency). We were starting a family and wanted to stay in the U.S., so the IHS opportunity was a great fit. The program didn't want internists (they preferred family physicians) so I agreed to practice as an FP in rural Arizona at a 60-bed hospital. I saw ER, pediatric, orthopedic, and trauma cases. Going into very rural clinics with a nurse practitioner led me to develop a lot of respect for mid-level practitioners.

The Clinical Director left, and no one wanted the job (administration was not seen as an attractive opportunity), so I split the role with a Family Physician. I was Chief of Staff of Medicine for the hospital. I loved the variety of patient care and administration – even if mundane (e.g., credentialing). It was refreshing to see patients after doing administrative work, so I even signed on for a third year. I found it very stimulating to impact patient care through both clinical and administrative leadership – running meetings, the Quality Improvement program, JCAHO surveys, etc. I went to a research-focused general medicine fellowship at **Brigham & Women's Hospital/Harvard Medical School. Partners Healthcare** was just being formed and a former mentor encouraged me to join them to work on several quality initiatives. I did a two-year research fellowship. Within five months I'd moved into an administrative role as Associate Medical Director within the Physicians Hospital Organization. I used skills to do medical management at the hospital level. Within one or two years, 80 percent of my focus involved administrative work and 20 percent was clinical. I became the Medical Director for the PHO, then Director of Primary Care Operations (in charge of 75 primary care physicians). It is exciting to have the variety of patient care, research, and teaching. I would become exhausted if I were to focus in only one of those areas.

One of the achievements that has been most gratifying is the total revision of the PCP compensation system. It required leadership, fairness, communication, due process. The benefits have been significant. Productivity has increased dramatically, which gives better access to more patients. No one left as a result of the change – which is personally meaningful to me as an indicator of the success of the transition to our new system. We also built in patient satisfaction, citizenship, and quality measures through a balanced scorecard approach. We brought in a consultant for the technical aspects.

When asked to identify the keys to my success as a physician leader, I would point to the fact that I've always asked for advice and listened to it. I'm very committed to asking for feedback from those affected by what I'm about to do and modifying my position to address others' concerns.

In my next role, a key challenge will be working at the hospital level – not just with my own division, but across departments. It will require leadership of people who don't report to me. I'll need to get people to collaborate on projects – to be a diplomat and facilitator as opposed to a

Continued

> supervisor. I'll do that by talking, listening, making proposals, and soliciting feedback. By nature I'm a consensus builder whenever possible. I like to find the common threads and build from there. I enjoy knitting people together, breaking down the silos. I use a systems approach to address challenges, by working with people all across the hospital."
>
> David G. Fairchild, MD, MPH
> Internist
> Chief of General Medicine, Tufts – New England Medical Center

We can see that Dr. Fairchild certainly understands the importance of working with others – not just other physicians, but other people in all types of clinical and administrative roles. By seeking others' suggestions, Dr. Fairchild is not only gathering great ideas, he is building others' commitment to the goals they now feel a sense of ownership over.

Points to Ponder

1 Think of a time when you felt a deep sense of collaboration with colleagues. What were the contributing factors?
2 What are you doing, or can you do, to create that type of experience with and for those you seek to lead?
3 How do people in cohesive, committed work groups treat each other differently than those in non-collaborative groups?
4 How often do you consciously consider the level of cooperation, respect for diversity, and shared commitment levels among the members of groups you seek to lead?
5 What are you doing to increase the morale, commitment levels, mutual respect, or synergies among people in the groups you lead?
6 What else could you do to enhance collaboration and thus the collective capacity for results?
7 What are the consequences of unresolved conflict among groups of colleagues?
8 How do groups that handle conflict effectively differ, exactly, from groups that don't?
9 What are you doing to help those you lead address and resolve the conflicts that inevitably arise? What else might you do?

Engaging Others to Work Well Together

Kieren P. Knapp, DO, FACOFP understands that engaging others to share in the work is more effectively done through enthusiasm than pressure. In "the old days" people sometimes explained this notion by saying "we can attract more flies with honey than with vinegar." The point is, effective leaders are magnets, drawing others toward the shared activity upon which the work will be completed.

> "Whenever I was given a task, I worked at it as if all else depended on the success of that task. When others realize that attitude and

share the enthusiasm of that success, they often will be motivated to join the effort and to do the same. It is hard to motivate others by eloquent speeches and smiles if they cannot see some sort of results over a period of time. That is how I see leadership."

Kieren P. Knapp, DO, FACOFP
Family Physician
Immediate Past President
American College of Osteopathic Family Physicians

Dr. Munzing also articulates this concept. He emphasizes the importance of influencing others through optimism – even, or perhaps especially – in difficult times.

"As a leader, be a positive and optimistic influence on others, especially in the most difficult times – be the conduit through whom others find a ray of hope – find strength or find vision."

Tim A. Munzing, MD
Family Physician
Director, Medical Education
Kaiser Permanente – Orange County

Another aspect of collaboration is the notion of shared accountability. As Doug Henley, MD, FAAFP explains, successful leaders ensure others get the credit when things go well, and accept full responsibility when they don't.

"Harry Truman has described a very potent method of leadership with this quote – 'You can accomplish anything in life, provided that you do not mind who gets the credit!' He realized that great leaders relish success by allowing others to get the credit.

I would add that when things go wrong, great leaders also look in the mirror for the person responsible."

Douglas E. Henley, MD, FAAFP
Executive Vice President
American Academy of Family Physicians

Collaboration Between Physicians and Administrators

"I believe the commitment of medical staff leadership to the hospital is enhanced by making physician leaders part of the hospital board. This, I believe, helps maintain continuity between the hospital board, administration, and the physician leaders.

The incentive for taking on leadership responsibility should be the desire to see your institution thrive. This is simple, but in many hospitals not realistic. As more physicians seek liberation from non-physician owned medical facilities, physicians and hospital administration must be ready to share the helm in order to assure smooth sailing and that their port of call remains vibrant."

Andrew M. Schwartz, MD
Cardiac Surgeon
Vice President, Medical Staff
Shawnee Mission Medical Center

How many physicians have you known who measure "success" in terms of "activity volume?" We all know they aren't always, or even usually, the same thing. That's why effective physician leaders understand the importance of "coming up for air" – or stepping outside the hectic day-to-day routine for rest, relaxation, rejuvenation and refocus. Amazing how your perspective can change when you stop long enough to see things from a different vantage point. How many of us, dealing with life and death every day, have the wisdom and insight to see things as clearly as did this taxi driver?

"I used to drive a cab for a living. One night, when I responded to a call at 2:30 am, the building was dark except for a single light in a ground floor window. Under these circumstances, many drivers would just honk once or twice, wait a minute, then drive away. But I had seen too many impoverished people who depended on taxis as their only means of transportation. Unless a situation smelled of danger, I always went to the door. This passenger might be someone who needs my assistance, I reasoned to myself. So I walked to the door and knocked. 'Just a minute,' answered a frail, elderly voice. I could hear something being dragged across the floor. After a long pause, the door opened. A small woman in her 80s stood before me. She was wearing a print dress and a pillbox hat with a veil pinned on it, like somebody out of a 1940s movie. By her side was a small nylon suitcase. The apartment looked as if no one had lived in it for years. All the furniture was covered with sheets. There were no clocks on the walls, no knick-knacks or utensils on the counters. In the corner was a cardboard box filled with photos and glassware. 'Would you carry my bag out to the car?' she said. I took the suitcase to the cab, then returned to assist the woman. She took my arm and we walked slowly toward the curb. She kept thanking me for my kindness. 'It's nothing,' I told her. 'I just try to treat my passengers the way I would want my mother treated.' 'Oh, you're such a good boy,' she said. When we got in the cab, she gave me an address, then asked, 'Could you drive through downtown?' 'It's not the shortest way,' I answered quickly. 'Oh, I don't mind,' she said. 'I'm in no hurry. I'm on my way to a hospice.' I looked in the rearview mirror. Her eyes were glistening. 'I don't have any family left,' she continued. 'The doctor says I don't have very long.' I quietly reached over and shut off the meter. 'What route would you like me to take?' I asked. For the next two hours, we drove through the city. She showed me the building where she had once worked as an elevator operator. We drove through the neighborhood where she and her husband had lived when they were newlyweds. She had me pull up in front of a furniture warehouse that had once been a ballroom where she had gone dancing as a girl. Sometimes she'd ask me to slow in front of a particular building or corner and would sit staring into the darkness, saying nothing. As the first hint of sun was creasing the horizon, she suddenly said, 'I'm tired. Let's go now.'

We drove in silence to the address she had given me. It was a small convalescent home, with a driveway that passed under a portico. Two orderlies came out to the cab as soon as we pulled up. They were solicitous and intent, watching her every move. They must have been expecting her. I opened the trunk and took the small suitcase to the door. The woman was already seated in a wheelchair.

'How much do I owe you?' she asked, reaching into her purse.

'Nothing,' I said.

'You have to make a living,' she answered.

'There are other passengers,' I responded. Almost without thinking, I bent and gave her a hug. She held onto me lightly.

'You gave an old woman a little moment of joy,' she said. 'Thank you.'

I squeezed her hand, then walked into the dim morning light. Behind me, a door shut. It was the sound of the closing of a life. What if that woman had gotten an angry driver, or one who was impatient to end his shift? What if I had refused to take the run, or had honked once, then driven away?"

Source unknown

Points to Ponder

1 What techniques or methods do you use to draw people in?
2 What do you do to encourage mutual self-respect?
3 How do you motivate people to put the greater good as a higher priority than simply individual self-interest?
4 In what ways can you give colleagues the credit for their accomplishments so that one benefit is greater cohesiveness?
5 What steps can you take to help those you lead promote greater collaboration with those they work with?
6 How can you role model, explain, or motivate those you lead to build respect for diversity *and* cohesion among collaborators?
7 How can you help others enhance their effectiveness in building collaboration – cohesive teams of otherwise diverse individuals, each of whom is strongly committed to their shared sense of purpose?

Build strong collaborations – even those that are brief or long distance

Physicians with strong interpersonal skills find ways of creating authentic, meaningful exchanges with others – whether the interactions are short term or ongoing, face to face or simply via phone or email. They use language that draws others in, conveys the sincere desire to find common ground, and creates opportunities for mutual benefit. One of the authors shares this story to illustrate the point:

Case Example by Dr. McKenna

Awhile back, I received an email message from a Dr. Donald Lurye – a physician executive in Indiana whom I'd never met. It seems I'd been quoted in a recently published article, and Dr. Lurye was concerned that my comments were misleading, perhaps downright inaccurate. Because Dr. Lurye's handling of the situation was such an excellent example of the power of clear communication and collaboration, I asked his permission to share the story with all of you. Here is an excerpt from the email I received from Dr. Lurye:

——-Original Message——-
Sent: Wednesday, April 14, 2004 5:38 PM
To: info@mindimckenna.com

Dear Dr. McKenna,

Thank you for your [comments in an] article in Group Practice Solutions comparing the various business degrees available for physicians. It was a cogent and necessary contribution to a very confusing topic. I struggled with this issue for months before deciding to pursue the Carnegie Mellon [Masters of Medical Management] MMM (Class of June, 2005).

I am curious about your characterization of the MMM. On the one hand, you refer to " ... dealing with change and looking at large-scale organizational dynamics." In the next sentence, however, you recommend the MMM for physicians who " ... plan to manage staff face-to-face as they would in smaller practices."

The former sounds an awful lot like leadership, whereas the latter sounds like day to day office management. The MMM curriculum at CMU features strategy, technology and organizational leadership (www.heinz.cmu.edu/mmm/index.html).

I am curious as to how you arrived at your perspective. I am early in the CMU MMM program, but so far it seems tilted much more towards leadership than you suggest. Most of the MMM grads I know hold senior positions in very large organizations.

I think all of us who pursue these degrees are forever haunted as to whether we've chosen the right one. I remain interested in this topic. If you don't mind a brief e-mail exchange, I would appreciate any further observations or clarifications you can offer.

I fully agree that the MBA does allow one to consider leaving health care – another scenario that haunts many a physician executive!

Thanks again for the excellent article.

Sincerely,
Donald R. Lurye, MD
Chief Medical Officer
Welborn Clinic

Well, I can assure you, that was one of the most effectively crafted emails I'd received in quite some time! So I immediately called **Dr. Lurye**, thanked him for contacting me, and went on to have a delightful and enlightening conversation with this new-found colleague and friend.

You see, the fact of the matter is that when I saw how my comments had appeared, I agreed with **Dr. Lurye** that they were misleading! The person who wrote that article wasn't at fault. I had been the one responsible for ensuring my comments were accurate and helpful. I was the one who hadn't stayed on top of the details.

What intrigued me about **Dr. Lurye's** gracious correspondence was that he knew my comments were misleading! And yet he didn't accuse me, or belittle me, or challenge my competence. Nor, I might add, did he simply ignore them, which many of us might have been tempted to do. **Dr. Lurye** took the initiative to address it – partly to satisfy his own curiosity, he later told me, and partly out of concern for the publication's readers, who he felt deserved not to be misled. Rather than offending or alienating me, **Dr. Lurye's** comments made me want to contact him, made me want him to share with me the benefit of his perspective. So I called him, and I think it would be fair to say we have both learned new insights from each other.

I appreciated hearing about his MMM experience, and telling him about the Health Care Leadership MBA program where I teach. Our communications served to remind us of several key leadership principles:

1 Even when you think your point of view is well founded, be open to changing your position.
2 Tact and respect go a long way in engaging others to collaborate with you.
3 The phrase "win-win" may be overused, but the concept of mutual benefit is indeed productive.

Strong Bonds are Built by Authentic Leaders

Throughout this book you've been reading about the importance of character as a foundation upon which credibility is built and trust is earned. No one in their right mind would "follow" the lead of someone they disrespect or distrust. The most influential, compelling, remarkable leaders are those whose integrity, generosity of spirit, reliability, and judgment are impeccable.

And yet, none of us can expect or hope to be "perfect." All of us make mistakes. We may, at times, disappoint ourselves and others. We may, at times, "lose our way" – become disoriented and unclear about our work, our relationships, our values, our priorities.

Those among us who aspire to be all we can be, to do all we can do – will engage in honest, inner-directed reflection. Only as we gain awareness of ourselves and others, can we be authentic leaders, authentic human beings. Dr. Gaillour explains:

"Effective leaders inspire others to be their best and act in a way that honors their values, or the values of their group. We do so by speaking from our essence, our heart, our values. Effective leaders are masters at using authentic personal power to attract people to their cause, at inspiring people to work together to accomplish results, and helping people feel good about being a member of the team. Authentic personal power comes from being who we are and feeling comfortable about it. It involves letting go of fear – fear of looking incompetent or feeling awkward – and all the fears that cause us to lose confidence in ourselves and lose the trust of others. We are most powerful when we are most real – when we play fair or walk our talk or get real.

Authentic leaders model character that inspires others to be their best, to act in a way that honors their values or the values of their group. Authentic leaders model courage, integrity, and accountability. We model courage by speaking up for what is right without greed or self-interest, accepting the consequences of our wholehearted commitment to ethical behavior, regardless of the opposition we may encounter from others. We model integrity by aligning our choices and behaviors with our highest values, by speaking honestly, and demanding that others speak honestly as well. We model accountability by accepting responsibility for our decisions and actions rather than blaming others as if we were victims.

Authentic leaders hold firmly to our vision of making a difference in people's lives. Thus when we 'fall on our faces' we view it not as failure, but as an opportunity to learn and grow. Our vision is bigger than our fear of appearing foolish, or making mistakes, or being scorned by skeptics. We do whatever is necessary to always speak and act in a way that is totally honest and consistent with who we are as individuals.

Authentic physician leaders recognize our responsibility to model the communication and interpersonal skills we want others to exhibit. We ask ourselves: 'How well have I communicated? How clearly have I set expectations? How consistently have I been modeling the behaviors I want others to adopt? How appropriately have I been holding myself and others accountable?'

This requires us to know ourselves – to separate who we are and want to be from what the world thinks we are. No one can teach us how to become ourselves, to take charge, to express ourselves. Only we can do that. We do so by engaging in honest reflection to increase our awareness of ourselves and those around us – of our deepest hopes and concerns, our needs and aspirations.

We uncover our personal power through self-reflection, by taking in the lessons we've learned from failures, by aligning our action with our values. We lead authentically as we allow ourselves to be guided by a higher purpose, to speak and behave in a manner consistent with our values, to project our very souls into our work. This requires an honest assessment of our underlying values and natural gifts, and a willingness to fully express them, rather than letting fear hold us back. To do our best work, most of us will benefit from committing to a personal development plan and enlisting a mentor, colleague or, coach to assist us in assuring our choices and behaviors are driven by our values and character."

Insights from Francine R. Gaillour, MD, MBA, FACPE

Internist

Founder and Director of Creative Strategies in Physician

Leadership™

Points to Ponder

1 Do you consider yourself to be an authentic leader? On what do you base that perception?
2 Would others consider you to be an authentic leader? Would they be "right?"
3 How important do you believe it is to build authentic relationships – with colleagues, patients, loved ones, those you lead?
4 What steps can you take to become more authentic – in your work, your relationships, your life?

References and Further Reading

Bettner M. and Collins F. (1987) Physicians and administrators: Inducing collaboration. *Hospital & Health Services Administration* **32**(2): 151–60.

Darves B. (2001) A growing number of physicians are finding satisfaction, reaping rewards by becoming physician executives. *NEJM CareerCentre* **June 20.**

Fernandez C.R. (1998) Make physician-administrator teams work. *MGM Journal* **45**(5): 12–14.

Frist W.H. (1989) *Transplant: a heart surgeon's account of the life-and-death dramas of the new medicine.* New York: The Atlantic Monthly Press.

Kagarise M.J. and Meyer A.A. (2004) Academic Medical Centers. In: Keagy B.A. and Thomas M.S. *Essentials of Physician Practice Management.* San Francisco: Jossey-Bass Publishers.

Kouzes J.M. and Posner B.Z. (2002) *The Leadership Challenge: how to keep getting extraordinary things done in organizations.* San Francisco: Jossey-Bass.

Lister E.D. (2000) Effective health care leadership requires well-organized team. American College of Physician Executives, *Click Online Medical Management Magazine* **July.**

McKenna M.K. and Pugno P.A. (2002) Strengthen physician relations by helping residents develop ACGME-mandated competencies. *The Society for Healthcare Strategy and Market Development Spectrum* **November/December.**

Montgomery K. (2001) Physician Executives: The evolution and impact of a hybrid profession. *Advances in Health Care Management* **2**: 215–41.

Shields M.C. (1994) The physician-administrator team revisited. *MGM Journal* **41**(5): 10, 110.

Sterns T.H. (1999) How physician/administrator teams work in small groups: Six steps to make it happen. *MGM Journal* **46**(3), 44–50.

Watson M. and Wooten K. (2000) An accidental team: Physician executives tackle teamwork. American College of Physician Executives, *Click Online Medical Management Magazine* **September.**

Chapter 13

Coordination of Decisions and Actions

"Nothing is particularly hard if you divide it into small jobs."

Henry Ford

"Yeah, right" you may be thinking, "Easy for Henry Ford to say, he never had to navigate this vastly complex system of medicine." True enough, but hang on a second and let's consider whether we can apply any pearls of wisdom that do apply principles of "divide and conquer" toward the effective leadership of healthcare delivery.

In a medical lecture, Dr. William Jessee (2004) described the current competitive tensions between many hospitals and physicians in terms his audience could understand – he framed the scenario as a clinical case.

> "The patients were an 89 year old couple, known as the 'hospital' and the 'hospital medical staff.' Their chief complaints were increasing tension in the relationship, failure to communicate or understand

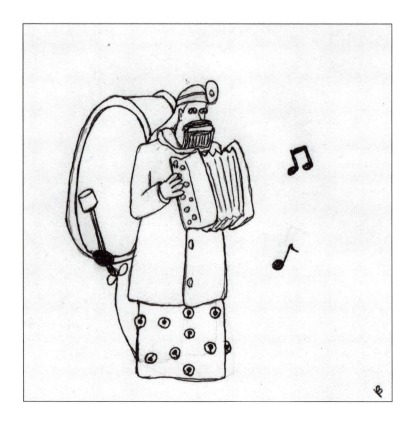

one another, frequent arguments, occasionally culminating in emotional or legal abuse. Both patients had at times threatened that they wanted 'a divorce.' Symptoms observed? Several hospitals that had revoked privileges of staff physicians who had invested in other hospitals.

An underlying cause or contributing factor to the physician/hospital relationship patho-physiology is the financial dilemma faced by physicians today. Research indicates that reimbursement revenues are not rising in proportion to the rise in expenses, and that without Congressional action, Medicare rates will actually decline significantly starting in 2006, even while professional liability expenses will likely continue to increase. The trend of shifting of financial responsibility from employers to patients is increasing providers' cost of collections.

The prognosis is grim – in fact, inability to generate new sources of revenue (e.g., not simply traditionally reimbursable services) will lead to practice insolvency.

The care plan includes two important components. First, stop the bleeding by identifying the revenue 'leakage' and fixing it. Second, get a transfusion by adding new revenue sources – such as ancillary services, complementary and alternative medicine, medication dispensing, online consultations, e-health services, boutique practices, charging administrative fees, and offering other non-insured health-related services.

Will this approach address the couple's patho-physiology? Can this couple's relationship be saved? Maybe. If they open a dialog of frequent, candid conversation, genuinely listening to each other's concerns. If they clearly define their vision and objectives. If they establish ways for measuring and rewarding attainment of their shared goals. If they seek win/win opportunities such as joint ventures, information technology collaboration, or passive investments – by hospitals in physician-controlled enterprises or by physicians in hospital-controlled enterprises. If they are flexible, willing to consider and adopt new approaches. If they build effective teams – teams that trust and mutually respect one another's knowledge, skills, strengths, weaknesses, similarities, and differences. If they invest in leadership education – including formal training programs, books and articles, 360° assessments, and informal coaching and debrief sessions. If they practice evidence-based management as well as evidence-based medicine.

Prognosis? The underlying issues are not going away any time soon. The challenges can be anticipated and addressed – but they require a new leadership style from all three legs of the traditional hospital leadership stool – the administrators, the physicians, and the hospital trustees."

William F. Jessee, MD, FACMPE
Pediatric, Preventive and Emergency Medicine Physician
President
Medical Group Management Association

We hope you agree by now that leadership and management are complementary but quite different activities. As you reflect back on the people you've worked for or with, odds are you would describe some of them as strong leaders and others as strong managers. We hope you've not had the misfortune of working for someone who neither leads nor manages well, although it does happen more often than any of us would like. In our many years of experience working with people of all professional backgrounds, we've observed that the people who exhibit strong leadership *and* strong management abilities are rare indeed. And yet, both leadership and management skills are needed for the consistent achievement of remarkable results. In fact, managing oneself is a necessary prerequisite to successfully leading others. And one aspect of managing ourselves that most of us find difficult is that ongoing challenge of managing our time.

Time Management Tips for Busy Physician Leaders

So, you decided to take the affirmative step and move into a leadership position. Somewhere along the line, the harsh reality strikes you, "When will I find the time to get done all the things I have to do and add all of these new responsibilities?" Managing your time well is a step in the right direction. Although this section is not intended to be a comprehensive treatise on time management, rather this is hoped to be an outline of basic principles which we have gleaned from multiple resources and which seem to be most pertinent for application by physician leaders.

First, you must answer the question of why this is important. In addition to increased productivity, managing one's time well has multiple other affirmative consequences. When time is managed well, job satisfaction increases and the work produced then serves as a source of personal enrichment. Managing time well also improves interpersonal relations. How? Leaders who manage their time well are able to give co-workers the attention they need and deserve. Managing time well also benefits the leaders themselves, by reducing pressure, stress and anxiety, thus resulting in a more pleasant day-to-day life and ultimately in better health.

In discussing these principles of time management, we also wish to articulate a few "truths," which lend perspective to the principles. First of all, in managing one's time, the techniques and steps that work are highly individualized. There are no magic formulas and there have been no time management "breakthroughs" in recent history. All of the key time management principles advocated these days have been around for a long time and have proven themselves valuable in a variety of settings. Obviously, to determine whether any particular time management suggestion will work for you requires that you actually try it. Remember the old television commercial that promised us "Try it, you'll like it." So too, we believe that all of the time management principles we're describing require at least some minimal initial effort. We hope many of you will find them easy to apply and maintain, and will as a result, experience the benefits of better time management. We offer, however, an important caveat to this claim. Please do not try all of them all at once. Time management is a skill, and like any skill, must be learned and mastered a step at a time. So review these principles and consider which you think will work best for you. Then try a couple of them to see if they work out and are compatible with your preferences and life style.

"Cleaning House"

The first basic principle is to simplify your life by getting your office in order. We recommend that you spend some "quality time with a large garbage can" to sort and discard many of the items you have stacked up in your office. Decide which items are really essential and which are actually garbage. If you come across a document that you know is kept on file by someone else, critically evaluate whether you need to keep it or whether you can recover it from someone else at some future point if you need it. Critically evaluate things you have on file that are more than five years old. Our present environment changes so rapidly; if you haven't used it in the past five years, its usefulness now may be debatable. We guarantee that once you have "cleaned house," you will have a better sense of what you have, and will make better use of those resources in the near future. To be perfectly honest, we must also admit (in fact, we guarantee) that once you have done a major clean out and discarded things previously saved for an extended period of time, you will find at least one of those items would have been "nice to have" within two weeks of when you threw it away. That is an unfortunate reality; but one you will survive.

Establish an Effective Filing System

Another principle is to establish an effective filing system. Do you keep personal files that are duplicates of those kept by your staff? For files that include non-confidential material, why not consider turning them over to your staff who can file and manage for you? For dealing with personal files, consider tips that are described in all major time management handbooks. Typically, such handbooks recommend that you file documents, based of course on your preferences, according to the dates they are due (especially appropriate for ongoing projects), according to their priority or importance, or according to any other approach that works best for you.

> "I've learned over the years to type brief notes summarizing the key points of an article, then discard the full article to save space. I also keep a bibliography of articles I find helpful, and categorize them under headings such as 'medicine tips' or 'electronic medical records.' All physicians need some type of organizational filing, storage, and retrieval systems to effectively deal with the vast quantity of information we need to be able to access quickly and reliably."
>
> M. Susan Kraft, MD, MRO, AMEt
> Family Physician
> Faculty Physician, Baptist-Lutheran Medical Center
> Goppert Family Medicine Residency Program

Use a Compost Pile

One filing principle, however, that is particularly useful is that of the "compost" pile. Undoubtedly, each day, you'll come across one or two pieces of paper or resources, the importance of which you cannot determine at the moment. Maybe this is just trash or maybe it is something that will be found to be important in the near future. May we suggest you immediately place these items on your compost heap, which is a small pile of paper immediately adjacent to your desk. Anytime you are unsure whether a document needs to be filed, discarded, given to someone else or acted upon, simply put on the compost pile. When your compost pile reaches the height of approximately six inches (which takes about three to four weeks), turn it upside down. Then briefly go through each page, taking what was on the bottom, looking at it, deciding whether it needs to stay in the compost pile because it may still become important, or its potential value has passed and it can be discarded. Going through the entire pile in this manner, you'll usually be able to reduce it to less than an inch in height. Then return it to its place adjacent to your desk, where it will sit, ready for additional contributions. Should one of the items in the compost pile be determined of importance, it is usually a simple manner to quickly go through the stack and recover that item.

Prioritize

Leaders who manage their time well are clear about their priorities. Much of the literature written by Stephen Covey, PhD takes the perspective that you should make a list of the priorities in your life, and avoid doing anything that doesn't move you affirmatively toward one of your top few priorities. Although some people will find that to be too restrictive, others may find it helpful to have a clear idea of what you hope to achieve in the short- and long-term future, and to distribute your energy and attention accordingly. Many of us make to-do lists. Those of us with poor memory capabilities use paper as a substitute. Once you've written something on your to-do list, you don't need to consume limited memory space in your head to recall it. That means you can direct your energies in more productive directions. Periodically review your to-do list, making a sub-listing of the critical items that must be done right away. Be very careful to include only those things with sufficiently severe negative consequences that you are motivated to accomplish them. Most leaders find it important to distinguish between what is truly important and that which merely presents itself as urgent but not necessarily important. Items that are both urgent and important should be your top priority. Finally, within the prioritization process, it's important to learn to say "no" to at least some of the many requests that will come in your direction. Sometimes, a "no" response can be modified to be "I can't do it all but if you will take the bulk of the responsibility, I'm willing to assist."

Delegate

Leading effectively and efficiently requires appropriate delegation of tasks. Nearly all resources available for improving one's time management emphasize the importance of distinguishing between delegation and abdication. You delegate when you retain responsibility for assuring completion of the task, and you enable those assigned the tasks to do them successfully. What is involved in successful delegation? First, you must provide clear direction for those to whom you assign tasks. You must ensure they understand the expected outcome or end product, and the time frame in which it will be accomplished. Successful delegation also requires that you provide those to whom tasks are assigned sufficient resources and sufficient authority to accomplish the tasks. Periodically check in with those to whom you've delegated. Help them measure and evaluate their progress. Help them decide whether additional resources or authority will be necessary. Help them make mid-course adjustments. We assure you, this is time well spent. Finally, when the task is completed, appropriately recognize the individuals involved. This is essential for assuring their willingness to offer further future assistance.

Manage Your Communications

In today's "Information Age" with 24/7 communications connectivity, any attempt to successfully manage one's time requires attention to the management of communications. This is an extremely high priority. To manage your *telephone* communications, provide your assistant with clear instructions as to those conditions under which you should be interrupted. This helps with prioritization of the flow of incoming calls. Permit your assistant the prerogative of scheduling call-back times for you. This minimizes the "telephone tag" phenomenon that can be both time-consuming and frustrating because it reduces the likelihood that you'll waste time returning others' calls only to find they are no longer available.

Manage your *email* correspondence. Teach your assistant to "clean out" your email inbox by discarding unnecessary items. This can significantly minimize the amount of time you'll spend on unimportant emails. Take advantage of email software to automatically file messages from specific sources or forward documents to others. Judiciously copy your communications to your staff and your management. This keeps them informed about what you are doing, enabling them to more appropriately respond when questions or concerns are directed to them.

Manage your *conventional mail* as well. Teach your assistant to pre-sort the mail and discard unwanted "junk." We assure you this investment of your time will prove to have been time well spent. Consider having your assistant provide you with color-coded folders including incoming mail. For example, you may benefit by separation of items that:

1 are time-sensitive and must be seen as soon as possible
2 require your signature
3 are important for you to at least briefly review before the end of the day and
4 are lower priority or can be addressed at a later time.

Not only do such communication management techniques enhance your personal productivity, they also keep your assistant better informed about the issues and projects coming your way, thus enabling them to be better prepared to respond as necessary. Perhaps you might also teach your assistant(s) to pass items on to others who are more appropriate than yourself for response or information gathering.

Maximize Your "High Productivity" Time

Successful leaders enhance their effectiveness by taking advantage of their personal high-productivity time. Are you a "morning person" for whom the early hours of the day are most productive? Or is late afternoon your "best time?" Schedule your tasks according to your "personal productivity clock" – the times of day when you seem best physically and emotionally prepared to deal with them. This will increase your productivity and reduce your stress. Consider blocking specific times on your calendar to work on specific tasks as if they were actual appointments. This will enable you to focus on important projects without being disrupted and distracted by short time frame demands.

Multi-Task

Another basic principle of time management is that of multi-tasking. For example, when traveling, consider carrying a folder of low-priority items that need to be read and discarded. In this way, you'll use your travel time productively while progressively reducing the amount of material you're carrying along.

Take advantage of "down time" – those short open spaces on your calendar – to respond to email. (Yes, email can be accessed these days via web-enabled phones and personal digital assistants in real-time or by synchronizing them periodically with your regular email system.) This increases your task completion without directly encroaching on more productive blocks of time in your day.

Enhance Your Personal Capabilities

Leaders who manage their time well also manage themselves well. We can all enhance our personal capabilities. Have you, for example, hired enough staff, invested in their training, and empowered them to help you make the most of your time? Have you trained your assistant to intercept requests for information, collect background data, and then draft initial responses? By doing so, you'll minimize the personal time required to produce a final product that meets your satisfaction.

Current technology can – if properly used – greatly enhance your personal capabilities. A slow computer with a slow Internet connection can waste enormous amounts by consuming many one-minute increments throughout each day. Failure to maintain current contact information for those individuals with whom you communicate regularly is certain to reduce your productivity – perhaps significantly. How often have we all said to ourselves, "I know I have her phone number here somewhere." Consider using cellular paging, voicemail, voice-recognition software, and other technologies that can help you maximize your productivity once you've invested some initial time in learning how to use these resources appropriately. Some find it useful to integrate their systems for managing appointments, communications, and contact lists. Whether you prefer integrated or distinct systems for each of these tasks, be sure you have an approach that you find effective.

While a thorough description of various calendar, communication, and contact tools is beyond the scope of this book, we do hope you'll make the commitment to explore and adopt approaches for efficiently managing each of these types of tasks.

Boiler plate

Another principle of time management involves what we call "boiler plating." Most of us have to produce memos, letters and reports on a regular basis. Many of these documents are similar in format, although the contents vary. Why not prepare a "boiler plate" template for standard reports, incorporating data fields that require only periodic updating to make the reports relevant and current? Similarly, consider using a standardized format for referral correspondence or letters of reference. The template might include, for example, an initial paragraph that articulates the reason for the letter and its subject, a middle paragraph that is individually customized to the specific focus of that letter, and a final paragraph that summarizes your position and offers more information should such be required.

Using a "boiler plate" approach will save you time. It also increases the feasibility of delegating such correspondence or reports to an assistant. This further reduces the amount of time required for you to communicate in written form.

Manage Your Calendar

Good time management of course involves good calendar management. Many calendaring systems are available on the market today, including both paper and electronic forms. We strongly recommend that you try multiple types of calendaring systems before selecting the one you'll use long term. Why? Some of us are "day-at-a-glance" people, others prefer "month-at-a-glance" formats for monitoring and managing our time commitments.

Regardless of which type of system you choose, be sure to parallel the system with that of your assistant, so some appointment scheduling can be done on your behalf, without double-booking or having time commitments "fall through the cracks."

Have you been following the steady stream of time management resources coming available on the market? If so, you have probably noticed that there is little "new" information on this subject. And yet, periodic review of time management principles can remind us of techniques that will help us tackle this perennially challenging area.

> "The trouble with the rat race is that even if you win you're still a rat."
>
> Lily Tomlin

In fact, effective leaders recognize the importance of organizational culture – the explicit and implicit norms and values that guide behaviors. We all know intuitively that people are likely to work harder and be more effective when they feel appreciated, respected, and needed in their work. Effective leaders enable people to do their best work by putting policies, procedures, and processes in place that minimize constraints and maximize opportunities for people to share ideas, suggest improvements, and benefit from the collective successes of the organization. Not only do effective leaders encourage opportunities for collaboration and teamwork, they eliminate bureaucratic structures and processes that hinder productivity.

> "A committee is a group that keeps minutes and loses hours."
>
> Milton Berle

Whether an organizational structure is designed around functional areas (such as purchasing, facilities or finance) or service lines (such as surgery, emergency department, or rehabilitation) effective organizations help, rather than hinder, the timely and efficient flow of information and other resources.

> "Vision without action is but a dream. Action without vision is drudgery. Vision and action can change the world."
>
> Joel Barker

Successful leaders recognize that vision and inspiration alone are insufficient to achieve the desired outcomes. Leaders collaborate with others who are gifted in the science of management. They do so to optimize coordination in the use of resources and activities. Such coordination is essential for ensuring that scarce resources (including time and energy as well as monetary and physical resources) are aligned with agreed-upon priorities. And frankly, to ensure that results are achieved on time and within budget. This notion applies to the provision and delivery of healthcare services as readily as it does to the production and delivery of tangible consumer products.

Are you still early in your professional development? That's great! Why? The earlier in your career that you're able to gain any type of knowledge, skill or credential, the greater the benefit you will extract from it. Have you already been working for many years? That's great as well! Why? The more work experience and life experience you have, the more likely you are to recognize what additional knowledge and skills you need.

> "Experience is a good school. But the fees are high."
>
> Heinrich Heine

One physician leader who uses her skills of coordination to enhance the quality of healthcare is Jeannette South-Paul, MD. As you'll soon discover, Dr. South-Paul recognizes how important it is for leaders to be well organized, because as leaders our time is never fully our own. See what she has to say about the mindset physicians must adopt when transitioning into leadership roles. She explains why developing the perspective and behaviors of a generalist, rather than a specialist, is so essential for physician leaders.

Insights from Jeannette South-Paul, MD

"There is a critical need for leadership in healthcare. This is the second time I've been a Department Chair in an Academic Medical Center, and I see the need every day. I was in the Uniformed Services University of the Health Sciences (Military Medical School) in Bethesda. The Army trains everyone to be a leader – they realize that no matter what your rank, you need leadership skills.

I believe leadership begins with teamwork. Teamwork is necessary for institutions of all types. That's what enables people to work well together. Unfortunately, that notion is foreign to the culture of medicine and the culture of academia. In both environments, the mindset is 'all about me, myself and I.' For example, universities consider whether faculty are promotion or tenure 'worthy' based upon what faculty members do by themselves, for themselves. That is what the institutions seem to value. They undervalue the notion of caring for your neighbor.

I mentored my sister through her MBA education, and noticed she had lots of team assignments, with time allotted for the teams to actually meet and work together! In medicine, I'm often asked to lead a team but the team participants aren't given adequate time to meet. Good team leaders bring people together in shared time and space relationships, encouraging everyone to bring insights and skills. At this point, I prefer to participate in, rather than lead, task forces because I know that I'll contribute by serving as a participant, but I can't be assured other participants will contribute if I'm the one leading the initiative.

Who do I know that demonstrates effective physician leadership? Certainly the elected officials of medical societies and other professional associations or trade groups. We don't have enough 'role models' in medicine – or at least, don't have readily available means of identifying them and learning from their example.

I stepped beyond the day-to-day role of running my department to seek higher visibility for my messages – by writing, speaking, lecturing. Leaders must find ways of championing their causes and spreading their messages. Leaders must also be well organized. Otherwise, no matter how smart they are, they'll find they simply cannot do it all. Once in a management role, your time is not your own. Managers go from meeting to meeting all day long. This is quite different from the work of those who specialize in a particular field. Focused expertise is important, but it does not equip anyone to be a generalist in management.

Leaders must be masters at managing conflict. They must do it well, and consistently. In an academic medical environment, we must resolve conflicts not just among faculty, but also among staff, and between faculty and staff, even between your own group and other parts of the institution.

My path to becoming a physician leader? When I was very young, I thought I wanted to be a social worker in order to help the underserved. My parents were great role models, but it seemed to me that most people didn't care. Over time, I realized that social workers are essentially facilitators, so I switched to medicine as a desired career path at the age of 12. My parents were poor, so I earned scholarships, including **ROTC** service during college. I went to the **University of Pennsylvania**, where my mother worked. Upon acceptance to several medical schools, I decided to go to the **University of Pittsburgh.** I liked the structure, camaraderie, and support of the military. My residency program offered many opportunities for responsibility and opportunities to be creative in solving problems. The

Continued

culture was 'if you're organized and do your due diligence, you can get support for your recommendations.'

I served on active duty for 22 years and then came to the **University of Pittsburgh** to build what was a very small department within a very large organization. Many opportunities exist for me to exhibit leadership. I've been here since July 2001. My focus is on developing ambulatory care programs as access points for the underserved. That's my passion. I'm also focusing on building an academic perspective within family medicine. That will improve the impact family medicine can have for patients. And ultimately, it's all about the patients."

Jeannette South-Paul, MD
Chair of the Department of Family Medicine,
University of Pittsburgh School of Medicine

As we can read from these comments by Dr. South-Paul, the importance of teamwork cannot be overemphasized. Without strong, cohesive teamwork, the risk of conflict is elevated, the likelihood of remarkable results is diminished.

"A team had four members called Everybody, Somebody, Anybody and Nobody. There was an important job to be done. Everybody was sure that Somebody would do it. Anybody could have done it, but Nobody did it. Somebody got angry about that because it was Everybody's job. Everybody thought Anybody could do it, but Nobody realized that Everybody wouldn't do it. It ended up that Everybody blamed Somebody when Nobody did what Anybody could have done."

Gibbs

Learning From Others' Example

Another physician who demonstrates the use of strong coordination skills for the enhancement of high quality healthcare is Mark H. Belfer, DO, FAAFP. As you'll see, Dr. Belfer concentrates on leading physicians through the performance of his organizational responsibilities as a Family Medicine Residency Program Director, and through his volunteer service on the Board of the American Academy of Family Physicians Foundation.

Insights from Mark Belfer, DO

"All leaders should be capable of being standard bearers, pioneers, activists and executives at various times, though each of us may be especially strong in one or two of those areas. Jonas Salk is a good example of a pioneer who made significant contributions to the delivery of healthcare. Throughout history there have been lots of standard bearers and pioneers, activists and executives. We can and should learn from their example."

Mark H. Belfer, DO, FAAFP
Family Physician
Residency Program Director
Akron General Medical Center/NEOUCOM

Clearly an 'action-oriented' physician leader, Dr. Belfer illustrates through his actions and comments the importance of coordinating optimal allocation of resources to keep costs down, results up, and people energetically involved in their roles as members of patient-specific care teams and organization-wide care providers.

> "Besides the noble art of getting things done, there is the noble art of leaving things undone. The wisdom of life consists in the elimination of nonessentials."
>
> Lin Yutang

Self-Mastery First

By contrast, Nancy Baker, MD, points out the importance of refraining from action in certain circumstances. In sharing her leadership journey as a female physician, Dr. Baker helps us recognize the fact that successful physician leaders must first coordinate their own personal and professional agendas, before they can effectively coordinate the activities of entire programs, departments or organizations.

Insights from Nancy Baker, MD

"I don't mind doing the wash, and folding the laundry, but where do we keep the towels?" This remark was made by the husband of one of my esteemed women physician colleagues as we were discussing how our partners' hard work and sacrifice had made our roles as leaders possible. We also acknowledged gender-related differences in both leadership and home-making. The distinctions may be due to men and women being raised with a different worldview; they may be due to our differing abilities to multi-task.

I don't see many women physician leaders living the life I've imagined. We know that women and men are significantly influenced by the presence of suitable role models and mentors. Though I've been blessed by having deep and sustaining friendships with a few male mentors, they don't understand how I balance my role in the workplace with my role in one of the most complex, purposeful organizations that exists – family. I am simply one of four individuals living in my household who feels called to a vocation. Each decision that any one of us makes has a profound influence on the others. **Adrian Barnwell, PhD**, a child psychologist with whom I worked during residency training, offered me these words of wisdom before my marriage, 'Remember, it's never 50/50 for you and your partner in terms of career satisfaction and fulfilling home responsibilities. Sometimes it will be 20/80 and other times it will be 80/20, etc. Just remember to take turns in order to be fair to one another.' Sometimes, it simply hasn't been 'my turn' to accept a leadership position that would entail added professional responsibility.

Continued

Power and prestige have never motivated me to pursue or accept leadership roles. Primarily, I've been drawn to leadership when I believed the work was meaningful and the added responsibility would magnify the significance of my work. More recently, I've accepted various positions of authority when I've simply become impatient with what appears to me to be ineffective leadership. I've been affirmed for my ability to help various groups in which I participate, articulate our core ideology and envision a clear future. **Collins** sees these as key steps for organizations he describes in his book *Built to Last* (1994). I'm simply not interested in being part of organizations that lack vision and a clear mission.

Only recently have I come to believe that I have the necessary skills to be an effective leader. For much of my career, I felt I lacked the business and management skills necessary to run an effective organization. Hearing experts now espouse emotional intelligence, or EQ, as a determinant of leadership success, I feel there may be an important niche for me and other women to fill. One of my PLC colleagues recently described EQ as the 'currency of leadership.' **Daniel Goleman** first described the concept in terms of a leader having a high degree of self-awareness and self-regulation, including a propensity for reflection and thoughtfulness, a high degree of comfort with ambiguity and change, and significant personal integrity. Emotional intelligence is also characterized, according to **Goleman** (1998), by a high degree of personal motivation, empathy, and social skill. I believe emotional intelligence is a quality reinforced in most women, repeatedly.

I've never believed there is only one way for me to accomplish my life goals. Awhile back, I said 'no' to an offer to be nominated for a national office in a professional medical organization. One of my closest friends, a male, urged me to reconsider. He said, 'You never know when one door closes, if another will open.' I had considerable difficulty explaining to him that such has not been my life experience. Thus far, new and unexpected opportunities have presented themselves every time I've said, 'no.' I have not seen my life journey as linear, nor have I seen it organized in five or ten year phases. For me, life really is about living each moment as though it may be my last. Knowing what I know, having the opportunities that are before me, I feel an urgency to make every moment count – both in my personal and my professional life. If I can also help someone else, male or female, on their leadership journey, then so much the better.

I recently agreed to join the **Physician Leadership College (PLC) at the University of St. Thomas**, in order to gain insight into my own 'call of service' as a leader. During my 20-year career as an academic Family Physician, I have been offered a number of leadership positions. Some, I have humbly accepted; others I have declined, much to the surprise of some of my male peers and mentors. My leadership journey, in both personal and professional arenas, may be different from that of my male friends and colleagues."

Nancy Baker, MD
Family Physician
University of Minnesota

Perhaps Dr. Baker is correct in stating that her leadership journey may be different from that of some male friends and colleagues. On the other hand, the principles that Dr. Baker proposes are universally applicable. All physicians – whether male or female, primary care or subspecialist – must decline many "good" opportunities in order to channel time, energy and attention toward the "best" opportunities that come along. That is the only way to fully realize your potential to make the significant, meaningful impact on healthcare that only you can make.

Making Decisions and Taking Action

Effective physician leaders understand that analysis is important, but even when insufficient information is available, leaders must sometimes go on and make decisions or take action.

> "When faced with the tough decisions, gather all the data, weigh and analyze it, and take counsel from your most trusted advisors. Objectively weigh each factor you can grasp. Then, at the end of the day, when the facts are all considered, decide with your gut. Intuition separates the good leader from the great ... the 'feeling' of knowing the right thing to do. Learn to trust that feeling."
>
> Leo J. "Lee" Baxter

Dr. McPherson points out that physicians' medical training offers an ideal training ground for managerial decision making.

> "Managers must make quick decisions, often on the basis of complex and insufficient data. And so, our medical education can be quite helpful, because physicians, too, must by necessity become comfortable with making difficult decisions quickly. The key difference has typically been in the degree to which decisions are made independently (in medicine) or collaboratively (in management). Either way, good communication skills are essential.
>
> Consider, for example, what all of us want from our physicians and our managers. We want them to listen to us, to understand us, to clearly convey to us what we should do. We want to believe that they are focused on our best interests; we can discern that by what they say, as well as by what they do."
>
> Deborah S. McPherson, MD, FAAFP
> Family Physician
> Associate Director, Family Medicine Residency Program
> Kansas University Medical Center

Dr. Munzing recognizes how important it is to seize opportunities for action. He gives this advice to physician leaders:

> "Avoid paralysis by analysis – don't miss opportunities waiting for all the information when you have a sufficient amount to make a good decision. Be careful to avoid being lulled by a good result or envi-

ronment, failing to take the risks to make a great result or environment."

Tim Munzing, MD
Family Physician
Kaiser Permanente – Orange County

Points to Ponder

1 In what way do organizations reflect their vision and values through their allocation of resources (including budgets and the use of time)?
2 What happens when leaders within an organization fundamentally disagree with those resource utilization decisions?
3 How do you (or would you) handle situations in which you are responsible to oversee coordination of resources in ways that you perceive to be suboptimal or down right inappropriate?
4 What specific activities or resources need to be more effectively coordinated within your organization, or among the people you seek to lead?
5 What exactly could you do to help those you're leading achieve significantly better outcomes, or achieve them far more efficiently?
6 What would it take for you to make that happen?
7 What prevents you from making it happen?
8 What knowledge or skills could you gain to more effectively coordinate the usage of resources for the achievement of the vision you share with those you're leading?

References and Further Reading

Allen D. (2003) *Ready for Anything: 52 productivity principles for work and life*. New York: Penguin Group.

Collins J. (1994) *Built to Last: successful habits of visionary companies*. New York: Harper Business Essentials.

Covey S.R. (2004) *The Eighth Habit: From effectiveness to greatness*. New York: Free Press.

Covey S.R. (1992) *Principle-centered Leadership*. New York: Simon & Schuster.

Covey S.R. (1989) *The Seven Habits of Highly Effective People*. New York: Simon & Schuster.

Covey S.R., Merrill A.R., and Merrill R.R. (1994) *First Things First: To live, to love, to learn, to leave a legacy*. New York: Simon & Schuster.

Fargason C.A., Jr., Evans H.H., Ashworth C.S., and Capper S.A. (1997) The importance of preparing medical students to manage different types of uncertainty. *Academic Medicine* **72**: 688–92.

Fiore N. (1989) *The Now Habit: a strategic program for overcoming procrastination and enjoying guilt-free play*. New York: Putnam Books.

Fisher R. and Ury W. (1991) *Getting to Yes: negotiating agreement without giving in*. New York: Penguin Books.

Goleman D. (1998) *Working with Emotional Intelligence*. New York: Bantam Books.

Jessee W.F. (2004) *From Competition to Partnership: A clinical case study of physician – hospital relations*. Paper presented for the L.R. Jordan Distinguished Lecture. Sandestin, Florida. August 4.

Kaplan S.H., Greenfield S., Gandek B., Rogers W.H., and Ware J.W. (1996) Characteristics of physicians with participatory decision-making styles. *Annals of Internal Medicine* **124**(5): 497–504.

Kindig D.A. (1997) Do physician executives make a difference? *Frontiers of Health Services Management* **13**(3): 38–42.

Stack L. (2004) *Leave The Office Earlier: the productivity pro shows you how to do more in less time ... and feel great about it.* New York: Broadway.

Stahl M. and Dean P.J. (1999) *The Physician's Essential MBA: what every physician leader needs to know.* Gaithersburg, MD: Aspen Publishers, Inc.

Chapter 14

Change: Enabling Resilience and Renewal

"I believe leaders in medicine and in any field have a goal that is more future-focused than others; and they just won't quit, even if their goal takes 10 or 20 years to achieve."

Monte L. Anderson, MD
Gastroenterologist and Hepatologist
Mayo Clinic Scottsdale

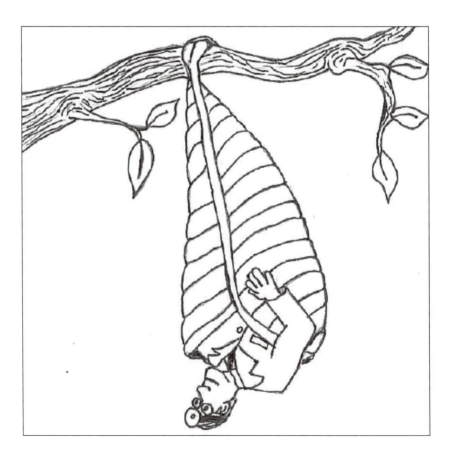

Imagine you've won the lottery! And your winnings include a free one-week vacation to a mystery destination. You pack for Tahiti – swimsuit, sun hat, flip flops and all ... imagining colorful umbrellas atop frosty, frothy cocktails on the beautiful sunny beach. Except – when you arrive at your surprise vacation destination and step off the plane ... yikes! You're in the Alaska tundra. Now there's nothing wrong with the Alaska tundra – it's beautiful, in fact. But where is your warm winter parka when you need it? Without mittens, or heavy socks, or a thick woolen muffler, you aren't at all prepared for this journey you've found yourself on. Forget the frosty Mai Tai – you need a cup of hot cocoa!

As we see it – that's the sort of dilemma most physicians are encountering today. You've packed and prepared for one sort of journey and found yourself having a very different type of experience altogether. Unprepared, and weighted down with baggage you don't need, what might otherwise be a fascinating, enjoyable adventure is ... well ... tough.

> "To endure is greater than to dare; to tire out hostile fortune; to be daunted by no difficulty; to keep heart when all have lost it; to go through intrigue spotless; to forgo even ambition when the end is gained – who can say this is not greatness?"
>
> William Makepeace Thackeray

Physicians today are well served by lightening the load – letting go of the baggage that weighs heavy upon them, and replacing old skills, old attitudes, old world views with ones that better suit the needs of the present situation.

What might you discard? That fine vintage wine, for one thing. That's right – no whining allowed. Same for your favorite candy – those habit-forming sour-balls you used to have in steady supply. You see, no longer are physicians accommodated or commiserated with when the complaining, blaming, victimization comments begin. And leave the ladder behind – climbing the status pole of hierarchical pecking-order structures is also passé. No more eggshells – you don't want those around you feeling the need to tiptoe around your temperamental moods. Dump the junk drawer and all the clutter stashed within it. Throw away the soap box – 'cause here's a news flash – folks (like patients, or residents or nurses, for example) no longer expect or want their physicians to be the brilliant and autocratic "sage on the stage" – they want you to be their trusted and involved "guide on the side" – using your expertise to help them join you in making good choices for their health. Won't need the wishbone – because "hope" is *not* a strategy. You can also drop the dice – the "new you" will gain skills and insights to make evidence-based decisions rather than leaving things to, well, a "roll of the dice." Unpack the bleach – no "whitewashing" or sanitizing of the truth for you. Your hammer has to go too – no more pounding your beliefs into others – it bruises them and just doesn't work very well in these contemporary times. Take off the blindfold and throw out the rose-colored glasses. Leading physicians today require clear vision and constant attention to ever-changing realities. No longer is it acceptable to keep your head in the sand, or delude yourself into seeing an idealistic picture that's, well, rosier than reality.

"Hmm," you're thinking to yourself, "then what will I need? What new tools are appropriate for this journey I'm on?" We're so glad you asked. May we suggest you'll want a mirror and a window. You'll use the mirror to look at yourself and see what others see (as Dan Goleman points out, self-awareness is a key to emotional intelligence, which in turn is a key to success).

The window is for looking into the world – what are others doing, hoping, wanting and needing from their leaders, from you? You'll definitely want a roadmap – to efficiently and effectively make use of the road signs and benchmarks, the lessons learned from those who've gone ahead. But you'll need a compass as well – for physician leaders today must traverse uncharted waters, going where no one has ever yet gone before. Bring along a magnet – you're going to want to draw folks in as a coalition of collaboration, working together toward the vision of a better, brighter future. Knitting needles will help as well – so you can get folks out of their functional "silos" and knit them together into a unified team. Leaders pave the way – so a flashlight will come in handy – part of your responsibility in guiding the team requires that you enable them to see where to go and what dangers lay ahead. When the going gets tough and the troops get tired, and believe us, that will happen, you'll need a source of power – a battery re-charger to tap into the source of continuous renewal that provides stamina and staying power for sustained ongoing results. And last, but certainly not least, you'll want a candle – to kindle the spark of passion, illuminate the vision, and warm the hearts of others who are by chance or by choice fellow pilgrims with you on this amazing adventure in healthcare.

> "Life is no brief candle to me. It is a sort of splendid torch which I
> have got a hold of for the moment, and I want to make it burn as
> brightly as possible before handing it on to future generations."
>> George Bernard Shaw

Physicians cannot expect to lead changes in healthcare without having a solid understanding of change management principles, and the skills necessary to bring change about. One physician who clearly understands this is Susan Kraft, MD, an experienced family physician, medical records officer, informatics consultant, and residency program faculty physician.

Insights from M. Susan Kraft, MD

"Physicians need to be in active management of change. Particularly with respect to the implementation of technology, change needs to be planned and implemented in advance of the implementation. The use of change management strategies at an early stage might save a great deal of money and organizational pain. In order to implement technology or *any* healthcare strategy successfully, physicians need to be involved in that change. The best technology in the world will be ineffective if system planning is not accomplished by careful attention to change management. (Austin and Boxerman 2003) Diligence, patience, and a positive attitude are keys to success, and leadership is essential.

Effective change management with regards to information systems/technology requires open communication and understanding of behavioral and cultural factors that may inhibit or lead to misunderstanding. A through, comprehensive staff orientation and training prior to initiation should include open communication about the technology, clear understanding of the goals, administrative support and leadership should be visible, and get buy-in from the users from the beginning. Every attempt should be made to avoid being cryptic or secretive. Physician leadership is a crucial element in change management because the physician is able to encourage, guide, and support the successful implementation from its inception to its completion."

> M. Susan Kraft, MD, CRO
> Family Physician
> Faculty Physician, Baptist-Lutheran Medical Center
> Goppert Family Medicine Residency Program

As pointed out by Dr. Kraft, all physicians are faced with chaos, complexity, and constant change in healthcare today. Thus successful physician leaders recognize the importance of equipping those they lead to persevere and stand firm on core values and principles, even while adapting to an ever-changing environment of complex laws, regulations, economic conditions, population demographics, and consumer expectations. Both resilience and renewal are necessary to embrace innovation and continuous improvement without experiencing burnout, stress, or fatigue. Successful leaders ensure innovation and continuous improvement by encouraging both *resilience* and *renewal*.

Overcoming Setbacks and Disappointments

> "Whenever God closes a door, He always opens a window. However, the door has to close first."
>
> Adapted from an old Quaker proverb

Three months ago, you were approached by a national organization inviting you to apply for one of its senior management positions. Since then, you've met and interviewed with most of the senior staff of that organization and the more you've learned about it, the more attractive the job opportunity seems. Although you are happy with your current position, this opportunity would be a substantial promotion and with time, you've come to want this job.

Unfortunately, a number of late applicants for it have substantially drawn out the timeline for a decision by the selection committee. Notwithstanding the delay, you have repeatedly received the tacit message that the organization really wants you for this position. As time goes on,

Continued

you become more and more hopeful that you will be selected. However, ultimately, you are notified that one of the late applicants has been selected for this job that you did not start out seeking but had come to really want. Your disappointment is profound.

The scenario just described is probably not an uncommon experience. Most people with ambition would be disappointed if, after having been invited to apply for a position, they were not ultimately selected. Accompanying the sense of disappointment can be a feeling of "failure" as an individual. "Where didn't I measure up? In what way were the selected applicant's qualifications better than mine? Did I do or say something during the application process that compromised my attractiveness as a candidate?" These and other questions commonly accompany a sense of decreased self-worth and "second guessing" behavior. Although these responses are entirely natural, such an experience can more than just hurt your feelings. It can also create a sense of depression and have other negative impacts on both your personal and professional life.

The question, then, is how to cope with this sort of experience? Are there ways of thinking about such occurrences that can be helpful in restoring self-esteem and re-engagement of your enthusiasm for the work and priorities with which you currently are involved? In actuality, there are several approaches, some of which may be more attractive to you than others. Each is, we believe, at least worth considering, in order to gain "perspective" from the experience.

"He who has never failed somewhere, that man can not be great."

Herman Melville

The first perspective to take away from an experience of "failure" is that it is okay to grieve over perceived losses. In fact, failing to acknowledge the normal grief experience can prolong its negative impact. Grieving helps us move toward acceptance and recovery. It can be a highly functional technique for getting over a negative event. For most of us, the pain of grief will subside over time. Reassurance of that fact can be quite comforting.

"Adversity does not build character ... it reveals it."

Successories

Another approach that can help when coping with the sense of loss is to attempt to put yourself in the place of the selection committee. Can you think of other qualities an applicant may bring besides the ones that characterize you which would be an advantage to the organization? Organizations' needs evolve with time. Is this a point in history where that organization has a specific need or an enhanced need for a specific experience or skill set, which has not been emphasized in your personal developmental history? For example, in the case of physician leaders, it may be politically advantageous for a physician in a particular leadership position to come from a medical discipline with which that particular organization has found more recent challenges. The special expertise and experience of working in a particular medical specialty can provide insights to dealing with challenges involving that discipline and ones similar to it, the advantages of which may far outweigh other qualifications.

A simpler perspective is this: we simply may not always know what is best for us. The spouse of a recent candidate for U.S. Surgeon General, who was not selected for that position, was known to remark: "In life, there are only two tragedies. The first is not getting what you want, and the second is getting it." In other words, we may not know the potential negative consequences that might have accompanied achieving the goal we had set for ourselves. Perhaps failing to be selected for a position will later provide an opportunity to be considered for something else even more attractive.

In a similar vein, a more spiritual perspective can be taken. Failure to get something that you want can be viewed as a simple message that God's plan for you in this world does not include that job which you sought, but instead is along another direction of which you are as yet unaware. Perhaps there are needs in the organization with which you currently work that only you can meet. Perhaps your life is to be directed along a completely different path that would result in more "good" than you can fathom at this moment. Such perspectives can significantly accelerate the acceptance of a perceived failure.

> "**Larry Weed,** MD is a hero to me. He was trained as an engineer, and then went to medical school. While at the University of Vermont in the 1960s, he looked at medical records and realized there must be a better way. He came up with the SOAP method – way ahead of his time. He makes astute comparisons like 'if the airline industry was like medicine we wouldn't have radar, we'd encircle airports with ICUs.' But **Larry** has been ineffective with over 90 percent of docs because they aren't ready to hear or accept his perspective. Effective leaders understand what they can (and can't) say to have an impact. They understand the culture – usually because they've been there. They can build bridges between the different cultures of medicine and management."
>
> Randall Oates, MD
> Family Physician
> Founder and President, Docs, Inc.

Another viewpoint to be considered is the reality that there are no guarantees in life. Competition for a job is a human process and such processes are likely to be affected by any number of forces, both large and small. In human processes, errors occur because no one has a right to expect perfection. In life, a situation such as this may demand a simple acceptance that sometimes things don't work out the way we want them to ... and that is just reality. In the words of one of the author's favorite clinical teachers, "Suck it up, get over it, and move on."

Everyone gets bad news from time to time, and failure to achieve a particular goal or be selected for a job you want is indeed bad news, but perhaps it is not such bad news. What if the news instead was: "You have a terminal illness." If you are reasonably satisfied and fulfilled in your job, maybe failing to get a new one is not such a terrible thing. Consider the many people who, each day, hear words like: "It appears that the chemotherapy has been unsuccessful." How many of those people are able to maintain their optimism in the face of adversity and loss? Maybe your situation isn't quite the tragedy you thought it was.

Keep in mind that in a thousand years it won't really make a difference whether or not you got that job. Stars are formed, exist for their natural life span, then disappear over the course of billions of years. Each of us, although important as an individual, is only a small piece of the puzzle of life on this planet. Our personal sense of failure or loss, though valid and individually important, may indeed be of relatively minor consequence in the grand scheme of things. Perhaps being a good person and doing our best on a day-to-day basis is the important and valuable contribution we're called to make in the world.

> "We should be careful to get out of an experience only the wisdom that is in it – and stop there; lest we be like the cat that sits down on a hot stove-lid. She will never sit down on a hot stove-lid again – and that is well; but also she will never sit down on a cold one any more."
>
> Mark Twain

Setbacks help us gain appreciation for the value of learning from life experiences. Research confirms that nearly all successful leaders have experienced at least one major loss or setback in their careers or their personal lives. Through them, we learn from the experience and emerge even better prepared to face the next challenges in life. Learning and growing from our personal experiences should be among our most highly valued opportunities.

Charles Jaffe, MD, PhD takes a different approach in his work to improve the quality of healthcare. By collaborating with individuals and organizations including healthcare providers, to regulators, pharmaceutical companies, and associations, Dr. Jaffe is an advocate for the utilization of clinical informatics by mainstream physicians because he believes proper use of information technology can "raise the bar" for the quality, efficiency, and effectiveness of all physicians. Dr. Jaffe's leadership in establishing universal clinical data standards is a necessary next step in order for informatics to become widely adopted by physicians in all fields of medicine.

Insights from Charles Jaffe, MD, PhD

"There is probably no secret to the successful transformation of a clinician. Many of the skill sets that prove essential for patient care can be translated directly into another workplace. Tireless devotion, the ability to accept change, and an abiding concern for others are invaluable assets. Of course, some of the traits of the physician as caregiver do not transfer well in the corporate environment. I've had some stunning disappointments, but I've never stopped believing in the inherent goodness of mankind, despite strong evidence to the contrary.

Some of the building blocks for corporate leadership are honed in the early years of physician training. Certainly, we honor intellectual honesty, true emotional courage, and the ability to empathize. Despite the success this bears within the clinical framework, the independence and individual resolve born in the critical care setting do not translate well into the hierarchical reporting structure and inherent delays of the corporate world. Strategic intervention outside of the pathways of the organization chart is disparaged, regardless of the level of achievement.

The complexity of corporate life does not parallel the demands of patient care. The patient interview has no equivalent, but good communication skills are well rewarded. On the other hand, a challenge to the status quo requires organizational substantiation. Activities are planned to coincide with business objectives and the serendipity of discovery can be easily overlooked. In contrast, the patient care plan, often the purview of the clinical nurse, is seamlessly translated into the structured timelines of business imperatives and team objectives.

Physicians entering the corporate world can expect to face surprising hurdles. Clinicians are almost always expected to be devoid of any business skills. Independence and self-reliance, usually essential in patient care, are rarely welcomed in corporations. Peer communication is anticipated, but there is surprisingly little support for leader-to-novice interaction that is so commonplace, and often prized, in academia.

Great challenges are often met with great rewards. At the same time, as my first mentor reminded me, an organization 'is not a meritocracy.' Much like the first days following completion of a training program, the initial experience in a corporate environment is likely to seem both frightening and exciting. Often physicians do not succeed in the transition because they are unwilling to accept the challenges that follow. I find it fascinating. Four years after transitioning into the corporate realm of healthcare, I still greet every day with the same enthusiasm that I once felt four years after residency."

Charles Jaffe, MD, PhD
Director of Clinical Informatics
Astra-Zeneca Pharmaceuticals

As Dr. Jaffe points out, physicians who aspire to make a difference in healthcare by moving beyond the traditional role of clinician can expect to encounter obstacles – not the least of which may be skepticism or even disdain from others. To find success and fulfillment in your calling you must persevere despite what anyone else may say or do.

Feeling discouraged? Unsure about whether the uncertain promise of potential outweighs the ego-bruising experience of inevitable setbacks? Take heart from someone who persevered over failure – not once, but many times – to eventually become a truly great leader.

He failed in business in '31.

He was defeated for the legislature in '32.

He was reduced in military rank from captain to private in '32.

He failed in business in '33.

He was sued for unpaid debts in '34.

His sweetheart died in '35.

He had a nervous breakdown in '36.

He was defeated for Speaker in '38.

He was defeated for Elector in '40.

He was defeated for Congress in '43.

He was defeated for Congress in '48.

He was defeated for Senate in '50.

He was defeated for Vice President in '56.

He was defeated for Senate in '58.

He was elected President in '60.

Who was this man? Abraham Lincoln.

Source unknown

Points to Ponder

1 What setbacks or obstacles have you encountered?
2 What have those experiences taught you about yourself? About leading well?
3 What obstacles have you not yet experienced that would be reasonable to anticipate – given your strengths and weaknesses, goals and aspirations?
4 What can you do to avoid or prepare for those challenges?
5 Reflect on a time that you didn't handle a situation as well as you would have liked. What might you have done, or not done, or done differently, to handle it more effectively?
6 Do you find yourself trying to avoid risk or failure?
7 How can you combat that natural tendency, and instead view failures as opportunities for growth?

Another physician, Bruce Bagley, MD, also offers insights for physicians who aspire to be compelling leaders. Dr. Bagley emphasizes that leaders are typically quite adept at lifelong learning. Leaders learn from family and friends, reading and mentors, trial and error, and last but not least, from encouragement and praise.

"With so much change occurring in our healthcare environment, the need for good physician leadership has never been greater. Group practice, hospital systems, managed care organizations, and hospital systems are all struggling to stay agile in a rapidly changing environment. Of course, leadership is needed at every level, but it is most important to realize that enlightened physician leadership is needed to effect physician behavior change.

There is a tendency in medicine to name the person who is the best physician of the group to a management or leadership position assuming that the skills required for success as a physician can be translated into organizational leadership and management expertise. The organization loses the best physician from clinical responsibilities and gains a mediocre manager.

Leaders are not born with everything they need. They learn the necessary values from family and friends; the necessary skills from reading and mentors; the necessary toughness from trial and error; and the necessary love for those they serve from encouragement and praise."

Bruce Bagley, MD
Family Physician
Medical Director for Quality Improvement
American Academy of Family Physicians

As Dr. Bagley so aptly demonstrates, physician leaders who advocate healthcare policy reform are likely to be proactive in mobilizing other medical professionals to make their voice heard on issues well before those issues are brought before Congress in the form of newly proposed laws or regulations. Physician leaders who are concerned with reforms that facilitate further medical advances are typically proactive in seeking information to understand where significant gaps exist between current medical practice and new approaches that will become technologically and economically feasible in the near future.

Daniel Durrie, MD, is another physician who is making a difference in healthcare. He uses his worldwide recognition for clinical excellence to bring about improvements in the quality of ophthalmologic care received by patients – his own and those treated by the physicians he mentors and educates.

Insights from Daniel Durrie, MD

"I think if you look at the role of physicians historically, it is not too surprising why we are in the situation we are in today. Back in the 1920s and 1930s, the system was very simple. There were patients who needed care and there were doctors – providers – who could provide that care. There was a very close partnership in decision making between the patient and the doctor on what to do – medication, therapy, surgery – and the cost of the care needed. The doctor was well aware of the inconvenience or cost of the procedure or medication, and together they made the decision. Then medicine began to get a more complicated. We needed specialized facilities to be able to provide care. Hospitals became more sophisticated,

Continued

so now patients were not only treated at home or in hospitals, but at a specialized facilities like nursing homes or even disease-specific facilities such as TB sanitariums. So now the system had three parts: the patients, the providers, and the facilities. That worked very well, and it was still a direct patient-to-provider relationship. The doctor would help the patient decide whether to go to the hospital or not, and certainly costs were part of that decision making.

The next thing that happened was the development of the third party payer system. Healthcare was getting more expensive and a safety net was needed. Doctors helped found Blue Cross and Blue Shield and other insurance companies to have a place to 'park the money' until it was needed. People could pay a small amount every month and build up a reserve, and then when something happened, healthcare would be paid for in that indirect way by the third party.

Then in the 1960s, the Medicare system was formalized and there was more third party paying. The government was starting to get more involved in wanting to provide care across the board without any consideration of financial need. Then employers, in order to attract good employees, started paying more of healthcare, and so today, 80 percent of all healthcare is paid by someone other than the patient.

The process became quite complicated, and doctors were willing to give up some of that decision making, either because of their lack of knowledge in management or because of the lack of leadership skills in the overall healthcare system, and that leadership need was provided by insurance companies, government, third party payers, and hospitals.

Now there are five players in the healthcare system of today: patients, providers, facilities, insurance companies, and payers (employers and the government). Who has taken over the decision-making power? Instead of the patient and the doctors making decisions, the power has shifted to the hospitals, insurance companies, and the payers.

How did this all take place? I think the doctors were part of helping the system develop in an effort to get better patient care and control costs, but physicians failed to recognize the importance of their role as the leaders in healthcare decision making. So now the healthcare system has changed so dramatically that the physicians find that not only have they lost control of the healthcare decision making, they don't have the leadership skills to really fight back into that system very well.

There is starting to be a lot more recognition that we need to develop physician leaders, involved at the hospital level, insurance companies, government, and we have seen a lot more physicians who are starting to use the leadership skills they have, or have a desire to fine-tune them. I am seeing more young physicians who recognize that the future of the medical practice is dependent on having good physician leaders, either those who will do it for themselves and learn the skills, or try to encourage other people to have those skills to move into that position.

I have always been involved in large practices since I went into practice over 20 years ago. I started in a practice in Omaha, Nebraska, a large practice that had a great style of management. We had a key physician leader and it was someone who was very good at it. I don't know where he learned how to do it, but he was good at managing our practice. He was very fair. He was a sort of a benevolent dictator. He was so fair and so good that no one else needed to or wanted to have the job. So there was not a lot of need for me in my first 12 years of practice to develop leadership skills. I was mostly watching and really admiring how someone else was doing it

Then when I came to Kansas City, I joined a physician who was established in the community and over the next 10–12 years, we grew a practice that was very large, and I was able to watch the management style of several people. We even associated with a national management company and then I was able to watch how management went on in multiple practices. I was learning all along which management styles worked and did not work, and then when I eventually had my own business, which I have had for about two years, the mentoring I had over such a long period of time made leading a practice fairly easy and it was almost natural to be more of a leader and have more decision making.

I think that physicians are very accustomed to learning to by mentoring. In medical school, we looked to our faculty, who clearly knew more than we did, and we wanted to learn from them. During internship, we learned a lot, not only about medicine, but how to manage people, and then through residency, watching the residents ahead of you and the chief resident. Then most people go out into practice, join someone or are involved in hospital groups. They always watch the people who are already leading others, and perhaps choose to emulate those who are doing it successfully, and reject the methods of those who are not as successful.

My mentors have all been positive influences on me, from medical school to my fellowship, where Jack Filkins, MD, who was the senior partner and mentor in Omaha, was a man I always appreciated learning from. He had great ways of making people work together. I think, and hope, I picked up some of those skills along the way. You also have to try to find what works for you. Just because someone else is successful in one way does not necessary mean you will be successful in the same way; you must work out your own style. That is done by trial and error, like medicine itself. I think we all realize we have to pursue a process – learn to do the surgery, learn to prescribe the medications, and learn to prescribe the diagnostic tests and what gives us the answer the fastest. We learn leadership the same way.

One thing I learned from Dr. Filkins is what I call the 'third alternative' theory. I don't think he had an official name for it, but I saw him do it all the time. He would be involved in a discussion between two parties – two physicians, two employees, or perhaps even two groups of people – who were having trouble making a decision because they had opinions which seemed

Continued

to be at odds. The topic could range from an office expansion, hiring of employees, patient flow alterations. He would enter the group discussion as a leader, and he would come up with another alternative that neither one of the parties had considered and get them to entertain discussion on this third alternative. It was fascinating to watch, because as people discussed the third alternative, they always came back and resolved the issues they had been discussing before. Maybe that third alternative was the best way to proceed, and the original arguments were discarded, but most of the time, they would return to their original arguments, but now having broken down some of the barriers, and they were able to make a decision and move ahead, and not be at a road block. I don't think this method is intuitive, but if you see someone do it and try it yourself, it works very well. I use this method all the time, because I don't like conflict, and so if I come into a room and an argument is going on, I am quite uncomfortable, so I use this method, and the easiest thing to do is to get them a little bit off their original subject, discuss a new alternative and let them come back around to the original discussion. It works great.

Mentoring is definitely my preferred style of learning, and I also think the medical community is made for it. It works for doctors, and I think when it is applied to other aspects of practices, both for the people who want to be leaders and those who are being trained to be leaders, it just fits. I think most physicians are more comfortable learning this way than going out and taking a business leadership class or trying to learn it off the Internet. I think this applies to physicians leading their staffs and also being leaders in the community.

One of the things I have found has been very helpful to me is my own fellowship training program that I have had for the last 18 years. I have had up to four physicians who spend the year with me in advanced post-graduate training. This has been a great program because they keep me on the ball because they are always asking questions about why I did something in a particular fashion, and challenging me medically. I also learned to help them grow into their career and I think a lot of them have appreciated that they have learned some leadership skills from being a part of that program. The other thing I really enjoy is that we have a fellowship reunion every year where everyone gets back together and share ideas with each other, having had similar training but diverse positions now. Everyone finds it very valuable with respect to business skills and leadership skills. I am very proud of them because they have given a lot back – in patient care, ophthalmology research, and also they are all fairly active in their communities and I think it is something I would like to see more of. This is a non-university based fellowship program that we have done in private practice. Most people don't do this, but it truly is an extension of the mentoring system and it has worked out very well for both me and those who have gone through the program.

I think physicians need to look at how they can get involved in their community in a leadership role. We get a lot from the community around us, and we should be giving back. I don't mean just writing checks to the charities, but also figuring out how to lead by example to our employees on how to be involved in the community. Donations of time are frequently harder to do than giving money, but I think it gives employees a better feeling about what medicine is all about – active participation in the community.

An example is a program that I started a few years also. My specialty in ophthalmology is refractive surgery and optical research. I have a lot of tools and skills that help get people out of glasses. Most of the time this is for people who have found out on their own that they don't like the inconvenience of glasses or contact lenses and they make a decision both medical and economical to pay for and have this elective surgery. But there is a very special group of people, easy to identify, that really *needs* refractive surgery. This group is made up of people who have a disease or injury where they have lost the ability of move their arms. The most obvious group is quadriplegics. These are patients who one day had a life which was basically normal, and the next minute, after the accident, they no longer can move their arms and legs, and their whole life changes. Imagine someone who wears contacts or wears glasses, who now have to ask a care giver every time they want to put their glasses on or off. This was an obvious need, and I needed to figure out a way to help this group of patients. I talked to my staff and discussed the general idea with them, answered their questions, and then we started finding patients within the community on whom we could do surgery at no charge as a give-back to our community. Over the last couple of years this program has not only been extremely successful in our helping a lot of people, but also it has shown the office staff that we really care and that we need to be and can be an active part of the community. This program has given back way more to all of us than the patients have received.

Now that the program is successful at a local level, I am working on how to make it into a national, and possibly international, program. I am working on figuring out how I can get other eye surgeons in other communities to provide the service to their patients and the leadership skills are necessary for that. I know that physicians have questions, and I want to respond to them ahead of time. I want to mentor others in how this has worked for us – good communications being foremost. It is fairly easy once you have done something successfully – you can 'write the manual' on how to apply a good idea to another community.

One of the issues that is a problem with physicians is time management. They are busy, and often they don't control their own schedule. So if they are going to try to lead, they must figure out how to become efficient enough to take care of patients, run a business, and also try to have some leadership within the medical community, whether that is working in politics, working on the hospital staff, or working in the community. One thing I have found is that I am not very good at narrowing the focus of projects. I have realized over the years that when I start a project, it will

Continued

grow and grow over a period of time. If it is successful, I will want to have it larger and larger. This, of course, creates a problem, in that there are only so many things you can do in a day.

I have an analogy I use. Every time I plant a tree in my 'garden,' I know that it is going to grow and eventually the branches from each tree are going to run into each other. So every few years, I have to cut down a tree or two and no longer do one or two of the activities. I either pass it on to someone else to do, or just narrow my focus. As an ophthalmologist, I was trained in corneal disease and performed corneal transplants as well as cataract surgery, and I also do a lot of research. When I moved to Kansas City, I quit doing cataract surgery and focused on just cornea and refractive surgery and research. Then as things got a little more complicated, I decided to stop doing corneal transplants because I had a new partner who could do that, and then I focused just on refractive surgery and research, and I can see a time in the future when I will just do research.

Another example of how I have 'cut down the trees' is how I have worked in professional organizations. Since I have been involved in refractive surgery since it first started, I have also been involved in several start-up professional organizations. I have been a founding member of the boards, a committee member, and occasionally an individual committee chairman. I know from experience that I am not very good at being chairman of committees or organizations. I like to start the process, be on the planning committee, see the organization grow and then move on. I know my own personality – I want to help get it started and get it going, but I am not very good at maintaining things. I liken it to the fact that in the spring I like to plant things in my yard, but I don't like pulling the weeds. The same thing applies to the projects I do. I am more interested in the founding of an idea and the moving along and then eventually, when it gets to the point where that idea has matured or that idea is past its prime, I will start looking for a new challenge.

My practice now has three parts. I have a business consulting division, in which I help industry develop new products for our specialty. I have a research division that does FDA clinical trials, both formal and informal, to try to improve the quality of refractive surgery locally, regionally, and worldwide. The third part is the surgical division that not only takes care of patients, but teaches surgical techniques to people who are doing some of the new procedures that are being introduced once FDA approval comes. I look at it as a complementary group of tasks. If we get involved in the ideas early with business development, then we can help companies to develop the right products at the right time in the future. Going through FDA approval process we can learn about the procedures during their critical development cycle. Then we can take what we learn and apply it to teaching people how to avoid the problems during their early adaptation of the new technology. Each of these has taken some structure and leadership within the office. They are not intuitive to begin with, and a lot of people ask me how I have the time to run all of this, and I think it is because of the people who are around me and the structure of the practice. You have to build leaders around you. The best way to teach your key personnel to be leaders is by example. It is amazing what you can accomplish with the right team.

We have a very low turnover rate in our employees. I think they have stayed with me for a long time because we are meeting what the employee's goals are which helps to make this a career rather than 'just a job.' I try to focus in on helping build on their strengths so that it is enjoyable and rewarding to work here. I don't even mind if people say it is fun to work here, because I think it should be fun to go to work. If you are going to spend the majority of your life at your job, which most of us do, it should not be drudgery, or we are going have high employee turnover. I like to see that – I like to see that people are meeting their goals. If I do have an employee leave because they are offered a 'better' job, or their spouse is transferred, or whatever the reason, I am always excited for them also. I am happy for someone to move to their next level, and I am glad to be a part of that process. You don't want to keep people working in a situation where they are unhappy and can't grow. I think that is what I want to continue to provide – for everyone within the team to have the opportunity to look at where they can go to the next level, either in the practice or in their next job.

If I were just starting out, knowing what I know now, I would do a couple of things differently. One thing is I would have tried to learn to speak another language. I wish I had pursued Spanish. It would really help me right now because I do a lot of research in other countries. I think that some more formalized business training would have also been helpful. Along the way, physicians usually make some bad investments or bad decisions, and it costs them financially. I see this all the time – a physician invests in something because their brother-in-law said it was a good idea, or they get things in the mail, and think they should invest. Most of the time it is a waste of time and money. It usually happens because of the physicians lack of knowledge in this area. We don't learn how to read a balance sheet or prospectus in Medical School. Training in business would be a good idea – some basic business training as part of the curriculum, but then on an as-needed basis, because some people are more interested than others.

I have been asked if I have a plan for the future. I am pretty happy with the way things are working out now. I am trying to fine-tune what I am doing, so I think I have learned enough along the way that now I am trying to hone some of the skills I have acquired. I think our practice is rather unique; I don't see other practices that are like ours. Unfortunately, when you look at mentors, you sometimes have to look backwards, and I do that, and hope I am passing along some of the things I have learned to my new partner. My daughter is going into ophthalmology; she is a fourth year medical student now, and is applying now for ophthalmology residencies, and she is married to my partner, who did a fellowship with me.

Continued

I can now see the future of the practice pretty easily. I think I now need to learn how the be the mentor for the future leaders of our practice.

I very much like to watch someone doing something at a very high level, at the top of whatever it is. I don't care whether that is an athlete, a musician, a dancer, or race car driver, a golfer, or it could be just watching someone be a great parent. I think that I learn something from every single one of those areas, even if they are way out of my field. That is something I enjoy looking for. If I go to a performance and see someone performing at their best, it gives me huge satisfaction, and then challenges me to go and work on trying to do something in my field in such an excellent fashion.

I had an experience years ago when I was associated with a man in Omaha who was a manager of a race car team. It was showroom stock racing and they ran 24-hour endurance races. There was a team of Saleen Mustangs. He asked me if I wanted to go and be on the pit crew. This had always sounded interesting to me, so I called with my two brothers-in-law, one a lawyer and one an auto dealer, and we went to Lexington, Ohio, to the mid-Ohio raceway and we were in the pit crew. Watching the teamwork for this was fascinating because my job for not only the 24 hours of the race, but also the practice session before and everything afterwards, was to lift the jack and the rear tire over the wall and then take it back. That was my whole job. I was awake for 40 hours. Someone else took care of fuel, someone else the other tires, etc. If I did not do that correctly, we were not going to win, so I concentrated on doing my job.

It was also interesting to see how the team worked. The drivers were well known – professional race car drivers. While we were out there working for hours on end, they would do their 2–3 hour stints and then they would go back to the luxury motor home and sleep, and eat, and talk to the press, and we just kept working. Then after we won the race, the press came over and all they wanted to do was talk to the drivers, and the drivers got kissed by the pretty girls, and they had their pictures taken, and we were down cleaning up the tires. We all knew that we had won the race just as much as the drivers had, but it was a team effort, everyone did their job. While I was returning to my home, I realized that on my surgical team, I am the driver. Without the whole team of the people who take care of the patients in check-in, post-op, the scrub nurses, and the people who make sure the instruments are sterile, this would not work. I can't just be the 'driver' and take all the credit. When I see patients one day post-op, they frequently tell me how great their vision is and how great I am, but I have to then turn around and thank all the people who got me there."

Daniel S. Durrie, MD
Opthamalogist
President, Durrie Vision Center

As we've seen from Dr. Durrie's example, being true to your calling requires a strong conviction, and a willingness to forsake "good" uses of your time to focus on "best" uses of your time. Doing so requires courage, and confidence that the choices you're making will ultimately be the best – for you and those you're called to serve.

> "Courage does not always roar. Sometimes, it is the quiet voice at the end of the day saying, 'I will try again tomorrow.'"
>
> Successories

Another physician who exhibits passion and courage in the service of her patients and colleagues is Alma Littles, MD. For her, physician leadership is mostly about advocacy – seeing changes that need to be made, and then being willing to bring the changes about.

Insights from Alma Littles, MD

"For me, physician leadership is all about serving as an advocate for patients – helping my patients access quality healthcare. As a practicing physician, I found myself in a position of responsibility, and I realized my patients were looking to me for help in more ways than just treating their medical problems. Many patients don't know how to navigate the health-care system. They need someone to assist them – to be their advocate.

I received my undergraduate and graduate education from the University of Florida in Gainesville. I'd grown up in Quincy, Florida – a small rural town in northern Florida with a population of around 8000. My parents both worked in tobacco farming – neither finished high school. My father died when I was 14 years old. Mom had raised 10 children to adulthood (two others died in infancy) I was the youngest, and the only one to go to college. Many of my brothers and sisters had the ability to be college graduates, but resources weren't available. Instead they all rallied to ensure I made it through successfully.

I completed my Family Medicine residency at Tallahassee Memorial Hospital, which is only about 22 miles from Quincy. I served as Chief Resident there – which was a natural for me, because of my active leadership roles in medical school, where I served as President of the minority student group and also became involved in the American Academy of Family Physicians at the national and state level. Through my volunteer leadership role in the Family Medicine Interest Group as a student, I learned about the specialty and about advocating for my peers.

As Chief Resident, I was an advocate for other residents – ensuring an appropriate allocation of vacation time and consistency in scheduling. I also helped residents have more input into the curriculum through several initiatives that were ultimately adopted by the faculty.

The people-oriented nature of Family Medicine was a great fit for me. Having grown up in a large family, I'd seen how one person's illness affects others in the family. What I do today I could see even way back then.

Continued

I returned to my native Quincy and started a solo private practice where I worked for five years. During that time, I had to force issues on behalf of my patients, so I appeared before legislative committees at the state capitol in Tallahassee to help legislators see how decisions they made would impact patients on a day-to-day basis. I also led and participated in committees within the community that focused on public health issues, and within the local hospital, where staff committees dealt with policies and procedures that impacted patients.

I enjoyed my involvement with colleagues. Networking gave me a platform to speak from a global view on behalf of physicians across the state, sometimes even across the country. Opportunities for participation were presented to me by my medical specialty society and I eagerly jumped at them.

I've always been a 'teacher' of sorts. Certainly, my role as Chief Resident involved a great deal of teaching. I also served as a preceptor for residents while working in private practice. It was a natural next step to join the faculty of the residency program, which I did in 1996. I became Director of the Residency Program in 1999 and fulfilled those responsibilities until 2002 when I joined the College of Medicine at **Florida State University**. Ours was the first new medical school to be launched in 20 years. Our first class began in 2001, for graduation in 2005.

My initial appointment in early 2002 was as Chair of the Department, but just six months later I was appointed Associate Dean for Academic Affairs. This position has oversight of the entire four-year curriculum, which involves many responsibilities such as ensuring adequate faculty to carry out the curricular goals, and evaluating course content and delivery. Our program follows a distributive model – students spend their first two years at the Florida State campus in Tallahassee, then their third and fourth years in regional programs – in Pensacola, Orlando, Tallahassee and Sarasota. There is a great deal of coordination involved in carrying out our curriculum. A big part of my focus is moving the program from provisional to full accreditation.

I miss patient care, and am working on developing a preceptorship forum for myself and other faculty who wish to remain active in medical practice.

I am fortunate to have a wonderfully supportive husband. He has given much to help me achieve success in my career. That helps a lot. I also have an 11–year-old son who brings perspective about who I am – his Mom – and how I should set my priorities.

Leadership brings with it certain responsibilities. Physician leaders must continually seek opportunities to enhance our skills. It's hard to lead if we are falling behind the curve. I have had several particularly rewarding experiences to continue my professional growth; one was a fellowship in faculty development at the University of North Carolina – Chapel Hill and another was a fellowship with the National Institute of Program Directors. Even if you aren't able to do a fellowship, find a way to keep learning and growing though the many resources that are available these days."

Alma Littles, MD
Associate Dean of Academic Affairs,
Department of Family Medicine and Rural Health
Florida State University

As Dr. Littles pragmatically points out, "The issues that need to be dealt with are usually easy to see. What's needed are people who are willing to do something about the issues – people who won't accept things the way they are."

What issues do you see that need to be addressed? If you're unsure, spend a few minutes contemplating what annoys you. Often, those matters that make us angry or restless are matters we want or need to tackle. Recognizing them for what they represent is an important early step. Having the energy, willpower or resolve to do something about them is important as well.

> "[Good leaders] always ask questions of others and themselves. In search of these answers there is a persistence and tenacity that will not stop when others may quit."
>
> Penny Tenzer, MD
> Vice Chair, Department of Family Medicine and Community Health
> Director, Family Medicine Residency Program
> University of Miami School of Medicine

Points to Ponder

---

1 How can you help those you lead learn to be concurrently resilient (persevering) and flexible (adapting) so they don't succumb to excessive stress and, ultimately, burnout?
2 What are you willing to give up in order to become a more effective physician leader?
3 Reflect back on some of the major changes you've initiated or been faced with in your professional life or preparation for your vocation. What do you plan to do differently next time you face similar changes?
4 What habits are you entrenched in so extensively that if you were to change them, could significantly enhance the effectiveness and fulfillment you experience in your work?

Don't Accept the Status Quo

At this point, let's presume, shall we, that you've made up your mind to invest some of your time and energy, perhaps also your money, into developing or enhancing your effectiveness as a physician leader. One decision down, lots of choices still to go. How will you create a professional path that truly reflects your passions and purpose? What contributions to healthcare do you want to make? What competencies do you need in order to make those contributions? Who will you lead? What will you lead them to do? What will be different (better) as a result of your leadership?

> "Leaders are never satisfied by the status quo ... they are always looking to improve, continually striving for excellence."
>
> Mark H. Belfer, DO, FAAFP
> Family Physician
> Residency Program Director
> Akron General Medical Center/NEOUCOM

Balance and Perspective

Ironically, when we are most committed to demonstrating excellence in our work – be it clinical excellence or technical expertise, organizational effectiveness or individual results – we are often most challenged to maintain balance and perspective. The passion and fervor with which excellence is pursued often makes it seem unnatural to set aside time for renewal, relaxation, revitalization, even re-training. Physicians who lead clinical excellence in their field make it a priority to ensure that the clinicians they're leading invest time and energy in re-training and renewal.

> "One of the symptoms of an approaching nervous breakdown is the belief that one's work is terribly important."
>
> Bertrand Russell

Points to Ponder

1 What planning competencies can you apply to help others achieve their goals?
2 In what ways can you help others set goals that are concurrently challenging and achievable?
3 What ground rules have you conveyed to those you seek to lead? What else could you convey that would benefit those you work with?
4 What exactly are you doing to help people plan their careers and set their goals in order to optimally align their activities with their individual values and priorities?
5 How can you help others persevere in some aspects and adapt in other aspects of their work?

References and Further Reading

Austin C.J. and Boxerman S.B. (2003) *Information Systems for Healthcare Management.* Chicago: Health Administration Press.

Berwick D.M. (2003) Disseminating innovations in health care. *The Journal of the American Medical Association* **289**: 1969–75.

Bowe C.M., Lahey L., Armstrong E., and Kegan R. (2001) Questioning the "big assumptions" Part I: Addressing personal contradictions that impede professional development. *Medical Education* 37: 715–22.

Bowe C.M., Lahey L., Armstrong E., and Kegan R. (2001) Questioning the "big assumptions" Part II: Recognizing organizational contradictions that impede institutional change. *Medical Education* 37: 723–33.

Christensen C. (1997) *The Innovator's Dilemma.* Boston: Harvard Business School Press.

Ferlie E., Fitzgerald L., Wood M., and Hawkins C. (2001) *The Diffusion of Innovation in Health Care: The impact of professionals.* Paper presented at the Academy of Management Annual Congress. August 2001.

Gelmon S. and Mickevicius V. (1984) Do physicians manage? A perspective on physician-managers in teaching hospitals. *Health Management Forum* 5(4): 55–65.

Laschinger H.K.S., Finegan J., Shamian J., and Wilk P. (2003) Workplace empowerment as a predictor of nurse burnout in restructured healthcare settings. *Longwoods Review* 1(3): 2–11.

Maguire P. (2001) Five strategies for physicians to overcome burnout. *ACP-ASIM Observer* March 2001 online at www.acponline.org.

Pugno P.A. (1981) Psychologic stresses encountered by resident physicians. *Family Medicine* 13(1): 9–12.

Schneller E., Greenwald H., Richardson M., and Orr J. (1997) The physician executive: Role in the adaptation of American medicine. *Health Care Management Review* 22(2): 90–6.

Shelton C. (1999) *Quantum Leaps: seven skills for workplace recreation*. Boston: Butterworth-Heinemann.

Swenson R.A. (2002) *Margin: the overload syndrome*. Colorado Springs: NavPress.

Swenson R.A. (1999) *Restoring Margin to Overloaded Lives*. Colorado Springs: NavPress.

Tabenkin H., Zyzanski S.J., and Alemagno S.A. (1989) Physician managers: Personal characteristics versus institutional demands. *Health Care Management Review* 14(2): 7–12.

Section IV

Becoming a Compelling Physician Leader

"How do physicians develop leadership effectiveness? Some physicians are born with natural gifts that enable them to get about the daily grind. They're fundamentally optimistic, often somewhat manic in the pursuit of their passions. They're able to think from a systems perspective, to get beyond 'me' and 'now.'

Many of the same attributes that drove them to become physicians can help them become effective leaders. Remarkable physician

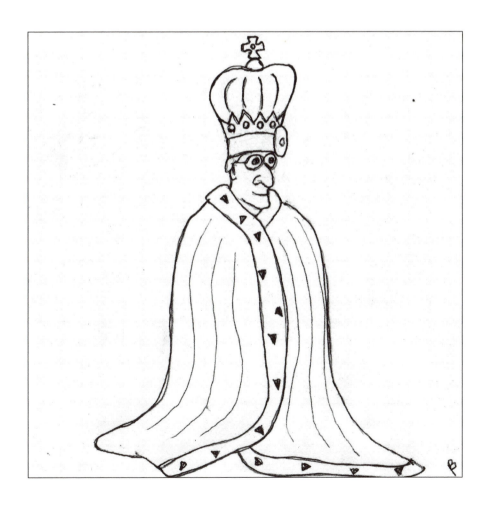

leaders care about the healthcare system and what happens to it and care about patients. Remarkable physician leaders leverage their unique insider's knowledge of what is wrong with healthcare in ways that help to transform it."

J. Peter Geerlofs, MD
Family Physician
Chief Medical Officer, Allscripts Healthcare Solutions, Inc.

A Challenging Journey

Suppose the pursuit of your life's vocation requires you to hop into a sporty little convertible for a drive down a long winding road on the journey toward the pursuit and attainment of your professional goals. You are excited to get started, anticipating an enjoyable, straightforward excursion. After all, you're bright, you're well-educated, your driving skills are impeccable.

Not long after you've set out on this journey you encounter several clues that your trip won't proceed as you'd planned. The road signs, you notice with a tinge of concern, are written in a foreign language – they're meaningless, entirely useless to you. Oh, you can recognize the fact that they're signaling danger – but you're unable to decode their messages and thus avoid the risks that lie ahead. To make matters worse, you quickly begin encountering many unexpected bends and bumps in the road. The bends and bumps are slowing you down, sometimes nearly causing you to veer off what is becoming an increasingly narrow, ever more winding path.

Pulled over for traffic violations you didn't even realize you'd committed, you realize that things are fast going from bad to worse. You unwisely waste precious time and energy railing against the law enforcement officials who are, after all, simply carrying out their orders. It seems you've forgotten, or perhaps don't really care, that they, too, have families to feed.

You can't help but wonder why you ever undertook such a foolhardy journey in the first place. Certainly there were easier, better paths you could have taken to "get ahead." Oh well, you're invested now. Too late to turn back – what would everyone say? Besides, you know for a fact that you aren't the only one experiencing unexpected difficulties. Other drivers, similarly anxious and tired, stressed and depressed are all around you. In fact, at times it seems they may run you right off the road.

By now, the sun has begun to set; the elements have become frightening and downright formidable. With the top down on your sporty little car, rain begins pelting you in the face. It doesn't take long before you're terribly cold and thoroughly drenched. What will you do? Drive faster, of course, in an understandable although futile effort to outrun the storm. Others have sought an exit ramp to find shelter from the storm. But not you; you're driven (literally) to stick it out. After all, you're smart, tenacious, and let's face it – a bit headstrong.

No longer certain you're even on the right course, anxiety flashes. You wonder whether your original goal is even still within reach. Your vision, once so alluring and clear, has been all but obscured by filters of fog and distractions of darkness. You'd like to consult a map, but don't believe you can afford the time. Besides, this road is so bad you can't imagine anyone else has ever gone down this path before. Sure, you have a dashboard, but it is so cluttered and complex, you couldn't possibly discern which gauges are most deserving of your attention.

By now, you know you need help, but you can't hear a thing – so who could you turn to for assistance? Sure, a radio is available, but you're hurtling along at such a frantic pace, you couldn't possibly take the time to dial in for a news and weather update. Windshield wipers would help – but they were one of many items sacrificed in your expense-reduction program. Gone, too, are the turn signals and horn – not just yours, but also those of everyone around you. It seems no one is prepared to signal a change in direction, or to forewarn others of impending disaster. How could someone as smart as you have let themselves become so vulnerable?

"Faster, faster," you think to yourself. Forget any notions of enjoying the trip. In fact, forget about reaching the original destination. At this point, you're fighting to survive against a formidable and unforgiving environment. You're hoping against hope that by keeping your head down, by refusing to give in or give up, you'll somehow survive – shaken, perhaps, but intact. As you continue hurtling down the road at record-breaking speed you realize this journey – what once began as a desirable journey – has become, without a doubt, your worst nightmare.

"Oh come on," you may be thinking as you read this. "Anyone with half a brain would know to pull over, look at a map, refocus their thoughts, turn on the radio to hear the forecast." Right. Unfortunately, you probably know physicians who've found themselves on just such a journey. Too seldom are physicians willing or able to "pull over," collect their thoughts, and come up with a plan to more effectively (and enjoyably) proceed on the difficult journey.

Reimbursement rates are declining, expenses continue to rise, labor market shortages are yielding too few workers with too few skills, and ever-more-burdensome legislation is enacted. The practice of medicine continues to evolve – it has gone from being an art, to a science, to a business, to a crime. Clearly, the path of the physician has become tougher than you could have imagined.

Can you relate? Then perhaps it's time to pull out of the fast lane, look at a road map and turn your radio to the news or the weather forecast. Will you take a few moments to clear your vision and collect your thoughts before resuming your journey? Who knows – you may find ways to make your trip more enjoyable. Or you may decide to take a different road altogether, or to pursue an entirely different destination.

> "Conviction is worthless unless it is converted into conduct."
>
> Thomas Carlyle

Prepare to Address Challenges

As Dr. McPherson points out, you have the essential prerequisite for becoming a compelling leader – because you know intuitively what people want from those whose lead they would follow. That's a good place to start.

> "The notions and terminology associated with 'physician leadership'
> may be unfamiliar to most physicians. But all of us are clear about

what we want from those whose lead we are willing to follow. Consider what you want from those whose lead you would follow, and be that kind of leader for others."

Deborah S. McPherson, MD, FAAFP

Family Physician

Associate Director, Family Medicine Residency Program

Kansas University Medical Center

Leadership advice for early-career physicians

"A great Hebrew sage once asked the following three questions: 'If I am not for myself, who will be for me? If I am only for myself, what am I? And if not now, when?' These three questions have tremendous implications for leaders.

All leaders realize they must accomplish difficult tasks. People often get to positions of leadership by using their personal charisma and energy to achieve their own goals. They therefore advocate for themselves. But clearly leaders cannot focus on what is good only for themselves; they must have the concerns of their organization in their hearts at all times. So leaders must go beyond self-serving interests to serve the needs of those around them. And finally, great leaders understand that 'timing is everything.' Successful leaders do not run from making decisions, but rather they know that making a bad decision (and taking responsibility for it) is often better than making no decision at all. So leaders learn to deal with problems 'now.'

Being a leader, in medicine or anywhere in life, is a great challenge. Being the leader of a successful organization, however, is one of the most rewarding experiences one can imagine."

Kevin Scott Ferentz, MD

Family Physician

Residency Director and Associate Professor

University of Maryland School of Medicine

Work well with others, and accomplish results

Leading physicians is tough, complicated, messy, heart-wrenching work. Don't let the challenges cause you to become scared or cynical. Do take heed, and build for yourself a strong foundation so you're equipped to avoid or overcome the pitfalls you'll encounter. Why? Because anyone who is serious about being an effective leader will inevitably encounter challenges. Such is the life of a leader.

"What advice would I give physicians who aspire to be compelling leaders? Figure out what gets people out of the gate, be seen as a 'good guy' – friendly, fun, enthusiastic. Great leaders are those who volunteer or say 'yes' to the challenges – not whiners. Leaders are good-natured people. They're team players. They say 'Yes, I'll work on that with you.' My advice is to be someone who gets things done. Follow through. Accomplish results. Credibility is earned by being fun, reliable, trustworthy, getting things done and then building momentum. Solicit advice, listen to people. Be willing to modify your views."

David G. Fairchild, MD, MPH
Internist and Chief of General Medicine
Tufts – New England Medical Center

Points to Ponder

1 Can you think of instances in which you've relied excessively on your intellect or sheer effort, versus seeking the expertise and assistance of others? What can you learn from the results of those choices? What steps can you take to make better choices in the future?

2 Are you ever distracted by a natural human urge for prestige or power, for fame or fortune? Has the pursuit of money or the adherence to ideology ever impaired your effectiveness as a physician leader?

3 Have ego, arrogance, intellectual superiority, self-righteous indignation, or stubbornness ever limited your effectiveness as a leader? We're all human, and as such, experience the foibles of our humanity. Which particular dysfunctions must you guard against so you don't jeopardize the trust and respect of those you seek to lead?

4 Have you ever found yourself in a compromised situation due to conflicts of interest or competing obligations? Have you felt unable to move forward due to loyalty to an individual or group? If so, what were the "best practices" you used to address the situation?

5 What pitfalls are faced by those you aspire to lead? What are you doing – we mean actively saying, deciding, or taking action – to help them overcome the pitfalls they're likely to encounter?

Chapter 15

Being a Leader: Reflection, Self-awareness, Focus, and Goals

"I have no idea whether leaders are made or born. I'm sure circumstances may awaken latent leadership qualities. We all know physicians who seem to have been born with natural gifts that enable them to get beyond the daily grind and focus on solutions rather than complaining about the problems. I believe a critical characteristic to look for is unbridled optimism and the ability to never feel like a victim. Leadership is all about having a clear vision and the certainty that one step at a time, that vision can be obtained."

J. Peter Geerlofs, MD
Family Physician
Chief Medical Officer
Allscripts Healthcare Solutions, Inc.

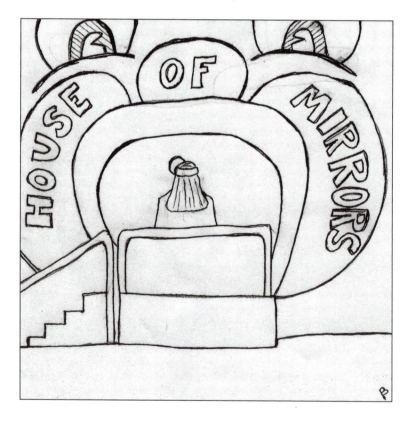

"The phrase 'I didn't learn that in medical school' has been exclaimed countless times, by nearly every physician who has ever gone into practice – or assumed a leadership role of some sort."

Perry A. Pugno, MD, MPH, CPE
Family Physician
Director, Medical Education
American Academy of Family Physicians

Gaining Awareness – of Yourself and Others

"After residency I was a flight surgeon in a rare Family Practice assignment and had the most fun a physician could have. I took care of an aviation population whose vested interest was to stay healthy so they could fly. I took care of pilots and support staff, delivered their babies and flew missions with them – some of them in the front seat. That experience taught me humility in that physicians are not the only highly skilled professionals on active duty and that delivering a baby in the middle of the night was a lot easier that hovering a helicopter. After my aviation tour I returned to the hospital as residency faculty and was mentored by a handful of family physicians who would later become national figures in our specialty and the Army. I learned more by listening than talking."

John R. Bucholtz, DO
Family Physician
U.S. Armed Services

Why do *you* want to be a physician leader? What choices do you need to make? Here are a framework and some considerations for deciding. First, determine whether your goals and aspirations involve clinical excellence (patient care), organizational excellence (practice management), reform (advocacy and activism), or innovation (discovery, invention or dissemination of innovation). Next, determine the constituency you intend to impact (e.g., the community, your professional organization, legislators and policy-makers, or the educational system). You'll then need to consider your preferences – what skills and knowledge do you wish to gain, how do you like to learn and develop, when is the optimal timing for you to fit it into your schedule.

"The average person thinks he isn't."

Father Larry Lorenzoni

Consider your constraints. How much time, money and energy do you have to invest in your development as a physician leader? What other priorities are also competing for your time and attention?

"We can't put our faults behind us until we face them."

Unknown

Marketing Yourself

We realize that many physicians have traditionally scorned marketing as unprofessional and self-promoting. Too often, it is seen as a means of generating additional income by making promises – sometimes unfounded ones. It seems the disdain for marketing may stem from a misconception of its purpose. Marketing is simply the means by which one aligns the needs and wants of a market (people who share similar characteristics or interests) with the products and services of an organization. It isn't just about advertising – in fact, that's only a very tiny tactic in the spectrum of activities involved in good marketing.

Market Research

Long before any advertising is done several decisions must be made and actions must be taken. You begin by conducting market research to profile the potential customers (prospects) whose needs/wants you might serve. This includes not only the patients, and their guardians or caregivers, but also the decision makers and gatekeepers who can facilitate or block their awareness of and preference for your services. Employers, health plans, and affiliated providers are what marketers call "stakeholders" – people or organizations who may significantly impact or be impacted by the services you provide. Market research also involves the analysis of the competitive alternatives. This includes not only those physicians who provide directly comparable services, but anyone else who offers what your "customer" might perceive to be a competitive alternative. For example, chiropractors are well served by considering as competitive alternatives such services as massage therapy and yoga classes and any other optional investment of time and money that patients might choose rather than seeking chiropractic services.

Market Segmentation

For optimal success – which in most businesses includes notions of profitability, competitive advantage, growth rate, and so on – it is important to clearly segment your market so that you don't offer too many services to address too many needs for too many types of people. Targeting certain market segments that best align with your organization's competencies and goals makes it far more feasible to continuously enhance the mix of services you provide and thus optimally meet the needs of those you serve. Primary care physicians may wish to target within a geographic area certain patient populations and the health plans who determine reimbursement for their services. Some may also target the benefits managers that work for large local employers, as those individuals can suggest medical practices to patients seeking care.

Subspecialists should consider primary care practices as a target market because those groups are in a position to send patients to you – or to your "competitors." Practices seeking rapid growth may target other "feeder channels" as well. For example, many orthopedic groups now market to sports team coaches; dermatologists, and cosmetic surgeons often market to beauty salons. Though we aren't aware of any ob/gyn practices marketing to and through maternity clothing or baby supply stores, we do know the marketing departments of hospitals with large maternity wards now offer email baby announcement services (with convenient online links to purchase gifts for newborns through the hospital gift shop). Preposterous? Hardly. New parents are delighted by the convenience of "one-stop shopping" during the overwhelming, albeit joyous, birth of their child.

Why target specific market segments? Doing so enables you to focus your advertising expenditures to reach the people for whom your services are most relevant. Who in healthcare doesn't welcome ways of increasing the beneficial impact of your expenditures?

Have a Clear Value Proposition (Brand Advantage)

Another important marketing concept involves branding. Once you've conducted market research and selected which target markets to focus on, you'll need to have a compelling message to share – a reason for them to choose your services versus those of some other practice. To do this, you'll need to have a powerful and clear value proposition – a compelling reason why people (patients, health plans, or anyone involved in the choice of providers) will choose your services rather than someone else's. What can you offer patients that is better than what they can expect elsewhere? Marketers refer to this as your sustainable, differentiated competitive advantage. In the business world, competitive advantage usually stems from offering the most innovative or highest quality product or service, the most personalized and responsive relationship and support, or the best value – not necessarily the cheapest, but the best value for the price. In most fields, prices aren't regulated as they are in healthcare with government or third-party reimbursement rates. So organizations that differentiate themselves with a competitive advantage based on "value" usually invest higher than average amounts in technology or equipment to streamline operational efficiency and thus keep prices low.

Competitive positioning has been a foreign concept to most healthcare professionals, for several reasons. The professional oath to serve the infirm has been difficult to reconcile with notions of for-profit enterprise. The idea of claiming your services are "better" than those of your colleagues has not aligned well with notions of professional collegiality. The fact that reimbursement rates are set by forces outside the providers' control have served as a disincentive to invest in efficiency-enhancing technology – why invest more than your "competitors" when you can't recoup that investment through price increases, even if those investments result in improvements that are beneficial for your patients?

"Satisfaction" Versus "Loyalty"

Another marketing concept involves the measurement and enhancement of customer satisfaction and loyalty. First, let's clarify both terms, because while customer satisfaction is a good thing and thus we strive to achieve it, satisfaction can be sometimes overrated in terms of its actual benefit. Here's what we mean. Suppose you're satisfied with the meal you had at Restaurant X. You may also be satisfied with meals from Restaurant Y and Restaurant Z. So next time you go out to eat, you may or may not return to Restaurant X, despite your satisfaction with it. On the other hand, "customer loyalty" is the strength of the customer's commitment to select one company's products or services rather than any other company's. Consider an organization to which you are highly loyal – perhaps a local bookstore, a fitness center, or a clothing store. You would leap tall buildings (translate: drive across town) for the products, or services, or that shopping experience. You're convinced it is so much better than any other alternative.

Now ask yourself the tough question – how loyal are your patients, or those who control their choice of provider, to your services, your organization? If they aren't as loyal as you'd like, or you don't know how loyal they are, beware. To reduce the risk of losing those relationships, you need to increase their loyalty level.

Pick Your Focus

The key to having a sustainable, differentiated competitive advantage – an advantage so meaningful that it ensures strong loyalty – is mostly a matter of focus. You see, middle-of-the-road, not-particularly-compelling service providers often make the mistake of trying to offer competitive advantage in all three areas – quality or innovation (e.g., the best place in town for X healthcare procedure) *and* customized service (e.g., the entire staff knows every patient's name, and their hobbies and interests) *and* best value – which, granted, applies more to free market environments than to healthcare with its reimbursement regulations and the professional obligations of medical necessity.

No organization can be equally strong in every aspect. Believe us (and the many experts who've researched this extensively) – it simply cannot be done. There simply isn't enough time, energy, or money in the world to "be all things to all people." That's why Wal-Mart invests millions to offer customers the best price/value; 3M holds firm to a number of policies and procedures that ensure it continues to earn its reputation for inventing a steady stream of "coolest stuff;" and Saturn makes cars that are simply "OK," but then sells and repairs them with truly extraordinary customer service.

Brand Positioning

Once you're clear about your value proposition, the next step is to develop very clear brand positioning. Your brand is not your logo (e.g., Nike's swoosh sign), or promotional "tag line" (e.g., "we bring good things to life"). Your brand is your promise to your customers. Amazon pledges to be the world's largest and most trustworthy online bookstore. Starbucks positions itself as the world's greatest coffee shop. Disney offers the world's best family entertainment. You get the picture.

(Pause for a moment to consider the "brand" attributes you associate with the leading healthcare providers in your town or country. Which physicians, medical groups, and hospitals are distinctively known for something? What is that "something?" How do you suppose they developed that brand positioning?)

Marketing Communication Tactics

Have you identified one or a few target market segments that align with your competitively advantageous services, defined your value proposition, and determined your brand positioning? Now, finally, you are ready to consider the marketing communication tactics (messages and venues) that will best serve your purposes in letting people know your services are available and ideal for them. There are four key marketing communication tactics in business. First is advertising.

Advertising

You advertise when you pay someone to convey your marketing message by embedding it into printed publications, websites, radio or TV programs, or disseminating it as a stand-alone message via the postal service (direct mail) or online (email campaigns). Advertising can be used to build awareness – simply letting people know your practice exists, or informing them of new services you offer. It can also be used to change or enhance people's understanding of your services, say to dispel misconceptions or to compare your outcomes relative to your competitor's.

Promotions

Advertising can also be used in conjunction with promotions – which are time-specific offers or events that are designed to spike purchases of your services. In the retail world, we think of promotions as buy one, get one free or buy this, get that, or buy this at X dollars or X percent less than the usual price. In health-care, promotions are appropriate only for services that are elective (for ethical reasons) and high margin (for economic reasons). Some innovative practices encourage patients to schedule annual check-ups by offering discounts on massage, facials, vitamins, or various exercise, nutrition, health, or beauty aids. Not to confuse you, but the word "promotion" has a broader connotation as well. Most organizations, including medical practices, invest some amount of money in the creation and production of collateral – a big word for the materials used in the promotion of your work. Printed promotional materials range from business cards to simple fliers and full-scale brochures. Some organizations even produce videos or CD-ROMs to promote awareness of or demand for their services among the public or the healthcare community.

Publicity

A third marketing communication tactic often used in business is publicity, also sometimes referred to as "public relations." Publicity differs from advertising in that the dissemination of news about your services is more or less free – someone else is "telling your story," perhaps because what you're doing is so innovative, or because of its interest and benefit to the community. And, of course, free is good. But if you're alert while reading this, you noticed that we said "more or less" free. You see, the dissemination of publicity – placement in a publication, or air time on radio or TV – is actually free. And because the costs of advertising in those media can be considerable, the economics of publicity can be quite appealing. But odds are you'll have to invest some time, and perhaps money as well, to get the media to notice you. Thus the term "public relations." Large medical associations often invest in public relations on a large scale – paying salaries of lobbyists or hiring consultants to conduct image campaigns. Typically, medical practices don't think much about publicity, though proactive groups may issue press releases announcing the addition of a new physician, expanded office hours, or the launch of a newly available service. Some even host press conferences, inviting members of the media to hear news of your work and to answer their questions. Such events don't need to be terribly costly, but will require some time and effort to arrange.

The "ABCD" of Marketing

By now, you realize that advertising is just one tiny piece of marketing. And you no doubt understand why it is much easier to decide which media (print or mass communication channels) you'll advertise in, how and when you'll promote your services, *after* your strategic foundation is clearly defined. You may find our ABCD acronym helpful as a way of remembering the basic steps in marketing communications. In order for someone to use your services, you must first create **Awareness** among your target market, so they know your organization exists and the services you provide. You'll need them to be convinced of the **Benefits** such services represent for them. This is particularly tough for patients whose medical conditions are chronic yet asymptomatic – such as hypertension. Getting those patients to recognize the importance of regularly scheduled check-ups can be challenging. Once they appreciate the need for the type of services you offer, you must convince them of the **Competitive advantages** your practice offers – why they'll be better off seeing you than someone else, or pursuing the procedures and treatments you offer rather than some alternative that may be less advantageous for their health. Finally, you'll need to create a sense of urgency or **Demand** for the service. Not only do you want them to think "One day when I get around to it, I'll schedule an appointment with you." That's not in their interest or yours, if the services you provide are in fact beneficial for their health.

An Example of the Marketing ABCDs

Let's look at a consumer product example to be sure we're clear about the marketing ABCDs. Suppose you want to market DVDs. You'd need folks in your target market to be *Aware* of DVDs – what they are (features) and what they can do (benefits). But you can't stop there. You'd want them to be convinced of the *Benefits* of DVDs – the relevance for them personally. The product must satisfy an unmet need, or be different from or better than anything they already have. You also want them to believe that your DVDs are better – more Competitive – than anybody else's DVDs. And last, but most importantly, you want to increase Demand for those DVDs – so people will get up out of their recliner and make the purchase today!

Final Thoughts

We realize many physicians provide services that are truly medically necessary, and may not find these marketing notions fit well with your practice. We readily acknowledge that these concepts are most applicable for the marketing of elective services such as lifestyle-enhancing, wellness and prevention, or anti-aging procedures. We also respectfully point out that such procedures and products are an ever-growing portion of what often falls under the broadly defined category of "healthcare" in contemporary society. As healthcare continues to become more "consumer-driven," an increasing number of physicians are offering optional and complementary products and services instead of, or in addition to, the traditionally recognized medically necessary procedures and services.

Marketing is About the Planning, not the Plan

A final important point about marketing. Despite what you may read or hear, the magic of marketing is *not* in marketing plans, but in the planning process itself. Decisions are made so actions will be taken, not as a result of a document, but because of insights gained through the thinking and discussing and debating and concluding what your assumptions and priorities and intended results are. Realizing that marketing is about aligning the needs or wants of your market with the services you provide, you can understand why it is such an important function for anyone who is committed to serving patients' needs.

Gaining Clarity

"All of us are 'brainwashed' in that we've adopted a view of the world that seems true and natural to use. We fail to see our own conditioning and cultural indoctrination. There is a paradox here in that we are most fulfilled when we strive for the truth and reality. However, there is not a single or true reality. Each of us creates our own reality.

We must ask ourselves: 'What am I doing? Does it work? Do the results reflect my intent? Is it meeting my needs?' In the end, this is really about asking, 'What meets the common good? If this doesn't, then what would?' We need to be willing to step back, throw out all our assumptions, and take a fresh look.

Culturally, most physicians have a tremendous victim mentality. That's what creates a lot of the craziness in medicine. We need leaders to help us get out of that mindset. We are in charge of our well-being and our life's experience.

My advice to aspiring physician leaders is this: stop right where you are now, step back a minute, and ask yourself 'How can I be better or more effective? How can I raise the bar?' Creativity comes into it – being able to look at your situation without being frustrated and simply ask what does and does not work. Is there a way of doing it better? We need to re-engineer our processes. We need skill in change management. We need to apply evidence to our personal lives and our profession. We need to take a dose of our own medicine.

Why are some docs fulfilled in their work while others are stressed out and resentful? It is all about boundaries. Physicians as a group generally don't have clear boundaries or understand what their true realm of influence is. I don't stress out over things that I cannot control. People who are optimistic, happy, satisfied have clear boundaries about what they can and cannot influence. **Dr. Covey** calls it our 'sphere of influence.' That description is basically another way of explaining the Serenity Prayer – 'God grant me the serenity to accept the things I cannot change, courage to change the things I can, and wisdom to know the difference.'"

Randall Oates, MD
Family Physician
Founder and President, Docs, Inc.

Investing Time and Energy

In his widely acclaimed book *The Seven Habits of Highly Effective People*, Stephen Covey, PhD tells the story of the man who was too busy chopping down trees to stop for a moment and sharpen his saw. We easily see the humor in Dr. Covey's analogy, perhaps because we realize the applicability of this in our own life's work. Realizing the need for skill improvement is just the beginning step. To enhance our skills we must continuously commit to seek training and to practice. Such training and practice may unfortunately require somewhat substantial investments of time or money, both of which are in scarce supply within most hospitals, clinics and medical practices.

"Virtually anyone in medical school was at the top of his undergraduate class. Obviously, 50 percent find themselves in the bottom half of their medical school class. That reality can be very hard on people who sincerely want to use their talents. But leadership skills are not restricted to one's rank in class. To advance in the field of medicine, leadership skills have to be developed."

Monte L. Anderson, MD
Gastroenterologist and Hepatologist
Mayo Clinic Scottsdale

Gaining Perspective

"Want to gain perspective? Walk through a nursing home. You'll see people living with strangers, often sharing a room with someone they hardly know, with a chest of drawers and a wall to look at all day long. What's on that wall? Not their diplomas or their stock certificates. What people put on that wall is photos of family, hand-drawn pictures from their grandchildren or great-grandchildren, perhaps on occasion a medal of honor for having served their country.

Mother Teresa used to say 'We're not called to success, we're called to faithfulness.' She understood that the important thing isn't success in the way the world judges success. The important thing is being true to who God has called us to be.

So each of us must decide – 'What am I going to do with what I have?' All of us can do something. What's important is that we do what we can. Is leadership about doing things? It's about doing the right thing. And that's about being who you were made to be. Universal principles transcend culture and time if they're true and right. They may be implemented and expressed differently, that's all.

My advice to those who aspire to be leaders is this: Do what you can with the gifts you have, and do things for the right reasons. Don't take yourself too seriously. Don't lose sight of who you are, and what life is all about."

Gary Morsch, MD
Family and Emergency Medicine Physician,
U.S. Army Reserves
Founder, Heart to Heart International

Be True to Yourself

"My advice for physicians who aspire to be great leaders? Be true to who you are. My model will not work for everyone. Some doctors find physical medicine and rehabilitation too slow, they prefer not to deal with the chronicity of conditions we treat in this field. We have different interests and passions, different goals and aspirations. Yet all doctors, regardless of specialty, can benefit by learning to listen more to our hearts than our heads."

Reverend Pamela S. Harris, MD
Physical Medicine and Rehabilitation Physician
Kansas City Veteran's Administration Hospital
Minister of Health, United Methodist Church of the Resurrection

Admit Mistakes and Learn From Them

"I don't chart a course for the next five years, or do formal long range planning. I do, however, reflect on what I've accomplished (and what I haven't) as well as what I've learned. For example, reflecting on the email guidelines I've disseminated, I appreciate the impact they are having. Reflecting on the website I created about electronic communication in patient care, turned out to be, I believe, a good move. On the other hand, I regret not having spent more time writing.

I learn from my mistakes. I've come to realize that I'm not very deferential. I'm frank with people. I say, 'This isn't working well, can we talk about how it can be better?' I make it a habit to be positive.

Some people are sourpusses constitutionally. They have to work especially hard because nobody likes a sourpuss or downer.

You asked about mistakes I've made. Years ago, I sent an open letter to our CIO, pointing out that he was a scoundrel and a liar (not my exact words) for diverting promised resources from a patient safety initiative in IT. I later regretted doing that, because it was not politically savvy. I should have said those comments face to face (I had, but apparently not strongly enough), or in a private letter; sending the open letter was not the right thing to do. It was a rookie move that came from inexperience."

Daniel Z. Sands, MD, MPH
Internist, Faculty, Harvard Medical School
Chief Medical Officer and Vice President, Clinical Strategies
Zix Corporation

Points to Ponder

1 How can comparing ourselves to others impede our likelihood of fulfilling our own unique capacity for contributions in healthcare?
2 With whom do you compare yourself?
3 How does comparing yourself to others help or hinder your progress toward becoming a more successful physician leader?
4 What awareness – of self or others – do those you lead need to further develop?
5 In what ways can you help them look in a mirror or look through a window in order to do so?

Design Jobs to Align With Strengths

"In order to have the time to be involved, you have to lead other people, but you also have to take care of your own time, and can't get so busy you can't take care of your family, your friends, your practice, and your patients. I have had to learn over the years that I am just not very good at certain things and one of them is narrowing down my focus. I have to pay attention when things get too complicated and everything starts going backwards.

I have read a few books on management styles, and they tend to fall into two categories. Either you are trying to make employees or coworkers fix their weaknesses, or, the philosophy I agree with, manage to strengths. I think you can get a lot more value from managing to someone's strengths than by trying to correct their weaknesses. I like to look at both employees and colleagues, and determine their strengths and what they really like to do. If they like to manage people and if they like to take on complicated tasks, you should give them more and more of that type of project to do. But you should identify early that there are some people who are better followers than leaders, and the leaders lead using different styles. If you can identify the styles and position it within your organization, I think that you can get a lot more out of people.

A management book entitled *Living Your Strengths* by Clifton and Wisenman is interesting to me. The co-authors purchased the Gallup organization several years ago and now have a tremendous database relating to the success of different management styles. Their findings really fits very closely with what I believe leaders should do: evaluate the people you work with as quickly as possible, whether formally through testing, or just from discussions to figure out what they are good at and what they are not good at. Then take those facts into consideration and manage to their strengths.

When I was looking for a key executive assistant, I was fortunate enough to hire Jean Kraushaar, who has worked with me for the last 10 years. I knew I needed someone who would complement me by helping me be more efficient. I needed to find someone who likes doing that – who was good at follow-through and good at some of the skills I lack. Then I had to match up my weaknesses with her strengths, and then we became a great team. I always jokingly said that I needed someone who would not only tell me that tomorrow is my brother's birthday, but also tell me what I got for him, because handling details like that is not one of my strengths. Jean is great at it, so matching her strengths with my weak area has really helped me.

I am fortunate to have my wife of 33 years, Anne, who also supports me in areas I am not good at. I have a partner in my office who supplies surgical skills and patient skills I don't have. It helps to round out the practice. I believe it is vital to determine what people's strengths and weaknesses are, and design their roles to leverage their strengths. This frees us up to do what we are good at."

Daniel S. Durrie, MD
Opthamalogist
Durrie Vision Center

Self-assessment

Having strong desires and clear cut aspirations are necessary but certainly not sufficient for the attainment of great physician leadership. You'll also need to take a candid inventory of your current competencies and contributions to healthcare. Assess your current effectiveness in each of the areas below by placing an X in the box that most accurately reflects your competency level at this time. Rate yourself according to your *actual* knowledge and skills, not what you would like them to be in the future.

	Highly Competent	Moderately Competent	Minimally Competent	Not At All Competent
Current competency levels:				
Clinical (diagnostic, prescriptive or procedural) skills				
Interpersonal and communication skills				
Professional ethics and social responsibility				
Ability to convey a clear, compelling vision for the future				
Ability to build coalitions of support for change				
Ability to address the needs of multiple stakeholders				
Financial acumen and resource management				
Continuous learning and improvement				
System-based decision making and problem-solving				

Find that sobering? We're not finished yet! You'll also need to assess your activity levels in several key areas of physician leadership. Rate your *current* involvement in each of the areas below by placing an X in the box that most accurately reflects the extent to which you are personally engaged in each of these activities.

	Extremely Active	Moderately Active	Minimally Active	Not At All Active
Current activity levels:				
Impacting other professionals' clinical effectiveness				
Influencing peers to adopt new approaches in medicine				
Conducting clinical research investigations				
Publishing empirical studies or conceptual articles				
Teaching in medical school, residency or CME programs				
Lobbying for policy, legislative, or regulatory changes				
Accountable for the administration of healthcare service delivery				
Volunteering within a professional society				
Discovering or inventing new advances in medicine				

"In the absence of clearly defined goals, we are forced to concentrate on activity and ultimately become enslaved by it."

Chuck Coonradt

Identify Areas To Improve

At this point, you're getting closer to having a game plan, but we still have a few steps to undertake. You must identify what areas you wish to improve, and then decide how you'll go about improving them. First, consider the types and levels of competencies that you will need in order to achieve your vision, mission and desired contributions to healthcare. Do so by completing the following statement:

Because I want to positively impact _____,
[clinical excellence, organizational excellence, medical advances or healthcare reform]
I need to be highly **competent** *in these areas* (place an X next to all that apply):

    _____ Clinical (diagnostic, prescriptive or procedural) skills
    _____ Interpersonal and communication skills
    _____ Professional ethics and social responsibility
    _____ Ability to convey a clear, compelling vision for the future
    _____ Ability to build coalitions of support for change
    _____ Ability to address the needs of multiple stakeholders
    _____ Financial acumen and resource management
    _____ Continuous learning and improvement
    _____ System-based decision making and problem-solving

I also need to be highly **active** *in these areas* (place an X next to all that apply):

    _____ Impacting other professionals' clinical effectiveness
    _____ Influencing peers to adopt new approaches in medicine
    _____ Clinical research investigations
    _____ Publication of empirical studies or conceptual articles
    _____ Teaching in medical school, residency or CME programs
    _____ Presentations for CME or non-accredited programs
    _____ Lobbying for policy, legislative or regulatory changes
    _____ Administrative responsibility in a healthcare organization
    _____ Volunteerism (e.g., leadership within a medical society)
    _____ Entrepreneurship (e.g., commercialize new medical device)

Now it's time for some "gap analysis." This means you will compare your *current* competency levels against your *needed* competencies as determined by your aspirations. Place an X next to the 1–2 items below that represent the biggest gaps between your current vs. needed competencies.

    _____ Clinical (diagnostic, prescriptive or procedural) skills
    _____ Interpersonal and communication skills
    _____ Professional ethics and social responsibility
    _____ Ability to convey a clear, compelling vision for the future
    _____ Ability to build coalitions of support for change
    _____ Ability to address the needs of multiple stakeholders
    _____ Financial acumen and resource management
    _____ Continuous learning and improvement

_____ System-based decision making and problem-solving

Next, do another "gap analysis," this time comparing your *current* activities levels against the activities that would be indicative of successful leadership contributions to healthcare in the way you aspire to make a difference. Place an X next to the 1–2 items below that represent the biggest gaps between your *current* vs. *needed* activities.

_____ Impacting other professionals' clinical effectiveness
_____ Influencing peers to adopt new approaches in medicine
_____ Clinical research investigations
_____ Publication of empirical studies or conceptual articles
_____ Teaching in medical school, residency or CME programs
_____ Presentations for CME or non-accredited programs
_____ Lobbying for policy, legislative or regulatory changes
_____ Administrative responsibility in a healthcare organization
_____ Volunteerism (e.g., leadership within a medical society)
_____ Entrepreneurship (e.g., commercialize new medical device)

Don't become discouraged, regardless of how many competencies you wish to improve, or how much change you ultimately want to make to the activities in which you're having an impact. At this point it is very important for you to accept yourself as you are today, and see the fulfillment of your vision and mission as an ongoing, lifelong journey. To bring your focus back toward a manageable list of areas to tackle over the next few months (or years), list below no more than three key areas you wish to focus on in order to improve your physician leadership effectiveness.

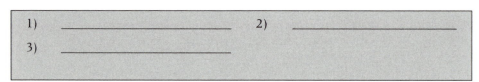

1) _____   2) _____

3) _____

Now ... armed with this information ... what are you waiting for?

Points to Ponder

1 How do your decisions and actions help those you lead achieve remarkable results?
2 What could you do more of, or less of, or do differently, in order to help them be even more effective and fulfilled in their work?
3 How can you help others learn to disagree without being disagreeable?
4 What steps could you take to help those you work with make better decisions or take more productive actions?
5 How can you help those you lead begin or complete their work on time, under budget, and with high quality?
6 How can you help others coordinate the alignment of resources and activities toward the achievement of key priorities?
7 What resources, abilities, or other means are available to you to help those you lead achieve their full potential?

References and Further Reading

Covey S.R. (1989) *The Seven Habits of Highly Effective People*. New York: Simon & Schuster Inc.

Henry R. (1988) *Roads to Medical Management: physician executives' career decisions*. Tampa: American College of Physician Executives Press.

Hirsch G. (2000) *Strategic Career Management for the 21st Century Physician*. Chicago: The American Medical Association.

Koska M.T. (1992) New approaches to developing physician leaders. *Hospitals* **66**(9): 76–8.

Linney B. (1996) *Hope for the Future: a career development guide for physician executives*. Tampa: American College of Physician Executives Press.

Lyons M.R., Ford, D., and Singer G.R. (1996) Physician leadership: How do physician executives view themselves? *Physician Executive* **22**(9): 23–6.

Tabenkin H., Zyzanski S.J., and Alemagno S.A. (1989) Physician managers: Personal characteristics versus institutional demands. *Health Care Management Review* **14**(2): 7–12.

Chapter 16

Learning About Leading: Self-study, Training Workshops, and Formal Education

"I think *Getting to Yes* is a wonderful book. It explains how to express negative opinions in a way that people won't find threatening or mean. It describes how to help people feel comfortable, not blamed. It teaches how to negotiate and express yourself.

All physicians should get some leadership training – even for running a solo office. All physicians need to lead, all physicians work with teams or groups. Even as residents, you'll lead medical service teams and have a context to learn leadership concepts and skills.

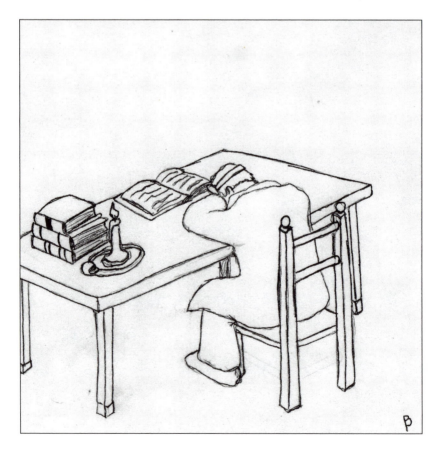

I subscribe to publications from the **American College of Physician Executives** but have never been to one of their courses. **ACPE** courses are frightfully expensive. I wish they would have an annual meeting."

David G. Fairchild, MD, MPH
Chief, Internal Medicine
Tufts – New England Medical Center

"I'm encouraged by the trend of more physicians going back to school to learn business and management skills. When physicians pair their clinical training and natural leadership aptitudes with business education, they can be a powerful force for change. However, getting a business degree doesn't necessary guarantee that a physician will be a good leader. If nothing else, it can help open doors for clinicians switching from clinical care to management. However, healthcare needs fresh new thinking. Anything that inculcates physicians in 'traditional' business-think could be counterproductive.

I'm a fan of **Clayton Christiansen's** ideas about disruptive innovation. I highly recommend both of his books – *The Innovator's Dilemma* and *The Innovator's Solution*. A professor at the Harvard School of Business, his theory describes how large, successful enterprises often are unable to successfully keep up with innovation, because most of their effort is on incremental changes requested by their demanding customer base. As a result, their products become ever more complex and expensive. This leaves room for tiny companies to do an end run around the larger business by producing products which are simpler, cheaper, and more in line with what the market as a whole, who can't afford the sophisticated products of the large company, wants. I'm greatly oversimplifying an elegant business theory – but the bottom line in my opinion is that healthcare needs disruptive innovation to transform itself quickly. This requires that physician leaders learn how to think out-of-the-box, getting beyond the delivery paradigms we have been living with over the past 30 years.

There are so many books that are relevant for physicians who aspire to become leaders. I would recommend **Regina Herzlinger's** book, *Market-Driven Healthcare*. Although somewhat dated, it's a wonderful example of re-thinking the whole system from the customer point of view. A perspective on the history of medicine is critical. A book by Paul Starr, MD, called *The Social Transformation of American Medicine* shows how far we've come in the science of medicine, and how far we must go in healthcare delivery."

J. Peter Geerlofs, MD
Family Physician
Chief Medical Officer
Allscripts Healthcare Solutions, Inc.

"I'm not familiar with many programs that help physicians learn to lead well. Physicians need those experiences and resources!"

Jeannette South-Paul, MD
Chair of the Department of Family Medicine,
University of Pittsburgh School of Medicine

"Why are dual degree programs becoming so prevalent? The practice of medicine is vastly different today. In the past, administration was mostly ignored by doctors who wanted to do their own thing. For example, when the U.S. government began funding medical care, the repercussions weren't quickly appreciated. When the government became the largest payer for medical services, it wasn't long before Washington began to dictate prices and standards. For better or worse, medical care in the United States was changed forever.

Another example is evidenced in technology advances. Doctors today must know about the business and the law of medicine. Pharmacists face similar challenges. They are scientifically oriented and running a pharmacy is a complex business. Many medical schools still avoid business topics – except as an option perhaps."

Monte L. Anderson, MD
Gastroenterologist and Hepatologist
Mayo Clinic Scottsdale

"I think these days it is not a bad idea for physicians to pursue an MBA along with their MD. A program for this is being developed in the Kansas City area, and I think that is great.

When we commit to medicine as a profession, we are also committing to some or all of the following roles: mentor, team leader, partner, employer, small business owner, accountant, and community leader, to name a few. Perhaps training for some or all of these roles should be included in the medical school curricula. But until that happens, those of us already in practice need to share our knowledge and experience with our younger colleagues. Perhaps doctors in training today will be better equipped to be leaders as well as physicians."

Daniel S. Durrie, MD
Opthamalogist
Durrie Vision Center

Successful physician leaders maintain competence in their ever-advancing clinical specialties even while developing competence in the art of leadership and the science of management. Doing so often involves mastery, or at least minimal comprehension, or management knowledge with regard to topics such as:

- **Accounting:** budgets, income statements, balance sheets, cash flow projections
- **Finance:** capital investments, lease vs. buy decisions, profitability and liquidity
- **Economics:** supply and demand, allocation of resources
- **Law:** legislation and regulation, contract law, liability
- **Ethics:** professional, organizational, social rights and responsibilities
- **Marketing:** attract and retain customers, strategies to grow and compete
- **Information Technology:** automation, decision support, data storage/transmission
- **Operations:** scheduling, facilities, procurement, resource utilization, quality control

- **Human Resource Mgmt:** hiring, training, compensation, performance management
- **Leadership:** setting direction, building commitment to achieve shared objectives
- **Organizational Behavior:** innovation, change, teamwork, job design, policies, values.

> "My organization decided to build an 'Academy' to train 25 to 30 physician leaders. I'm also involved with the **Healthcare Advisory Group**, an organization that is linking with the Masters Degree program of a local university."
>
> Richard B. Birrer, MD, MPH, MMM, CPE
> Family, emergency and sports medicine physician

Management knowledge can be gained through a variety of degree and non-degree approaches. For example, a Masters of Business Administration degree will likely encompass all of the knowledge areas listed above, and do so in the context of both commercial and not-for-profit settings, both production (manufacturing) and service firms. A Masters of Health Administration will likely also cover many of those areas, but may focus more extensively on health policy while de-emphasizing the quantitative or relational aspects of leadership. A Masters of Public Health is often sought by those planning to work in or through governmental agencies. The MPH is likely to focus extensively on public health concerns including epidemiology, disease prevention, and community wellness initiatives.

All over the United States, and in some instances around the world, medical schools and business schools are partnering together to offer "dual degree programs" in medicine and management. In fact, as of mid-2004, the AAMC listed 41 schools that offer MD/MBA combined degree programs, 61 MD/MPH programs and 1 MD/MHA program. There is a rise in the number of osteopathic medical schools that offer dual degrees as well – some in partnership with the business schools of other universities, such as the DO/MBA program launched by the Kansas City University of Medicine and Biosciences (formerly known as the University of Health Sciences – College of Osteopathic Medicine) and Rockhurst University's Helzberg School of Management.

Practicing physicians who have already completed their medical education are returning to school in record numbers to earn graduate degrees in management or business administration. Though many enroll in general MBA or executive EMBA programs, nearly 2,000 have opted for the physician-specific Masters in Medical Management (MMM) degree through one of three ACPE-affiliated programs at Carnegie Mellon University, Tulane University, or the University of Southern California. The ACPE also collaborates with the University of Massachusetts Amherst's completely online MBA program.

Insights from Dr. Lurye regarding the MMM degree program for physicians

"I decided to pursue a degree that would strengthen my knowledge of business in healthcare and technology, and that would offer me the credentials I would need to be seen as capable of fulfilling the responsibilities of healthcare leadership.

When considering whether to pursue a Masters of Medical Management degree, I asked several executive recruiters for advice. They all told me that experience trumps a degree, and yet, the candidate who has progressive, quantifiable experience *and* a degree has a definite advantage. Why? The answer is because a degree demonstrates a commitment to leadership and the willingness to acquire business skills. It also increases the likelihood (though without offering complete assurance) that the candidate has broader insights. Which degree the candidate holds is less important.

It seems to me that managed care organizations sometimes perceive a MBA to be more business-oriented than the more provider-specific MMM degree. And anyone considering a career move outside of healthcare will find a MBA offers greater options. It is certainly more portable, more widely recognized (better known) and more widely available in virtually all cities across the country. And of course, the MMM is designed specifically for experienced physician leaders.

I believe many physicians who intend to remain involved in the delivery of healthcare will find the MMM degree to be more appropriate. With its targeted focus, highly selective admissions criteria, and unique set of faculty resources, the degree is a true differentiator for physicians.

Regardless of which degree is sought, think hard before undertaking a totally online program. Personally, I found that a key advantage of the educational experience stemmed from the network of relationships I developed with my peers. And those types of relationships are typically best developed when supported through some forum for face-to-face interaction and dialogue. My Carnegie Mellon colleagues were all very bright, and were great people to collaborate with.

I would also caution against degrees that compress the training into too short a time frame. I took an 18-month program – and I found I needed time between onsite sessions (held every six months) and distance learning courses (four to six weeks each) in order to apply and assimilate what I'd learned. Within the first few months, I could clearly see that my experience in the program had begun benefiting my organization.

Any physician who is considering a degree will be well advised to explore a variety of programs. Visit their websites and request their information packets. Speak with the program staff and faculty – perhaps even speak with a few alumni.

It is important to ensure that you are selecting the optimal program for your needs and interests. Each of the three MMM programs offers a unique focus. Tulane is especially oriented toward public health and epidemiology. The University of Southern California has a strong focus on entrepreneurship. Carnegie Mellon's emphasis on technology was of particular interest to me.

I believe that the 'best' degree programs are the ones that attract physicians who actually want to learn leadership so they will be better equipped to make a difference in healthcare, not because they are burnt out on patient care and expect administration to be easier. Management is not easier, it's just different."

Donald R. Lurye, MD, MMM
Family Physician
Chief Medical Officer
Welborn Clinic

Formal degree programs naturally require a significant investment of time and money. In recent years, the number of physicians seeking such degrees has risen dramatically. And yet, not all agree that formal education in business is essential for physicians.

"The MD is far more important than the MBA."

John R. Musich, MD, MBA
Obstetrician and Gynecologist
Past Chair, Council for Resident Education in Obstetrics and
Gynecology

"Experience is the name everyone gives to their mistakes."

Oscar Wilde

Why then, is there such growth in the number of physicians seeking dual degrees? The trend may be fueled in part by the attrition rate of physicians who wish to cease active involvement in patient care, and in part by the rise in physicians who aspire to govern large integrated healthcare delivery systems.

"Is there a need for a book on physician leadership? Yes. The topic would certainly make a good CME presentation. Physicians need to learn about leadership. It is important to realize that management is not the same thing as leadership. Both are important. The American College of Physician Executives offers good resources on executive management. And many books are available that address the subject of executive management – in healthcare and in general. For example, Collins' book *Good to Great* is one I have recommended other physician leaders read."

Mark H. Belfer, DO, FAAFP
Family Physician
Residency Director
Akron General Medical Center/NEOUCOM

"My experience is that one cannot learn leadership from the written word."

Michael Scotti, MD
Internist
Retired Senior Vice President
American Medical Association

Various non-degree certification options such as the Certified Physician Executive or Certified Healthcare Executive can be earned through professional associations/societies.

"The American College of Physician Executives is a good resource for physician leaders. They offer certification for Physician Executives. I'm certified as a Masters in Medical Management and as a Physician Executive. Another route some physicians choose is to earn a masters degree in business or administration. Such educational credentials are not sine qua non, but the insights and experiences they offer help to tear down the blind spots and see life through the perspective of those we seek to lead.

The **American College of Healthcare Executives** tends to focus on the needs and interests of healthcare professionals who are not medically trained physicians. The ACHE has a different focus than that of the ACPE, which exists to meet the needs and interests of physician executives. The ACPE made me much of what I am. Its programs and resources are very expensive, but the ACPE offers essential training.

Becoming an effective physician leader doesn't happen automatically. It requires investment in training and accumulation of experiences."

Richard B. Birrer, MD, MPH, MMM, CPE
Family, Emergency, Sports and Geriatric Medicine Physician

"My advice for docs wanting to be leaders? I'd give them a couple of books to read. One is *The Seven Habits of Highly Effective People* by Stephen Covey, PhD (1989). The other is *The Four Agreements* by Miguel Ruiz (2001). The latter deals more with the 'spiritual' and gets at the 'why,' not just the 'how' of leadership. The former focuses more on how to lead. They both emphasize the importance of having integrity, of always being your best, and not making assumptions. Those are the characteristics of effective physician leaders.

Back in the 1980s I read *The Road Less Traveled* by **Scott Peck**. I also studied the reality therapy and rational emotive therapy research by **William Glasser**, MD and **Albert Ellis**. The authors all advise not to make assumptions, just look at what works and what does not. I became involved with **Scott Peck's** work because I was doing a lot of work with alcoholics and drug addicts. I saw that just like most alcoholics, I (and most docs) had a tendency to experience guilt and shame over things we couldn't control. Once we accept what we can and cannot control, our stress level drops way down. For me, it is a bit of a spiritual matter. We're just humans, but are part of a bigger picture.

Don't laugh – but another person whose work I am excited about is **Dr. Phil**. That's right – the frequent guest speaker on **Oprah** who now has his own TV show. I'm excited by the impact he's having which is a bit counter to traditional counseling and pop-psychology. Dr. Phil's fame is a refreshing phenomenon in my opinion. He advocates accountability and taking appropriate action rather than making excuses and playing the victim. We're only victims if we choose to be, and he points out that we are where we are because of the choices we've made. I see him as a current, pop-culture form of the reality therapy and rational emotive therapy movement begun by Glaser and Ellis."

Randall Oates, MD
Family Physician
Founder and President, Docs, Inc.

"There are multiple pathways to develop leadership skills. Having an MBA – or some other advanced degree in business, management or leadership – isn't necessary for everyone. Depending on what point a person is at in their career, it may or may not be a good investment of time, money, and energy. Clinicians do tend to sanctify credentials, so having the degree can be helpful – especially for those aspiring to lead within the context of a large organizational hierarchy.

My advice to physicians who aspire to make leading contributions in healthcare? Read a lot! Especially early in your career. Many wonderful thought leaders have published some very good books and articles. (In fact, this book will be a terrific resource for physicians just out of training and for physicians in leadership positions.) Second, seek formal training courses – through professional organizations, universities, and other educational institutions. I'm not an advocate of MBA degrees for everyone, but I do believe many physicians will benefit by attending two to five day workshops in order to learn a particular aspect of business, management, or leadership that you need."

Ronald N. Riner, MD
Cardiologist
President, The Riner Group

"Some people gain skills via workshops – for example, workshops on speaking, writing, leadership, communication, giving presentations and so on. Such workshops are offered by medical societies and institutes at the national and state level. For example, Harvard Medical School offers seminars on communication. **The Bayer Institute** offers programs on provider–patient communication.

There is probably a need for a book on physician leadership. Whether there's a market for it is another question. I'm amazed by the number of self-help leadership books on the market – books like *The One Minute Manager, Good to Great, Inside the Tornado, Who Moved My Cheese*, and *Re-Engineering the Corporation*."

Daniel Z. Sands, MD, MPH
Internist, Faculty, Harvard Medical School
Chief Medical Officer and Vice President, Clinical Strategies
Zix Corporation

Where Traditional Management Education Can Go Wrong

Without criticizing or minimizing the value of traditional management education, we do want to provide some perspective for physicians seeking additional training from business education resources. Some of the classic principles deemed important for success in the business environment can run afoul in the physician-led environment. Several key differences exist between the environment of physician leaders and that of business leaders.

Traditional business literature and training programs often emphasize the importance of the "appearance" of power and how it can impact the influence potential of individuals in less powerful positions. Behavior that communicates "presence" and "authority" may help the traditional business-oriented middle manager in being perceived as a leader. Similar behavior by a physician leader, however, is too easily interpreted as arrogance and pomposity, negative characteristics to which physicians are particularly vulnerable. Because there is somewhat of an inherent assumption of power by physicians in leadership positions, behavior in a more down-to-earth and approachable manner will serve to greatly improve the potential impact of and tendency to follow a physician leader.

Traditional business education also typically emphasizes the importance of communicating a sense of dedication and commitment to your profession and institution as a way of establishing a leadership role. Once again, physicians are particularly vulnerable to a dedication to a profession that can decimate any semblance of a personal life. The balance of personal and professional life is important. Balance is essential for maintaining an appropriate context for decision making, a reality-based framework for prioritizing those decisions, and the social sustenance for the physical and emotional energy needed by physician leaders.

Finally, traditional business education commonly includes extensive training and negotiation skills. Business education that presumes a market environment functioning on a "win/lose" framework of finite resources and transient market advantages will emphasize skills to maximize personal benefits in negotiations. For physician leaders, however, the moral dimension that accompanies the environment in which they work demands an emphasis on "win/win" negotiation strategies. Rather than using the strategies for success in automobile sales, physician leaders must emphasize negotiation tactics more appropriate for marriage counseling. Physician leaders' success stems from establishing and sustaining long-term relationships built on trust and mutual benefit. Physician leaders whose negotiation skills are oriented toward maximizing mutual benefit will be the ultimate winners.

Points to Ponder

1 Why is it important to discern where traditional management education can go wrong?

2 What ways have you been influenced – for better or worse – by your own beliefs and actions, or the beliefs and actions of those you work with?

3 Think of a lesson you've learned from an educator, or an educational experience that has *not* served you well. What other traditional mind-sets would you benefit by letting go of?

4 What have you read or been told that defies your intuitive judgment?

5 How do you go about deciding which conventional wisdom or widely promoted practices to follow or to challenge?

References and Further Reading

Appleby J. (2002) Doctors earn MBAs to tackle ills of health system. *USA Today* **July 5**: 1–2.

Binius T. (1998) Medical business acumen: The growing number of physicians seeking business skills can find MBA programs tailored to their needs. *AMNews* **November 23/30**.

Blanchard K. and Johnson S. (1983) *The One Minute Manager.* New York: William Morrow & Company.

Collins J. (2001) *Good to Great: why some companies make the leap and others don't.* New York: HarperCollins Publishers.

Covey S.R. (1989) *The Seven Habits of Highly Effective People.* New York: Simon & Schuster Inc.

Dye C.F. (1996) Cultivating physician talent: Five steps for developing successful physician leaders. *Healthcare Executive* **11**(3): 18–21.

Ellis A. (2004) *Rational Emotive Behavior Therapy: it works for me – it can work for you.* New York: Prometheus Books.

Ellis A. and Harper R.A. (1997) *A Guide To Rational Living.* 3rd edn. Hollywood, CA: Melvin Powers Wilshire Book Company.

Ettore B. (1996) When an M.D. just isn't enough. *Management Review* **85**(3): 9.

Fisher R., Ury R.L., and Patton B. (1991) *Getting to Yes: Negotiating agreement without giving in.* New York: Penguin Books.

Glasser W. (1989) *Reality Therapy: a new approach to psychiatry.* New York: Perennial Publishing.

Greene J. (1997) Marcus Welby, MBA. *Hospitals & Health Networks* **7**(15): 36–8.

Guthrie M.B. (1999) Challenges in developing physician leadership and management. *Frontiers of Health Services Management* **15**(4): 3–26.

Hammer M. and Champy J. (2001) *Reengineering the Corporation: a manifesto for business revolution.* New York: HarperBusiness.

Johnson S. and Blanchard K.A. (1998) *Who Moved my Cheese? An amazing way to deal with change in your work and in your life.* New York: Putnam Publishing Group.

Koska M.T. (1992) New approaches to developing physician leaders. *Hospitals* **66**(9): 76–8.

Larson D.B., Chandler M. and Forman H.P. (2003) MD/MBA Programs in the United States: Evidence of a Change in Health Care Leadership. *Academic Medicine* **78**: 335–41.

Levin A. (2000) Medicine and MBAs. *Annals of Internal Medicine* **132**: 1015.

Lipson R. (1997) Back to school. *Health Systems Review* **30**(6): 49–51.

McGraw P.C. (2003) *Self Matters: creating your life from the inside out.* New York: Free Press.

McKenna M.K., Gartland M.P., and Pugno P.A. (2004) Defining and developing physician leadership competencies. American College of Physician Executives, *Click Online Medical Management Magazine* **February/March.**

Moore G.A. (1995) *Inside the Tornado: marketing strategies from Silicon Valley's cutting edge.* New York: HarperCollins Publishers.

Peck M.S. (2003) *The Road Less Traveled: a new psychology of love, traditional values, and spiritual growth.* New York: Simon & Schuster.

Propp D.A. and Uehara D.T. (2001) Creating a model physician executive. American College of Physician Executives, *Click Online Medical Management Magazine* **February**.

Ruelas E. and Leatt P. (1985) The roles of physician-executives in hospitals: A framework for management education. *The Journal of Health Administration Education* **3**(2): 151–69.

Ruiz M.A. (2001) *The Four Agreements.* Carlsbad, CA: Hay House, Inc.

Schneller E., Greenwald H., Richardson M., and Orr J. (1997) The physician executive: Role in the adaptation of American medicine. *Health Care Management Review* **22**(2): 90–96.

Schwartz R.W., Pogge C.R., Gillis S.A., and Holsinger J.W. (2000) Programs for the development of physician leaders: A curricular process in its infancy. *Academic Medicine* **75**: 133–40.

Shalowitz J., Nutter D., and Snarr J. (1996) Medicine and management: A combined educational program. *The Journal of Health Administration Education* **14**(3): 305–14.

Stahl M. and Dean P.J. (1999) *The Physician's Essential MBA: what every physician leader needs to know.* Gaithersburg, MD: Aspen Publishers, Inc.

Swartz H.M. and Gottheil D.L. (1991) The need to educate physician-scholars for leadership in the health care system (editorial) *Annals of Internal Medicine* **114**(4): 333–4.

Vinson C. (1994) Administrative knowledge and skills needed by physician executives. *Physician Executive* **20**(6): 37.

Williams S.J. (2001) Training needs for physician leaders. *The Journal of Health Administration Education* **19**(2): 195–202.

Chapter 17

Learning by Leading: On-Job Experience and Volunteer Leadership Roles

"Tell a man there are 300 billion stars in the universe and he'll believe you. Tell him a bench has wet paint on it and he'll have to touch to be sure."

Jaeger

We realize that physicians, perhaps more than any other group of professionals, are accustomed to *learning by doing*. That's why we predict you will refer to this

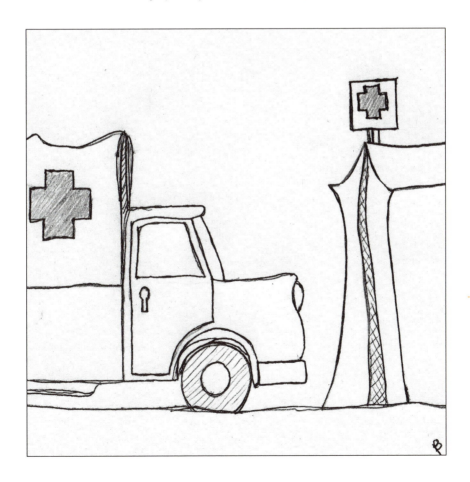

section again and again as you continue learning *about* leading physicians *by actually leading* physicians. This section is full of practical tips and techniques for applying the book's insights toward the achievement of your own aspirations and purposes.

> "The relationships between MGMA staff and our members in many ways parallel the relationships between physicians and administrators in medical group practices. Our members – volunteer leaders – are typically time-pressed; their first priority is quite naturally their 'day job,' which is both challenging and time-consuming. As volunteer leaders, they are dependent upon our staff to do things they do not have time to do themselves. To help our volunteer leaders maximize their impact, we encourage them to focus on policy setting and strategic decision making, and to delegate operational/organizational implementation of those policies and strategies to the staff. Strong leaders should give direction with sufficient clarity that staff can execute. Strong leaders delegate without abdicating or micromanaging.
>
> MGMA offers a workshop on volunteer leadership that is very popular. In it, we help leaders learn how to identify potential future leaders, how to get others to commit the time necessary to develop their skills, how to get others to volunteer. Many of the skills required for successful volunteer leadership are similar to the skills required for successful organizational governance. But volunteer leadership also includes a qualitatively different challenge as well – it requires an ability to influence other volunteers. When those you seek to influence do not work for you, relying on 'position power' just doesn't work. The ability to successfully lead volunteers – whether in a professional association, or a peer-to-peer context – requires a different style. It requires persuasion and teamwork to convince others to embrace ideas and work together."
>
> William F. Jessee, MD, FACMPE, FACPM
> Pediatric, Preventive and Emergency Medicine Physician
> President
> Medical Group Management Association

"If the opportunity exists, a fellowship after residency can be useful for developing leadership skills and learning about finance, statistical tools, quality improvement research and management."

> David G. Fairchild, MD, MPH
> Internist and Chief of General Medicine
> Tufts – New England Medical Center

"Physicians are often put into situations where failure is inescapable. How could that be? Physicians are smart and logical, and we care about being successful. Physicians wouldn't begin caring for patients after the first year of medical school before possessing the necessary tools or skills needed to properly care for patients. That would doom anyone to fail.

Why then do physicians enter leadership positions or administrative posts without the training or skills needed to do the job properly? 'Sink or swim' is not a good management approach, but it happens all too often.

Physicians need to mentor future leaders by providing learning opportunities. We need to put future leaders into leadership training courses and then provide ever-expanding leadership positions. We need to provide a mini-residency for future leaders – that might be more palatable."

Kevin J. Soden, MD, MPH
Emergency Medicine Physician
Medical Correspondent, NBC News
Soden Consulting Services

"Physician leaders should ideally have been in practice for at least 8–10 years. There is no substitute for the perspective that can be gained only through practicing medicine – perspective both on what is fundamentally wrong from the physician's perspective, but also on the incremental changes which would be acceptable by physicians with limited emotional room for change."

J. Peter Geerlofs, MD
Family Physician
Chief Medical Officer
Allscripts Healthcare Solutions, Inc.

"Physician leaders evolve out of their experiences. I don't see how someone could simply aspire to be one and go to school for it."

Randall Oates, MD
Family Physician
Founder and President, Docs, Inc.

"An important component of leadership is the ability to manage people. This is best done by creating a 'learning environment' where people are provided the knowledge, tools (especially information technology), and other resources to excel – for the good of the organization and the individual.

Also important is the creation and expectation of an environment where 'informed risk' is seen as of great value to the creativity and dynamic of an organization. In such an environment, leadership encourages an appropriate degree of risk in decision making that is informed by the best knowledge and data – and with the important understanding that if the decision is later found to be incorrect, the accountability for this outcome is to learn from the process, apply the learning to future decisions, and move on."

Douglas E. Henley, MD, FAAFP
Executive Vice President
American Academy of Family Physicians

"Becoming a medical staff leader is a process. The length of time needed from entering leadership roles to becoming a medical staff president is debated. Efforts should be taken to educate physician leaders – whether by chairing a quality improvement committee, serving as section chief or medical staff president. Individuals should be schooled so they will be prepared to take on their respective leadership roles.

While 'on-the-job-training' cannot be avoided, it should be minimized. Understanding the process of hospital governance and the relationship of your hospital in a health system (if it applies) is important. Going into a leadership role unprepared is just as bad as going into the operating room unprepared for the procedure you are about to perform."

Andrew M. Schwartz, MD
Cardiac Surgeon
Vice President, Medical Staff
Shawnee Mission Medical Center

"There is a large body of literature about leadership, organizational dynamics, analytical thinking, conflict management, and strategic planning. The wise new physician manager will want to get some training either through a formal course such as an executive MBA or through a disciplined plan of reading and interactive course work."

Bruce Bagley, MD
Family Physician
Director, Quality Improvement
American Academy of Family Physicians

"On the job experience is often as valuable – or more so – than a formal degree."

Tim Munzing, MD
Family Physician
Kaiser Permanente – Orange County

"**Cinda Johnson, MD, MBA** earned her business degree while serving as a Department Chair. She is now the Dean at **East Carolina School of Medicine**. She is a real role model. Many physicians would find her path too challenging, though, and not feasible economically or schedule-wise.

I believe formal training is best when nested in a real-time work environment. That way people can apply the theories and concepts they're learning into their actual work experiences, and draw from their work experiences to better understand the concepts and theories. I'm not sure all medical students or residents would appreciate leadership development courses even if they were offered during medical training."

Jeannette South-Paul, MD
Chair of the Department of Family Medicine,
University of Pittsburgh School of Medicine

Some physicians choose to develop or enhance their leadership competencies through on-the-job experiences such as special projects or assignments; outside-the-job volunteer experiences – for example, volunteering in one's professional medical society or community; or formal developmental experiences such as one to five day leadership skill building workshops offered for healthcare specific and general audiences.

> "How do physicians develop their leadership skills? They learn the territory by participating in committees – developing cogent communication skills. They read books on leadership and relationships. Some doctors find that it comes easier for them – they have more natural ability in that regard. All doctors, though, can develop leadership skills if they're willing to work at it."
>
> Monte L. Anderson, MD
> Gastroenterologist and Hepatologist
> Mayo Clinic Scottsdale

There are of course advantages and disadvantages to learning "on-the-job." For example, once you're practicing medicine and on call, you may lack the time. This is especially true when you also have family and community responsibilities. Keep in mind that not knowing what you don't know (but need to) can be costly.

Thoughts on "Managing Up"

Chances are good that the term "managing up" is not one you've heard before. Those with many years of experience in administration, however, understand its importance. The majority of management books you might read tell you how to affect the behavior of and influence those over whom you have supervisory responsibilities or who otherwise report to you. Managing up refers to the periodic need to "manage" those further up the administrative ladder than ourselves. For most people, this involves modifying the behaviors and influencing those to whom we report.

Why This is Important

Why is this important? For physician leaders or those moving up the administrative ladder, many find themselves reporting to senior administrators or other individuals who are not physicians. Consequently, the individuals to whom those physician leaders report, although otherwise extremely capable, will necessarily lack the experience and perspective of a physician who has worked in the clinical setting. This issue, of course, extends beyond clinical expertise, however, as many working professionals possess unique knowledge that those to whom they report do not have. When your supervisor is faced with decisions for which you have unique knowledge, it is important to find ways to bring that knowledge to bear or otherwise impact your supervisor's decision.

Going beyond knowledge, in your role as a physician leader you may indeed have extensive contact with constituencies with which your supervisor never has any such contact. Consequently, you may indeed understand issues or the implication of decisions in unique ways and must find avenues for imparting that information to those charged with the responsibility for making decisions that affect those constituencies.

Another reason why it's important to periodically "manage up" is simply to demonstrate your capabilities. A physician leader seeking additional responsibilities would do well to make sure that those to whom they report are well aware of *all* their capabilities and the breadth of skills they possess. Ostensibly, you were hired for those abilities your boss knew about. You may indeed retain your job or be promoted for those abilities you possess that you have yet to demonstrate.

Managing up is also an important skill because it's part of your overall obligation to further the vision, interests, and priorities of your organization. In other words, this is part of doing your best for your organization. Managing up not only allows you to demonstrate your capabilities but can make your boss look good and allow you to use the position power of others to facilitate the accomplishment of your goals. This is also one of the ways in which you can enhance your leadership for those constituencies depending on you, and to do so beyond the narrow confines of your current job responsibilities.

Four Dimensions of "Managing Up"

Four dimensions to managing up will help you accomplish your goals and help you keep the peace when your goals turn out to be unattainable. Those dimensions of managing up are:

> 1 establishing and building trust
> 2 communicating clearly
> 3 addressing the priorities of others
> 4 agreeing to disagree when necessary.

To be successful as a physician leader, you must earn others' trust – in you as an individual and in your integrity. In fact, the first step in becoming an effective leader is that of establishing and building trust. You must be consistently honest, even when it seems disadvantageous to you personally. Others must be able to depend on you for straight answers with no hidden agendas. Consistent honesty and concern for the best interests of your organization will command respect from others, even from those who may occasionally disagree with you on various matters. Trust is earned through the consistent demonstration of competence and character. A corollary to this is the overt and consistent willingness to support team efforts. Never miss an opportunity to help a peer or to provide a co-worker with pertinent information to which you have access.

Integrity can be demonstrated in many ways. In budgeting, for example. Resist the temptation to "pad" budget requests. Instead, submit annual budgets that are based on facts and realistic forecasts. This will command respect from conscientious finance officers. Integrity can also be demonstrated through strict adherence to ethical management practices. Stand your ground in this area, even if, on occasion, it involves personal sacrifice. Leaders of integrity are willing to risk losing their jobs rather than issuing directives they know to be ethically wrong or harmful to the organization. Ethical leaders realize that no job is worth keeping in that sort of environment.

A second dimension to managing up is clear communication. This includes excellent verbal and written communication skills. It also includes the capacity to present information in ways that can be readily assimilated by listeners or readers. Give your boss information the way your boss needs the information.

Given how busy we all are these days, respecting others' time by communicating succinctly and with appropriate focus will always be to your advantage. Clearly differentiating between opinion and evidence-based recommendations is similarly important, because it strengthens the reliability of the information you communicate, and thus your overall credibility.

A third dimension to managing up involves addressing the priorities of others. This is a corollary to the clear communication principle. If, for example, your organization is facing financial pressures, you will enhance the attractiveness of your recommendations by framing them in terms of cost savings or revenue generation. Similarly, your recommendations will likely be more favorably received to the extent that they minimize legal risk and position the organization in the most favorable light. Whenever possible, make your organization, and all involved in it, "look good." In other words, ensure that your recommendations reflect not only your priorities, but those of your supervisor as well.

A fourth dimension to managing up successfully involves recognition that there may be times when you and your supervisor will agree to disagree. This point is essentially a reality check. It would be unrealistic to expect that your recommendations will always be accepted, or that your attempts to influence will always be embraced with enthusiasm. Sometimes, you and your supervisor must simply agree to disagree. In those situations, it is your responsibility to accept the disagreement as gracefully as you can. With time, one of two outcomes will likely occur. Either the merits of your recommendation will eventually be appreciated, or you will learn the weaknesses within your recommendation and gain a perspective your supervisor had but you didn't. This is how we grow and learn.

Tips for "Managing Up"

Wondering how exactly physician leaders can consistently and successfully manage up? Summarized below are several tips we hope you will find useful:

1 Meet regularly with your supervisor. Always be prepared for those meetings with an agenda and use the opportunity to establish trust. Take advantage of the time to offer opinions and recommendations, especially those that you can support with facts and other evidence.
2 Keep your boss informed. Convey what you are doing, how you are prioritizing work, and how you approach decisions. Alert your boss to any areas of potential risk. For example, if you have reason to anticipate that an employee may soon leave the organization, share that information promptly (and privately) with your supervisor. Keeping your boss informed about what you are doing and what's going on is an effective way of conveying your capabilities and priorities.
3 Demonstrate your abilities by producing quality work, meeting deadlines, and committing due diligence to the tasks assigned to you. Everyone appreciates people whose personal standards for performance are high.
4 Put things in writing. Keep a record of meetings and conversations with supervisors. Establish a paper trail for decisions – including those delegated and those you've made personally. This is not a defensive self-protection notion. Rather, it is a means of enhancing efficiency – yours and your super-

visor's. By communicating recommendations to your boss in writing, you are providing an opportunity for review and reflection, rather than demanding instant reaction. Construct a "one side of one page" brief memo with three parts:

a concise articulation of the challenge or question at hand

b a short bullet-point list of pertinent facts related to the decision

c a clearly stated recommendation based upon those facts.

This structure increases the likelihood that your recommendation will be supported, or that you will be given an explanation of why it is not approved (which offers you an opportunity to learn).

5 Anticipate the needs of your supervisor. Doing so may allow you to "frame" projects in ways that you find most comfortable, rather than waiting for your supervisor to decide how things should be done, and perhaps choosing an approach that you find particularly difficult. Anticipating the needs of your boss also conveys that you have the organization's best interests in mind, and that you are putting in extra time and effort to support its success.

6 Successful leaders can be depended upon – even, or perhaps especially, during difficult times. Routinely volunteer to help find solutions to the challenges at hand. Do not shy away from challenging situations or tasks. This is one of the best ways to demonstrate your leadership capabilities.

7 Have the courage to set limits. During busy times, when asked to take on an additional task, spend a little time with your supervisor prioritizing the new assignment relative to your other current responsibilities. At such times, you'll be especially glad that you have been keeping your supervisor well-informed about the scope of what you are doing.

8 Don't forget to say "thank you." Over time, most of us will find that we have learned a great deal from our supervisors. We may discover many ways in which we have reaped the benefits of their support. Never neglect an opportunity to let your supervisors know how much you appreciate their support and the opportunities they have provided you. Because so few people express appreciation these days, such behavior is refreshingly unusual and will stand you in good stead.

Managing up is an important skill. It is equally important as managing those whom you supervise. Many of the characteristics that you make you an effective supervisor will also make you effective support staff. By consistently demonstrating these concepts, you will be modeling the behaviors you value most for others with whom you work.

A Case of "Managing Up" by Dr. Pugno

It was a time of change. The hospital administrator had been its CEO for more than 15 years, unusual longevity in the turbulent environment of healthcare administration. Although the moderate-sized community hospital remained fiscally solvent, reductions in reimbursement rates and the providing of poorly compensated services to a large indigent population had significantly reduced the hospital's operating margin in recent years. Now the old CEO was retiring . . . and the medical director was worried.

The new CEO was recruited from a large hospital system. With a background in accounting, he had worked his way up the administrative ladder by demonstrating exceptional skill at financial management and cost control. The medical director knew that one look at the financial reports would make the hospital's education program, an annual cost of several thousand dollars, a target for elimination. He needed to help the new CEO make the "right" decision in this case.

It was at the new CEO's first meeting with the hospital's governing board that the medical director implemented his plan. On the agenda was a brief report about the education program. The medical director began by acknowledging that the hospital had subsidized the education program from its inception. The chief financial officer, however, pointed out that when compared to similar education programs in other hospitals like theirs, the one they conducted was well within financial performance expectations. Then followed the presentation of the many benefits the hospital had gained from the education program, including the recruitment of some of the region's best surgeons and intensivists, and the establishment of an efficient outpatient clinic that minimized the inappropriate use of the emergency department and provided the majority of care for the community's most needy patients in a cost-effective manner.

It was demonstrated that education program graduates made up a substantial proportion of the medical staff and its referral patterns, and was directly responsible for bringing to the community hospital subspecialty consultants who provided both teaching and clinical services to it on a regular basis. Finally, with the medical director's pre-meeting encouragement, one of the members of the governing board pointed out how the education program's outreach services to the local community had resulted in substantial increases in charitable giving to the hospital foundation, including the recent gift of a major library expansion and the purchase of new diagnostic equipment. In essence, the case was made that the education program, although superficially a cost-center of the institution, was in fact a major asset whose benefits far surpassed the subsidy needed for its operation, and that the governing board of the hospital was well aware of those benefits.

At the next meeting of the governing board, the new CEO outlined his plan for the future development of the community hospital ... including enhanced support for the education program. That night, the medical director slept well.

Questions for Discussion

1 What elements of "managing up" are illustrated by this case?
2 What level of sophistication in financial management did the medical director need in order to make the case that the benefits of the education program outweighed its direct costs?
3 How important was "preparation" in the medical director's strategy to influence the new CEO's decision making?
4 Are there other examples of hospital operations that "don't make money," but may play a substantial role in its ultimate fiscal performance?
5 How does "managing up" differ from just 'manipulation' of others? (Makes the ethical point of benefit for self versus benefit for others ...)

Advanced Leadership Skills

Considering that the MD/MBA and DO/MBA dual degree programs are designed for medical students and residents, and the ACPE's MMM degree programs are designed for practicing physicians, what resources and experiences are available for physicians who've already earned graduate level degrees, yet want to continue enhancing their leadership capabilities? This field is so new, that question cannot yet be answered. Perhaps over time executive education programs will emerge for senior physician leaders, much as such programs became popular in the 1980s and 1990s for senior leaders in other industries.

In-house Leadership Development Programs

Perhaps healthcare will follow the lead of large companies that have developed in-house "Corporate Universities." In fact, some of the large and leading healthcare organizations already offer advanced leadership development programs for their staff physicians who have administrative responsibilities.

References and Further Reading

Chappelow C. and Leslie J.B. (2001) *Keeping Your Career On Track: twenty success strategies.* Greensboro, NC: Center for Creative Leadership.

Lombardo M.M. and Eichinger R.W. (1989) *Eighty-eight Assignments for Development in Place.* Greensboro, NC: Center for Creative Leadership..

Tangalos E.G., Blomberg R.A., Hicks S.S., and Bender C.E. (1998) Mayo leadership programs for physicians. *Mayo Clinic Proceedings* **73**(3): 279–84.

Treister N.W. (1995) Development of a local physician executive leadership program. *Physician Executive* **21**(4): 22–24.

Versel N. (2003) Hand in hand: VHA's physician leadership builds a bridge between suits and coats. *Modern Physician* **May**: 16–18.

Chapter 18

Learning From Leaders: Relationships, Mentors, and Teamwork

"I enjoy training fellows and working in academia. I believe mentoring is very important in medicine. Doctors are accustomed to learning from mentors – during residency, during internships, throughout practice. So mentoring is a natural learning system for us.

While practicing in Omaha, I was fortunate to learn from the 'perfect' leader – **Jack Filkins**, MD. He was active in research and in the community; he also ran the office very well. He helped everyone achieve far more than we otherwise would have. He was a 'benevolent dictator' – very tough on us! Eighteen months ago I found out Jack's wife had passed away so although I no longer worked with him, or even lived in the same city, I of course made it a point to

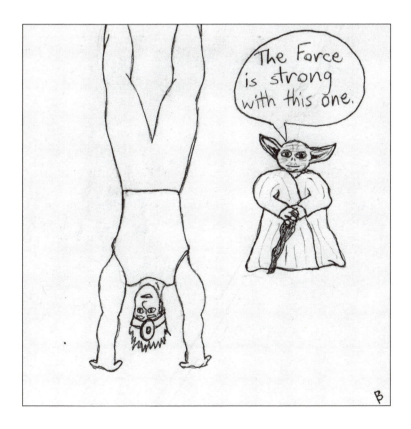

attend her funeral. When Jack looked up and saw me there, he gave me a certain look. I could tell he still considered himself my mentor, he still expected me to always do the right thing. I was so glad I'd rearranged my plans to be there. Relationships like that are very special.

Part of everyone's personality is innate; we're better off not fighting it. One responsibility of a mentor is to help people identify and build upon their innate gifts and interests. Good mentors offer insight; they instill confidence in those they're mentoring. Good mentors are good role models.

I've trained 30 fellows, and believe me – they're always watching! They expect me to do the right thing. And I expect them to do what's right as well. I find it intriguing that a very high percentage of them are still married to their first wives; and that 95 percent of them changed jobs within the first couple of years after training. I believe the former is an indication of their values; the latter is a sign of their confidence. As I said earlier, one of the key responsibilities of a mentor is to build confidence in those with whom they work."

Daniel S. Durrie, MD
Ophthalmologist
President
Durrie Vision Center

"Identify people who are doing work similar to yours, or to the work you aspire to do. Learn from them. Learn from the experiences of others any time you can. And tap into available resources. For example, the American College of Physician Executives, many hospitals, and nearly all of the medical specialty societies offer many books, articles, training workshops, and other resources."

Ronald N. Riner, MD
Cardiologist
President,
The Riner Group

"To grow leadership skills successfully requires a learning laboratory. In the ideal scenario, emerging physician leaders are given progressive responsibilities in finance and management under the guidance of an experienced mentor. Leaders should constantly seek feedback from their mentors and their organizations in order to foster introspection and personal growth."

Bruce Bagley, MD
Medical Director, Quality Improvement
American Academy of Family Physicians

"Having mentors is important – in all stages of your professional career. It helps to have colleagues to talk with, to watch and see what they do, to emulate successful styles, and avoid poor styles."

David G. Fairchild, MD, MPH
Internist and Chief of General Medicine
Tufts – New England Medical Center

"Good leaders get people the equipment, tools and training they need to succeed; and take care to shape people's expectations. The regulatory requirements in the federal system are tough, and resources are scarce. But if we keep stressing our resources, people quit. Then we lose the collective knowledge of people's historical perspective that comes only from experience. That requires even greater investment of time and money in hiring and training people. So we work hard to keep people through use of rewards, recognition, and incentives. For example, I gave everyone one hour paid time off before the holidays – telling them 'I know you've been working hard and I appreciate what you do.' Gestures like that go a long way.

It is important to carefully select middle managers and executives who show concern for others, who understand the vision of the organization, who are organized and get things done. Then train them well – not just on job procedures, but also time management and other broad skills. Mentor people, and demonstrate that you do what you're asking them to do. Selecting and training managers is time intensive up front, but essential for long-term success. So is the operational work of setting up systems and eliminating variability. After ensuring people are clear about the rules and regulations, give them the tools they need and empower them to make front line decisions by granting them the authority to make decisions within broad parameters. My employees know if they hit a snag or need my help they can get me involved."

Reverend Pamela S. Harris, MD

Physical Medicine and Rehabilitation Physician

Kansas City Veteran's Administration Hospital

and Minister of Health, United Methodist Church of the

Resurrection

"Hospital administration and medical staff must accept the responsibility of grooming medical staff leaders who are eager to serve, loyal to both hospital and staff, and able to conceptualize a vision of the future in which competitive holistic medicine is encouraged to take root and grow. The 'good ole boy' mentality is clearly a handicap. A 'hands on,' motivated, creative physician who is unaccepting of the status quo will best serve the hospital's needs and goals.

Most physicians are driven and goal-oriented. Not all are leaders; nor should they be. Ascension to medical staff leadership should not be haphazard. But the process should be all-inclusive in evaluating physicians for leadership positions. Leadership has no known genetic foci. Instead, leadership is a groomed trait, influenced by role models and mentors. Of the many people who witness a crisis unfold, only some will respond, and those who respond may do so in different ways. Leadership is not defined by those leading the charge, but by how the assessment of the past, critique of the present, and preparation for the future are handled by those out in front.

Hospital leaders must clearly understand that both patients and the physicians providing their care are important customers.

Dissatisfaction in either group is damaging to the stability of the hospital and poses a risk to quality. Dictatorial leadership is often patronizing at the very least, and invites disillusionment. Proactive is better than reactive."

Andrew M. Schwartz, MD
Cardiac Surgeon
Vice President, Medical Staff
Shawnee Mission Medical Center

"Too often, people believe they won't 'win' if they help others, they'll 'win' if they're better than others. That stimulates individuality and competition which are appropriate to some extent, but not when focused on excessively.

My advice for those who aspire to be compelling leaders? Look for someone whose style and results you respect, then contact them for advice and coaching. Take your problems to them and ask them for recommendations or confirmation of your plans."

Jeannette South-Paul, MD
Chair of the Department of Family Medicine,
University of Pittsburgh School of Medicine

More physicians every year are seeking out the services of qualified professional coaches who can help them set and achieve their career goals. Dr. McKenna is a Certified Physician Leadership Coach™, collaborating with others who have been trained through the Certified Physician Leadership Coaching Institute founded by Francine Gaillour, MD, MBA, FACPE. Visit www.physicianleadership.com for more information.

Thoughts on Mentors and Mentoring

It's probably safe to say that most physicians in leadership positions are able to readily identify multiple individuals they consider to be their mentors. In many dimensions of today's society, the affirmative role of a mentor in someone's life is gaining increasing appreciation. But what is mentorship, and what makes that relationship different from consultants, content experts and other advisors? Let's begin by attempting to define a mentor.

A mentor has several qualities. Most mentors are identified because they have special skills, experience, or unique perspectives from which others want to learn. What makes mentorship different from advisors and consultants, however, is the development and evolution of a personal relationship over time with the individuals they are mentoring. This affirmative willingness to generously share time helping someone else grow in knowledge and experience through a long-term personal relationship is the essence of mentorship. An important distinction is that mentors cannot be assigned. Doing so would be like "picking my friends for me." No, our mentors are those who we select and whose advice and counsel evolves over time as the personal relationship matures.

It may be useful at this point to address several of the issues surrounding mentorship using the format of frequently asked questions (FAQs). These are among the most common:

1 *Do I need to ask someone to be my mentor?* If you feel the need to ask someone formally to be your mentor, it probably means that you don't already have the kind of relationship that will evolve into that individual being a true mentor to you. Such a relationship is one more like that of a consultant to whom you ask questions and they provide you with answers. A mentoring relationship develops over time. Good mentors give freely of their time to those who seek it. Seeking the advice and counsel of people you respect, and sharing back with them how it has impacted you is one of the ways a mentoring relationship develops.

2 *Should I seek mentors?* Absolutely. Learning from the experience and expertise of others is one of the best ways in which we can grow. For many of us, a mentoring relationship has developed over time simply by our staying in touch with leaders and supervisors with whom we've worked in different settings. As our careers evolve and change, staying in touch with those whose judgment we respect and with whom we've already established an initial personal relationship is a good way to plant the seeds that will germinate into mentoring relationships.

3 *How many mentors should I have?* The answer to this question is highly individual. Many people can point to a single good mentor upon whom they depended for years, but most leaders readily admit that they have many mentors whose diverse perspectives and knowledge they've called upon periodically to help them as different situations arise. It may be helpful to think of mentors as members of a team that you assemble. Those are the people with the array of skills and knowledge that will help you over time. With time, if you identify an unmet need within your team, then seeking the counsel of someone with those particular skills will help you design and build the most functional team for your personal needs.

4 *As an emerging physician leader, is mentoring something I should do?* Yes! What better way to "lead" than by contributing to the development of others, especially those who are motivated to grow and learn themselves? In my experience, I actually feel that I learn more from the emerging leaders with whom I work than I can contribute back to those who consider me a mentor.

5 *How do I mentor someone?* Be there and be responsive. When you find yourself having repeated contact with someone who is clearly personally motivated to learn from you, do not neglect the opportunity to get to know them a little better, understand their aspirations and personal priorities. It will help you frame the advice you give them to be most compatible with their individual needs. Over time, it is important to stay in touch in order to continue to understand the path and preparation of the individuals seeking mentorship from you. Most importantly, be candid and forthright. A mentoring relationship is not a situation for political correctness. Those who seek your counsel as a mentor need your honest advice and the benefit of your experience, even if that advice is: "Don't go there; you'll be sorry."

Mentoring relationships benefit both individuals. Mentors learn from those they advise, and mentoring other emerging leaders is the essence of leadership. In the long run, it will undoubtedly be one of the most gratifying things you do.

For the mentee, the benefits are equally broad. Mentors provide a diverse perspective and the benefit of experience that may be very different from that of the advisee. Many of us have benefited from the years and breadth of experience of those who have mentored us. Perhaps most importantly, a relationship with a mentor provides a reality check against which you can measure what you think from the opinion of those with more experience whom you respect.

References and Further Reading

Lanser E.G. (2000) Reaping the benefits of mentorship. *Healthcare Executive* **15**(3): 18–23.
Perrone J. (2003) Creating a mentoring culture. *Healthcare Executive* **18**(3): 84–5.

Chapter 19

Launching Other Leaders: Publishing, Speaking, and Advocacy

"We can all be leaders. We can all impact others. We can all leave a legacy. Any of us can choose not to live for ourselves alone, but to give of ourselves in service to others."

Gary Morsch, MD
Family and Emergency Medicine Physician,
U.S. Army Reserves
Founder, Heart to Heart International

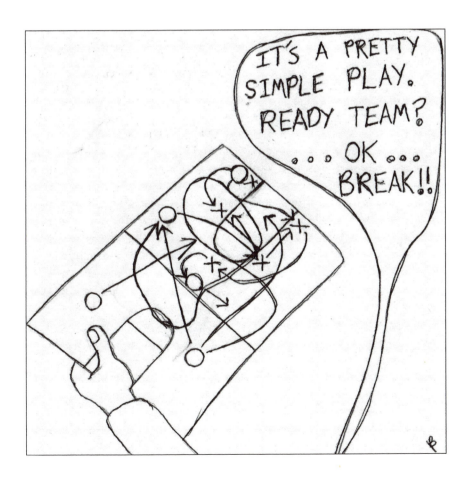

To help other physicians become leaders requires an investment of time, energy, and sometimes financial expenditure to support their development. Certainly, one way of doing this involves personal investment in relationships with the physicians we work with directly.

> "When teaching, it is important to ensure your audience gets the message. Effective presenters don't just show fancy graphics; good speakers make sure their points are clearly conveyed. I even teach courses to help people improve their presentation skills."
>
> Daniel S. Durrie, MD
> Ophthalmologist
> President
> Durrie Vision Center

We can support other physicians' development as leaders by encouraging them to read books, attend workshops, and enroll in educational programs. To extend our influence beyond that relatively limited reach, however, requires that we find means of sharing our insights more broadly. Dr. Durrie continues:

> "Not only am I passionate about contributing to advances in my clinical specialty through my research and speaking, and mentoring other physicians, I am also quite determined to help physicians regain their appropriate role in healthcare, and helping the public understand the leadership contributions that physicians can and do make in their communities. Doctors have a bad image, often times, and too many community leaders are critical of them. Sometimes the tension occurs because of misunderstandings. Physicians are concerned about their declining incomes, so when expected to 'make a difference' by giving money to the ballet, they (rightfully) become frustrated.
>
> Here in my own town, I believe people don't realize the extent to which so many physicians are serving as leaders and contributing to our community. Healthcare represents 14 percent of the gross national product in the United States, but it represents far less than that here in Kansas City. Healthcare organizations are ideal for any community – they do important, 'clean' work, offer valuable services, and provide strong employment opportunities. This town is great in cardiology, ophthalmology, and stroke. **The Kauffman Foundation** does a lot to support entrepreneurial endeavors, but I believe they're missing the boat by not bringing doctors into the initiatives.
>
> It was no accident that nearly all the ophthalmology companies ended up being based in Irvine, California. The community leaders consciously determined to seek them out. In our town, **Cerner Corporation**, and years ago **Marion Laboratories**, each became great healthcare organizations despite of, not because of, this community. I'd like the **Kauffman Foundation**, **Stowers Institute**, **KC Catalyst**, **the Community Foundation** and others to involve doctors and do so in a holistic, comprehensive strategy, not just by focusing on various pieces of the puzzle.

That's why I'm working now to identify a core base of physicians across a variety of clinical specialties who have experience doing research with companies and who really understand product development. For example, **Marilyn Reiner, MD**, has that expertise in neurology and stroke. I know several cardiologists who are involved in research and product development. I'd like to bring together physicians from various specialties and talk about this. I'll ask them 'Does this seem like a good idea? Is it important? Do you want to be involved?' I will be happy to represent the physician community – if they want me to. Imagine the possibilities if the community really knew when someone has an idea in such and such a field, they should call in so and so.

I can help physicians understand how to negotiate equity positions in product development firms. A friend in Colorado Springs taught me a lot about stock options, strike prices, understanding the implications of information such as the number of shares outstanding. More doctors could contribute to medical advances and gain economic advantage and enjoy the intellectual challenge if they were prepared to take the risks by equipping themselves with the knowledge it requires, and by committing to focus their time and energy on it."

Daniel S. Durrie, MD
Ophthalmologist
President
Durrie Vision Center

Some physician leaders actively support the development of physician leaders by publishing books and articles, speaking at conferences and symposia, and through advocacy – championing policies and funding to enable significant progress in this important arena.

One example of how this can be pursued even while maintaining an active clinical practice is provided by Bill Frist, MD. Even while he was busy building the transplant program at Vanderbilt University Medical Center, Dr. Frist set aside time in order to educate other physicians (and patients) about the importance of organ donation. In his book *Transplant* (1989), Dr. Frist describes how he used to travel around the country giving "little talks" to community hospitals, schools, civic groups and community clubs. He did so to champion his cause by building awareness among physicians and patients regarding the progress being made in transplantation and the urgent need for more organ donations.

> " . . . while I would much rather have spent my time with patients, I felt that no one could present the case of donor need to other physicians as well as one of their own. And it did not hurt for potential donors to hear a surgeon talk about the organ shortage. I was the one who watched waiting people die; I felt an obligation to speak for this group. Since closing the gap between available organs and dying recipients was essential if transplantation was to reach its lifesaving potential, I told myself I had no choice but to be a major part of the education project. The talk varied a bit given the nature of the audience . . . but my main points were always the same. I gave a brief history of transplantation . . . I also usually included the legal and political history of the field, which

was especially important to the physicians ... I always discussed the goals of transplantation, the quality of life issues ... I always stressed that the therapy was viable and effective, that patients lived full and productive lives ... I would mention costs, pointing out that heart transplants were expensive, but that those costs were coming down rapidly as more experience was gained ... I also drove home the team approach of transplantation and showed a slide with the patient and family at the center of a circle made up of the transplant surgeon, the referring physicians, social workers, psychologists, nurses, physical therapists, financial counselors, pathologists, and community support groups. I made the point that the cure wasn't the surgery, but the overall commitment to the continued care of these recipients. Sometimes I would turn to the future, showing the LVAD [left ventric-ular assist device, or 'balloon pump'] and explaining its uses, describing how we were trying to increase the specificity of immunosuppression and look for a less invasive alternative to the frequent heart biopsies. I also suggested to the audience that they consider the benefits of a resumed-consent law that might alleviate some of the donor shortage. I always ended with the donor shortage, hitting that point hardest of all ... I talked about donor cards, how important they were, not so much as legal documents, but as indications of a willingness to donate ... And finally I gave the telephone number for UNOS, a number they could call 24 hours a day to ask any question whatsoever about organ donation ... Then I stepped back and waited for the questions."

William H. Frist, MD
Cardiothoracic and General Surgeon and
Senate Majority Leader, U.S. Congress
in his book *Transplant* (1989)

Another example of ways physicians can have an impact beyond that of caring for individual patients is explained by Dr. Jessee:

"The number of physicians who belong to the Medical Group Management Association continues to grow. They are involved in all of our key focus areas, including education, research, advocacy, creden-tialing, alliances, and professional networking. Interestingly, most physicians tell us they did not join MGMA to exert influence as leaders in the organization, but rather to take advantage of our many resources they feel they need in their practices. For example, our physician compensation data and our many educational products and programs are quite helpful for any healthcare professional – clinician or adminis-trator – who seeks to differentiate best performing operational practices from those that are just average, or even struggling.

MGMA has also been fortunate to have the involvement of some outstanding physicians who have served as volunteer leaders in our organization. For example, Michael L. Nochomovitz, MD, a pulmonolo-gist at University Hospital in Cleveland, joined MGMA because of the relevance he found in our data on how physicians get paid and how much they get paid. He soon became active on our national survey committee and then on our educational committee. Realizing he wanted to help shape public health policy, Dr. Nochomovitz became even more involved with MGMA, and now serves on our Board of Directors. In fact, we've noticed that physicians, more than administrators, often join MGMA in order to help influence health policy."

William F. Jessee, MD, FACMPE

Pediatric, Preventive and Emergency Medicine Physician

President

Medical Group Management Association

Though some physicians may feel they are too busy to help develop other leaders, Dr. Littles points out that advocacy will benefit the leader, not just those the leader is seeking to serve.

> "There are many ways for physicians to become leaders on behalf of their patients, or to enhance the delivery of healthcare overall. Advocacy and education are two key ways.
>
> Being actively involved in your community is important also. Community involvement makes you accessible to people, and enables them to see you as a whole person, not just a physician. Physician leaders will also benefit from active involvement in your local medical society, and in the hospital or medical group staff where you work. I truly believe that as we focus on helping others, we ultimately benefit in some way."

Alma Littles, MD

Associate Dean of Academic Affairs, Department of Family

Medicine

Florida State University

References and Further Reading

Curry W. (1994) *New Leadership in Health Care Management: The physician executive*. Tampa: American College of Physician Executives Press.

Epstein R.M. and Hundert E.M. (2002) Defining and assessing professional competence. *The Journal of the American Medical Association* **287**(2): 226–35.

Fox R.D. and Bennett N.L. (1998) Learning and change: Implications for continuing medical education. *British Medical Journal* **316**: 466–8.

Frist W.H. (1989) *Transplant: a heart surgeon's account of the life-and-death dramas of the new medicine*. New York: The Atlantic Monthly Press.

Moon J. (2004) Using reflective learning to improve the impact of short courses and workshops. *Journal of Continuing Education in the Health Professions* **24**: 4–11.

Nash D.B., Markson L.E., Howell S., and Hildreth E.A. (1993) Evaluating the competence of physicians in practice: From peer review to performance assessment. *Academic Medicine* **68**: 19S–22S.

Reinertsen J.L. (1998) Physicians as leaders in the improvement of health care systems. *Annals of Internal Medicine* **128**: 833–8.

Schultz F.C. (2004) Who should lead a healthcare organization: MDs or MBAs? *Journal of Healthcare Management* **49**(2): 103–17.

Steinert Y., Nasmith L., McLeod P.J., and Conochie L. (2003) A teaching scholars program to develop leaders in medical education. *Academic Medicine* **78**: 142–9.

Williams S.J. (2001) Training needs for physician leaders. *The Journal of Health Administration Education* **19**(2): 195–202.

Section V

Your LeaderLauncher™ Tool Kit

We've designed this section of the book to serve as your own personal **Leader Launcher Tool Kit™**. And more resources are available at our website: www.PhysiciansAsLeaders.com. It includes an array of questions that can be used to *assess* your physician leadership *capacity*, to *enhance* your physician leadership *effectiveness, and* to *set and achieve goals*. In other words, tools to help you – and those you lead – achieve truly remarkable results.

You see, we aren't content to have you simply read about leading physicians. We hope you'll actually take steps to use the practical guidance we're providing in this book. Why? Because we're confident that you will enhance your effectiveness and fulfillment in the work that you do as you gain the insights, skills,

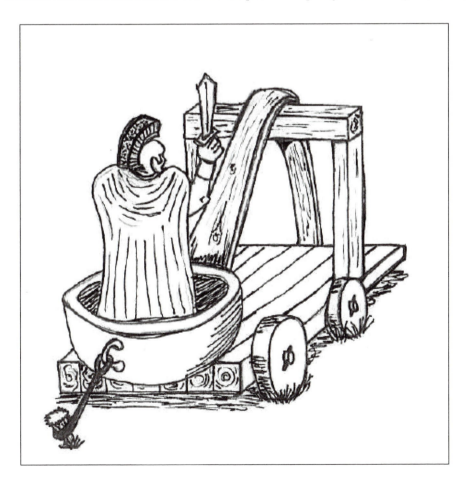

relationships, and experiences you need to become the physician leader you know you're capable of being.

You'll find that these assessment instruments can be quite useful. Simply by answering the questions and reflecting on your responses, you will gain insights regarding your:

- current:
  - perceptions, attitudes, or beliefs
  - attributes, traits, styles, preferences, interests, values, motives or characteristics
  - knowledge, skills, abilities, behaviors, or habits
- need for improvement in one or more areas of responsibility
- progress made in improving your proficiency level or performance
- opportunities to practice or reinforce various skills, behaviors or attitudes.

To grow and succeed, leaders need a realistic understanding of their behaviors, motivators and competencies. The brief assessments on the pages that follow are not fully validated, professionally administered instruments, but simply tools for reflection.

If you would like to learn more about yourself, we suggest you complete assessment instruments offered through a certified coaching professional. For more information, you may wish to call The KENNA Company at (816) 943–0868 or visit www.kennacompany.com/physicians.pdf. Joe McKenna, President of The KENNA Company and husband of Mindi McKenna, has over 30 years' experience working with professionals inside and outside of healthcare.

Leadership COMPETENCE Assessment

Instructions

Read each of the statements in the left column and indicate the extent to which you (or whomever you are assessing) *currently* exhibit those leadership practices by circling the corresponding number to the right of each statement. Reflect on the insights revealed from your perceptions.

	Have not appreciated the importance of this	Have sought to do this on rare occasions	Do this at times, but not well or often	Do this fairly well when focused on it	Do this routinely and reasonably well	Do this consistently and effortlessly	Focus on helping others do this well
Keep up with ongoing developments in the field through reading, discussions with colleagues, continuing medical education, and other activities that support lifelong learning	1	2	3	4	5	6	7
Involvement in medical specialty societies and professional associations – for continued growth and for contribution to others' development	1	2	3	4	5	6	7
Advocate through comments and behavior a strong, unwavering commitment to excellence	1	2	3	4	5	6	7
Contribute to the field through the conduct, application, and dissemination of new learning	1	2	3	4	5	6	7
Translate new learning into practical guidance for application by novice and emerging leaders	1	2	3	4	5	6	7
Practice new behaviors, attitudes, and skills with focused attention toward increasing mastery	1	2	3	4	5	6	7
Recognition by experts as having significantly impacted the field by affecting positive change in others' behavior	1	2	3	4	5	6	7

Leadership CHARACTER Assessment

Instructions

Read each of the statements in the left column and indicate the extent to which you (or whomever you are assessing) *currently* exhibit those leadership practices by circling the corresponding number to the right of each statement. Reflect on the insights revealed from your perceptions.

	Have not appreciated the importance of this	Have sought to do this on rare occasions	Do this at times, but not well or often	Do this fairly well when focused on it	Do this routinely and reasonably well	Do this consistently and effortlessly	Focus on helping others do this well
Behave honestly and ethically regardless of personal cost	1	2	3	4	5	6	7
Express genuine concern for others' well-being	1	2	3	4	5	6	7
Admit mistakes and apologize as appropriate	1	2	3	4	5	6	7
Accept responsibility for decisions and actions and for their consequences	1	2	3	4	5	6	7
Persist despite obstacles and setbacks	1	2	3	4	5	6	7
Maintain optimism and a sense of humor	1	2	3	4	5	6	7
Avoid conflicts of interest or compromises that result from competing obligations	1	2	3	4	5	6	7
Exhibit dependability, fairness, generosity, confidence, humility, patience, and wisdom	1	2	3	4	5	6	7

Leadership VISION Assessment

Instructions

Read each of the statements in the left column and indicate the extent to which you (or whomever you are assessing) *currently* exhibit those leadership practices by circling the corresponding number to the right of each statement. Reflect on the insights revealed from your perceptions.

	Have not appreciated the importance of this	Have sought to do this on rare occasions	Do this at times, but not well or often	Do this fairly well when focused on it	Do this routinely and reasonably well	Do this consistently and effortlessly	Focus on helping others do this well
Maintain awareness and curiosity about unfamiliar fields, perspectives, bodies of knowledge, and experiences	1	2	3	4	5	6	7
Notice trends, unmet needs or changes that signal potential opportunities or threats	1	2	3	4	5	6	7
Collect information from diverse sources	1	2	3	4	5	6	7
Recognize and interpret implications of information and events	1	2	3	4	5	6	7
Focus on future possibilities, identifying, and exploring previously unaddressed considerations	1	2	3	4	5	6	7
Devise ways to achieve the interests of all involved	1	2	3	4	5	6	7

Leadership COMMUNICATION Assessment

Instructions

Read each of the statements in the left column and indicate the extent to which you (or whomever you are assessing) *currently* exhibit those leadership practices by circling the corresponding number to the right of each statement. Reflect on the insights revealed from your perceptions.

	Have not appreciated the importance of this	Have sought to do this on rare occasions	Do this at times, but not well or often	Do this fairly well when focused on it	Do this routinely and reasonably well	Do this consistently and effortlessly	Focus on helping others do this well
Listen attentively, noticing what others convey through what they say and what they do not say	1	2	3	4	5	6	7
Ask questions to explore, clarify, confirm, or refute current understanding	1	2	3	4	5	6	7
Propose ideas and suggest new approaches	1	2	3	4	5	6	7
Instruct others with clear and comprehensive explanations	1	2	3	4	5	6	7
Express beliefs and opinions directly	1	2	3	4	5	6	7
Persuade others through compelling, convincing messages, focusing not on the mere transfer of information but on actual transformation	1	2	3	4	5	6	7
Encourage discussion and debate, even when disagreements arise, in order to increase understanding and involvement	1	2	3	4	5	6	7
Use appropriate means and media to communicate with optimal frequency, reach, impact, and cost-effectiveness	1	2	3	4	5	6	7
Inform others of news in a timely, accurate, and appropriate manner, even when the news may be unfavorably received	1	2	3	4	5	6	7

Leadership COMMITMENT Assessment

Instructions

Read each of the statements in the left column and indicate the extent to which you (or whomever you are assessing) *currently* exhibit those leadership practices by circling the corresponding number to the right of each statement. Reflect on the insights revealed from your perceptions.

	Have not appreciated the importance of this	Have sought to do this on rare occasions	Do this at times, but not well or often	Do this fairly well when focused on it	Do this routinely and reasonably well	Do this consistently and effortlessly	Focus on helping others do this well
Invite others to participate in tasks, fueling their enthusiasm by appealing to their values and interests	1	2	3	4	5	6	7
Welcome newcomers, providing needed information and opportunities for interaction	1	2	3	4	5	6	7
Explicitly describe how attainment of collective goals will enable attainment of individual goals	1	2	3	4	5	6	7
Demonstrate confidence in others by sharing decision-making authority	1	2	3	4	5	6	7
Persevere in commitment to the goals despite distractions, resource constraints and other obstacles that may arise	1	2	3	4	5	6	7
Show interest in the hopes, concerns, values, interests, and needs of others	1	2	3	4	5	6	7
Celebrate individual and collective successes with tangible rewards and other forms of recognition	1	2	3	4	5	6	7
Refrain from expressing personal views until others have had opportunity to contribute their perspectives	1	2	3	4	5	6	7

Leadership COHESION Assessment

Instructions

Read each of the statements in the left column and indicate the extent to which you (or whomever you are assessing) *currently* exhibit those leadership practices by circling the corresponding number to the right of each statement. Reflect on the insights revealed from your perceptions.

	Have not appreciated the importance of this	Have sought to do this on rare occasions	Do this at times, but not well or often	Do this fairly well when focused on it	Do this routinely and reasonably well	Do this consistently and effortlessly	Focus on helping others do this well
Disagree without being disagreeable, by expressing contrary views without criticizing other individuals	1	2	3	4	5	6	7
Share resources and help others succeed	1	2	3	4	5	6	7
Thank others and acknowledge their contributions	1	2	3	4	5	6	7
Align tasks in accordance with individuals' unique interests and diverse abilities	1	2	3	4	5	6	7
Identify common ground and shared values among individuals	1	2	3	4	5	6	7
Arbitrate disputes and resolve issues by facilitating agreements that benefit all involved	1	2	3	4	5	6	7
Discourage non-cooperation and unhealthy competition by confronting it directly when it occurs	1	2	3	4	5	6	7
Request advice, suggestions, and help	1	2	3	4	5	6	7
Put others at ease by offering reassurance, guidance, and appreciation for their involvement	1	2	3	4	5	6	7

Leadership DECISION MAKING Assessment

Instructions

Read each of the statements in the left column and indicate the extent to which you (or whomever you are assessing) *currently* exhibit those leadership practices by circling the corresponding number to the right of each statement. Reflect on the insights revealed from your perceptions.

	Have not appreciated the importance of this	Have sought to do this on rare occasions	Do this at times, but not well or often	Do this fairly well when focused on it	Do this routinely and reasonably well	Do this consistently and effortlessly	Focus on helping others do this well
Establish criteria by which priorities will be determined and options will be evaluated	1	2	3	4	5	6	7
Establish processes for implementing decisions that enable ways of monitoring their effectiveness and adapting as appropriate	1	2	3	4	5	6	7
Set specific, measurable, actionable, realistic, time-delineated goals	1	2	3	4	5	6	7
Generate and investigate options with consideration for their likely impact on all involved	1	2	3	4	5	6	7
Analyze and synthesize information, maintaining a willingness to alter views or processes if appropriate	1	2	3	4	5	6	7
Review and discuss mistakes or mishaps in order to learn from them	1	2	3	4	5	6	7
Involve others in decision making by soliciting their ideas, inviting their reactions, and informing them of new developments	1	2	3	4	5	6	7
Recognize the futility of trying to keep up with all available information; instead, establish a system for filtering inputs according to the results sought	1	2	3	4	5	6	7

Leadership ACTION TAKING Assessment

Instructions

Read each of the statements in the left column and indicate the extent to which you (or whomever you are assessing) *currently* exhibit those leadership practices by circling the corresponding number to the right of each statement. Reflect on the insights revealed from your perceptions.

	Have not appreciated the importance of this	Have sought to do this on rare occasions	Do this at times, but not well or often	Do this fairly well when focused on it	Do this routinely and reasonably well	Do this consistently and effortlessly	Focus on helping others do this well
Allocate resources in accordance with agreed upon values and priorities	1	2	3	4	5	6	7
Achieve goals within time and resource constraints	1	2	3	4	5	6	7
Encourage development of new skills by allowing opportunities to practice under the guidance of someone with more experience or expertise	1	2	3	4	5	6	7
Confront wrongdoing despite personal repercussions that may result	1	2	3	4	5	6	7
Resolve conflicts by identifying common ground and negotiating mutually beneficial agreements	1	2	3	4	5	6	7
Empower others to achieve results by addressing obstacles and providing necessary resources	1	2	3	4	5	6	7
Explore and test new approaches to tackle occasional and ongoing challenges	1	2	3	4	5	6	7
Establish coalitions of support, forums and processes to achieve the goals	1	2	3	4	5	6	7
Represent the interests of others, by advocating on their behalf	1	2	3	4	5	6	7

Leadership RESILIENCE Assessment

Instructions

Read each of the statements in the left column and indicate the extent to which you (or whomever you are assessing) *currently* exhibit those leadership practices by circling the corresponding number to the right of each statement. Reflect on the insights revealed from your perceptions.

	Have not appreciated the importance of this	Have sought to do this on rare occasions	Do this at times, but not well or often	Do this fairly well when focused on it	Do this routinely and reasonably well	Do this consistently and effortlessly	Focus on helping others do this well
Recognize that it is not possible to know, do or review everything and so establish criteria and processes for filtering inputs in support of intended results	1	2	3	4	5	6	7
Set and convey boundaries regarding non-negotiable commitments of time, energy, or attention	1	2	3	4	5	6	7
Maintain commitment to agreed upon values and priorities in alignment with the vision and goals	1	2	3	4	5	6	7
Conserve energy and resources by focusing attention and action toward key priorities, surrendering control of non-essentials	1	2	3	4	5	6	7
Resist the temptation to apply resources, energy, or attention to tasks or opportunities that do not support the vision and goals	1	2	3	4	5	6	7

Leadership RENEWAL Assessment

Instructions

Read each of the statements in the left column and indicate the extent to which you (or whomever you are assessing) *currently* exhibit those leadership practices by circling the corresponding number to the right of each statement. Reflect on the insights revealed from your perceptions.

	Have not appreciated the importance of this	Have sought to do this on rare occasions	Do this at times, but not well or often	Do this fairly well when focused on it	Do this routinely and reasonably well	Do this consistently and effortlessly	Focus on helping others do this well
Break away from routine responsibilities to engage in activities that replenish energy and perspective	1	2	3	4	5	6	7
Affirm and appreciate the intrinsically gratifying aspects of the work	1	2	3	4	5	6	7
Let go of outdated, counterproductive attitudes, beliefs, expectations, thoughts, and behaviors	1	2	3	4	5	6	7
Re-commit to the values and vision by remembering how and why they were originally established or agreed upon	1	2	3	4	5	6	7
Seek exposure to diverse and unfamiliar ideas, people, experiences and approaches in order to learn and grow	1	2	3	4	5	6	7
Re-design processes to adapt to changing realities and possibilities	1	2	3	4	5	6	7

References and Further Reading

Adrienne C. (1998) *The Purpose of Your Life: finding your place in the world using synchronicity, intuition, and uncommon sense.* New York: William Morrow & Company, Inc.

Albanese M.A., Snow M.H., Skochelak S.E., Huggett K.N., and Farrell P.M. (2003) Assessing personal qualities in medical school admissions. *Academic Medicine* **78**: 313–321.

Albanese R. (1989) Competency-based management education. *Journal of Management Development* **8**(2): 66–76.

Alcorn, Baum, Diamond and Stein (1996) *The Human Cost of a Management Failure.* New York: Quorum Books.

Allen D. (2003) *Ready for Anything: 52 productivity principles for work and life.* New York: Penguin Group.

Anderson D.J., Moran J.W., Brightman B.K., and Scheur B.S. (1998) *Transforming Health Care: action strategies for health care leaders.* Chicago: American Hospital Publishing, Inc.

Andreas C. and Andreas T. (1994) *Core Transformation: reaching the wellspring within.* Moab, UT: Real People Press.

Anonymous (1997) Leadership survey. *Hospitals & Health Networks* **71**(15): 26.

Anonymous (2002) Physician leadership: More than clinical excellence. *Health Leaders* Sponsored Supplement, October. RT2–RT15.

Anonymous (2001) Where did DISC start? (n.d.) Retrieved November 28, 2001, from www.conistondisc.demon.co.uk/what-is-tti-disc.htm.

Appleby J. (2002) Doctors earn MBAs to tackle ills of health system. *USA Today* **July 3**: 1–2.

Arond-Thomas M. (2004) Resilient leadership for challenging times. *Physician Executive* **vol**: 18–21.

Arygyris C. (1991) Teaching smart people how to learn. *Harvard Business Review* **69**(3): 99–109.

Asch E., Saltzberg D., and Lakser S. (1998) Reinforcement of self-directed learning and the development of professional attitudes through peer and self-assessment. *Academic Medicine* **73**: 575.

Atchison T.A. and Bujak J. (2000) *Leading Transformational Change.* Oak Park, IL: Atchison Consulting Group.

Atchison T.A. (2001) *Leading Transformational Change: the physician-executive partnership.* Chicago: Health Administration Press.

Atkins S. (2001) The LIFO Success Profile. (n. d.). Retrieved November 28, 2001, from www.stuartatkins.com/successprofile.asp.

Atkins S. (2001) *The Name of Your Game: four game plans for success at home and at work.* Los Angeles: BCon LIFO® International, Inc.

Austin C.J. and Boxerman S.B. (2003) *Information Systems for Healthcare Management.* Chicago: Health Administration Press.

Baber A. and Waymon L. (1992) *Great Connections: small talk and networking for businesspeople.* Manassas Park, VA: Impact Publications.

Babka J.C. (1997) The most important role a healthcare executive can play in easing this transition to managed care is that of a coach. *Healthcare Executive* **12**(3): 49.

Badaracco J.L., Jr. (2002) *Leading Quietly: an unorthodox guide to doing the right thing.* Boston: Harvard Business School Publishing.

Baker S.K. (1998) *Managing Patient Expectations: the art of finding and keeping loyal patients.* San Francisco: Jossey-Bass Publishers.

Baldwin G. (2001) Putting up a new shingle: Physician entrepreneurs learn that starting a dot-com company involves long hours and high risk. *Internet Health Care Magazine* **June**: 26–32.

Barnett P.A. and Gotlieb I.H. (1988) Psychosocial functioning and depression: Distinguishing among antecedents, concomitants, and consequences. *Psychological Bulletin* **104**: 97–126.

Barrick M.R. and Mount M.K. (1991) The big five personality dimensions and job performance: A meta-analysis. *Personnel Psychology* **44**: 1–26.

Barsky A.J. (1988) The paradox of health. *New England Journal of Medicine* **318**: 414–8.

Barzansky B. and Etzel S.I. (2003) Educational programs in US medical schools, 2002–2003. *The Journal of the American Medical Association* **290**(9): 1190–1196.

Barzansky B. and Etzel S.I. (2002) Educational programs in US medical schools, 2001–2002. *The Journal of the American Medical Association* **288**(9): 1067–1072.

Basile C.M. (1998) Advance directives and advocacy in end-of-life decisions. *Nurse Practitioner* **23**(5): 44–6, 54, 57–60.

Becher E.C. and Chassin M.R. (2002) Taking health care back: The physician's role in quality improvement. *Academic Medicine* **77**: 953–962.

Beckley E.T. (2003) Movers and shakers: These physician executives are changing society and the system. *Modern Physician* **vol**(no): May, 26–27.

Beckman H. (1994) The doctor-patient relationship and malpractice: Lessons from plaintiff depositions. *Archives of Internal Medicine* **154**(12): 1365–670.

Beckman H.B. and Frankel R.M. (1984) The effect of physician behavior on the collection of data. *Annals of Internal Medicine* **101**(5): 692–6.

Begun J.W. (1985) Managing with professionals in a changing health care environment. *Medical Care Review* **42**(1): 3–10.

Begun J.W. and Luke R.D. (2001) Reshaping the health professions in the new marketplace. *Advances in Health Care Management* **2**: 189–213.

Bell A.H. and Smith D.M. (2003) *Learning Team Skills*. New Jersey: Prentice Hall.

Belton D.G. and Baron C.R. (1987) Profile of the HMO medical director. *MGM Journal* **34**(2): 17–22.

Benbassat J., Baumal R., Borkan J.M., and Ber R. (2003) Overcoming barriers to teaching the behavioral and social sciences to medical students. *Academic Medicine* **78**: 372–80.

Benedict G.S. (1996) *The Development and Management of Medical Groups*. Englewood, CO: Medical Group Management Association.

Benko L. (2000) New leaders drive managed care. *Modern Healthcare* **March 13**, vol: 28–32.

Benson H. (1996) *Timeless Healing: the power and biology of belief*. New York: Scribner.

Benner P. (1984) *From Novice to Expert*. Menlo Park, CA: Addison-Wesley.

Bennis W.G. (1987) Four competencies of great leaders. *Executive Excellence* **vol**: (12)

Bennis W.G. (1989) *On Becoming a Leader*. Boston: Addison-Wesley.

Bennis W.G. and Cummings T.G. (2001) *The Future of Leadership: today's top leadership thinkers*. San Francisco: Jossey-Bass Publishers.

Bennis W.G. and Nanus B. (1997) *Leaders: strategies for taking charge*. New York: HarperCollins Publishers, Inc.

Bennis W.G. and Townsend R. (1995) *Reinventing Leadership: strategies to empower the organization*. New York: William Morrow and Company, Inc.

Berger W. (1999) Physician leadership in the new millennium. *Annals of Allergy, Asthma, and Immunology* **82**(6): 507–10.

Berwick D.M. (2004) *Escape Fire*. San Francisco: Jossey-Bass Publishers.

Berwick D.M. (2003) Disseminating innovations in health care. *The Journal of the American Medical Association* **289**: 1969–1975.

Berwick D.M., Godfrey B. and Roessner J. (2004) *Curing Health Care: new strategies for quality improvement*. San Francisco: Jossey-Bass Publishers..

Berwick D.M. (1998) Developing and testing changes in delivery of care. *Annals of Internal Medicine*, **128**(8): 651–6.

Berwick D.M. (1997) Medical associations: Guilds or leaders? [Editorial]. *British Journal of Medicine* **314**: 1564–5.

Berwick D.M. (1994) Eleven worthy aims for clinical leadership of health systems reform. *Journal of the American Medical Association* **272**: 797–802.

Berwick D.M. (1992) Heal thyself or heal thy system: Can doctors help improve medical care? *Quality of Medical Care*, **1**(Suppl): S1–S7.

Berwick D.M. and Nolan T.W. (1998) Physicians as leaders in improving health care: A new series in *Annals of Internal Medicine*. *Annals of Internal Medicine* **128**(4): 289–92.

Betson C. (1989) Physician managers: A description of their job in hospitals. *Hospital & Health Services Administration* **34**(3): 353–69.

Betson C.L. (1986) *Managing the Medical Enterprise: a study of physician managers*. Ann Arbor, MI: UMI Research Press.

Bettner M. and Collins F. (1987) Physicians and administrators: Inducing collaboration. *Hospital & Health Services Administration* **32**(2): 151–60.

Bialk J.L. (2004) Ethical guidelines for assisting patients with end-of-life decision making. *Medsurg Nursing* **13**(2): 87–90.

Biggs R.R. (2002) *Burn Brightly Without Burning Out: balancing your career with the rest of your life*. Tennessee: Thomas Nelson Publishing.

Binius T. (1998) Medical business acumen: The growing number of physicians seeking business skills can find MBA programs tailored to their needs. *AMNews* **November 23/30**.

Birrer R.B. (2002) The physician leader in health care: What qualities does a doctor need to be an effective organizational leader? *Health Progress* **83**(6): 27–30.

Birrer R.B. (2003) Becoming a physician executive: To be effective leaders, clinicians must first adopt a new mind-set. *Health Progress* **84**(1): 16–20.

Blair J.D., Fottler M.D., and Savage G.T. (2001) *Advances in Health Care Management*. New York: Elsevier Science Inc.

Blanchard K. and Bowles S. (1998) *Gung Ho! Turn on the people in any organization*. New York: William Morrow & Company.

Blanchard K. and Johnson S. (1983) *The One Minute Manager*. New York: William Morrow & Company.

Bodenheimer and Casalino. (1999) The unintended consequences of measuring quality on the quality of medical care. *New England Journal of Medicine* **341**(15): 1147–50.

Bogdewic S.P., Baxley E.G., and Jamison P.K. (1997) Leadership and organizational skills in academic medicine. *Society of Teachers of Family Medicine* **29**(4): 262–5.

Bolman L.G. (1995) *Leading with Soul: an uncommon journey of spirit*. San Francisco: Jossey-Bass, Inc.

Bolton R. and Bolton D.G. (1984) *Social Style/Management Style: developing productive work relationships*. New York: American Management Association.

Bonnstetter B.J., Suiter J.I., and Widrick R.J. (2001) *DISC: A reference manual*. Scottsdale, AZ: Target Training International, Ltd.

Bottles K. (2001) The good leaders. *Physician Executive* **March/April**: 74–6.

Bowe C.M., Lahey L., Armstrong E., and Kegan R. Questioning the "Big Assumptions" Part I: Addressing personal contradictions that impede professional development. *Medical Education* **37**: 715–22.

Bowe C.M., Lahey L., Armstrong E., and Kegan R. Questioning the "Big Assumptions" Part II: Recognizing organizational contradictions that impede institutional change. *Medical Education* **37**: 723–33.

Bowlby J. (1973) *Attachment and Loss, vol. 2: separation: anxiety and anger*. NY: Basic Books.

Bowlby J. (1980) *Attachment and Loss, vol. 3: sadness and depression*. NY: Basic Books.

Boyle P.J., DuBose E.R., Ellingson S.J., Guinn D.E., and McCurdy D.B. (2001) *Organizational Ethics in Health Care: principles, cases, and practical solutions*. San Francisco: Jossey-Bass.

Bradford and Cohen. (1984) *Managing for Excellence*. New York: Wiley & Sons.

Brand P.W. and Yancey P. (1993) *The Gift of Pain*. Grand Rapids, MI: Zondervan Publishing House.

Braithwaite J. (2004) A empirically-based model for clinician-managers' behavioural routines. *Journal of Health Organisation and Management* 18(4): 240–61.

Bridges W. (1991) *Managing Transitions: making the most of change*. Sherbrooke, Quebec: Perseus Publications.

Brooke P.P., Jr., Hudak, R P., Finstuen K., and Trounson J. (1998) Management competencies required in ambulatory settings. *Physician Executive* 24(5): 32–8.

Brooks K. (1994) The hospital CEO: Meeting the conflicting demands of the board and physicians. *Hospital & Health Services Administration* 39(4), 471–85.

Buchbinder S. (1999) Estimates of costs of primary care physician turnover. *American Journal of Managed Care*. 5(11): 1431–8.

Buckingham and Coffman. (1999) *First break all the rules: what the world's greatest managers do differently*. New York: Simon & Schuster.

Bujak J.S. (1998) Can physicians lead other physicians into the future? *Physician Executive* **September/October**.

Burton R. (ed.) (1998) *The Physician Leader's Guide*. 2nd ed. Alexandria, VA: Capitol Publications, Inc.

Callahan D. (1998) *False Hopes: why America's quest for perfect health is a recipe for failure*. New York: Simon & Schuster.

Calloway J. (2005) *Indispensable: how to become the company your customers can't live without*. New York: John Wiley & Sons.

Campbell C.M., Parboosing J., and Gondoz T. (1999) Study of the factors influencing the stimulus to learning recorded by physicians keeping a learning portfolio. *Journal of Continuing Education in the Health Professions* 19: 15–24.

Campbell J.D., Trapnell P.D., Heine S.J., Katz I.M., Lavallee L.F., and Lehman D.R. (1996) Self-concept clarity: Measurement, personality correlates, and cultural boundaries. *Journal of Personality and Social Psychology* 70: 141–56.

Canfield J. and Switzer J. (2005) *The Success Principles: how to get from where you are to where you want to be*. New York: HarperCollins Publishing.

Chapman T.W. and Confessorre S. (2002) The dominant influence of social context on CEO learning in health care: A challenge to traditional management continuing education and development. *Journal of Health Administration Education* 20(2): 123–34.

Chapman T.W. and Confessore S.J. (2000) Learning at the top. *Health Forum Journal* 43(2): 56–8.

Chappelow C. and Leslie J.B. (2001) *Keeping Your Career On Track: twenty success strategies*. Greensboro, NC: Center for Creative Leadership.

Chin E.L. (ed.) (2003) *This Side of Doctoring: reflections from women in medicine*. Oxford: Oxford University Press.

Christensen C.M. (1997) *The Innovator's Dilemma*. Boston: Harvard Business School Press.

Christensen C.M. and Armstrong E.G. (1998) Disruptive technologies: A credible threat to leading programs in continuing medical education? *Journal of Continuing Education in the Health Professions*. 18: 69–80.

Christensen C.M., Bohmer R.M., and Kenagy J. (2000) Will disruptive innovations cure health care? *Harvard Business Review* **September/October**: 102–17.

Christensen C.M. and Raynor M.E. (2003) Why hard-nosed executives should care about management theory. *Harvard Business Review* 81(9): 66–74.

Clarke-Epstein C. (2002) *78 Important Questions Every Leader Should Ask and Answer*. New York: AMACOM, division of the AMA.

Clement D. and Wan T. (1997) Mastering health care executive education: Creating transformational competence. *Journal of Health Administration Education* **15**: 267–73.

Clement J.P., Dodd-McCue D., White K.R., Clement D.G., and Mick S.S. (2001) Going the distance: The evolution of VCU's executive distance learning program over 12 years. *Journal of Health Administration Education* **19**(1): 33–50.

Cockerill T. (1995) Managerial competencies: Fact or fiction. *Business Strategy Review* **6**: 1–12.

Coddington D.C., Fischer E.A., Moore K.D., and Clarke R.L. (2000) *Beyond Managed Care: how consumers and technology are changing the future of health care.* San Francisco: Jossey-Bass.

Cohn L. (2000) Becoming a surgical leader. *Journal of Thoracic and Cardiovascular Surgery* **119**(4 Pt 2): S42–44.

Cohn R. (1988) Hospital management's linchpin: The medical director. *Physician Executive* **14**(2): 18–20.

Coile R.C., Jr. (2002) *The Paperless Hospital: healthcare in a digital age.* Chicago: Health Administration Press.

Coile R.C., Jr. (1996) Leaders of the future: Seven trends for 21st century health care executives. *Russ Coile's Health Trends* **9**(2): 1–6.

Collins J. (1994) *Built To Last: successful habits of visionary companies.* New York: Harper Business Essentials.

Collins J. (2001) *Good To Great: why some companies make the leap and others don't.* New York: HarperCollins Publishers.

Cordes D. (1988) Management roles for physicians: Training residents for the reality. *Journal of Occupational Medicine* **30**(11): 863–7.

Counte M.A. and J.F. Newman (2002) Competency-based health services management education: Contemporary issues and emerging challenges. *Journal of Health Administration Education* **20**(2): 113–22.

Covey S.R. (2004) *The Eighth Habit: from effectiveness to greatness.* New York: Free Press, a division of Simon & Schuster.

Covey S.R. (1992) *Principle-centered Leadership.* New York: Simon & Schuster.

Covey S.R. (1989) *The Seven Habits of Highly Effective People.* New York: Simon & Schuster Inc.

Covey S.R., Merrill A.R., and Merrill R.R. (1994) *First Things First: to live, to love, to learn, to leave a legacy.* New York: Simon & Schuster.

Crooks G. (2000) *Creating Covenants: healing health care in the new millennium.* Old Lyme, CT: Medical Vision Press.

Cummings K. (1998) Building trust in contentious times. In: LeTourneau B. and Curry W. *In Search of Physician Leadership.* Chicago: Health Administration Press

Curry W. (1994) *New Leadership in Health Care Management: Physician Executive.* Tampa: American College of Physician Executives Press.

Daaleman T.P. and Nease D.E. (1994) Patient attitudes regarding physician inquiry into spiritual and religious issues. *Journal of Family Practice* **36**: 564–8.

Daft R.L. (2002) *The Leadership Experience.* 2nd edn. Orlando: Harcourt, Inc.

Daft R.L. and Lengel R.H. (2000) *Fusion Leadership: unlocking the subtle forces that change people and organizations.* San Francisco: Berrett-Koehler Publishers.

Dagi T.F. (1995) Prayer, piety, and professional propriety: limits on religious expression in hospitals. *Journal of Clinical Ethics* **6**: 274–9.

Dalston J.W. and Bishop P. (1995) Health care executive education and training. *Journal of Health Administration Education,* **13**(3): 437–52.

Damasio A.R. (1994) *Descartes' Error: emotion, reason, and the human brain.* NY: GP Putnam's Sons.

Darling J., Walker E., and McKenna M.K. (2002) Keys to Organizational Excellence: Leadership Values and Strategies. *The Journal of Business and Society* **15**(2): 132–47.

Darling J.R. and Walker W.E. (2001) Effective conflict management: Use of the behavioral style model. *The Leadership and Organization Development Journal* **22**(5): 230–42.

Darves B. (2001) A growing number of physicians are finding satisfaction, reaping rewards by becoming physician executives. *NEJM CareerCenter* **June 20**.

Daugherty R.M., Jr. (1998) Leading Among Leaders: The dean in today's medical school. *Academic Medicine* **73**: 649–53.

Davis D.A. and Fox R.D. (eds.) (1994) *The Physician as Learner: linking research to practice.* Chicago, IL: American Medical Association.

Davis D.A., Lindsay E.A., and Mazmanian P.E. (1994) The effectiveness of CME interventions. In: *The Physician As Learner: linking research to practice.* Chicago, IL: American Medical Association.

Davis D.A., O'Brien M.A., and Freemantle N. (1999) Impact of formal continuing medical education: Do conferences, workshops, rounds, and other traditional continuing education activities change physician behavior or health care outcomes? *The Journal of the American Medical Association* **282**: 867–74.

Davis D.A. and Taylor-Valsey A. (1997) Translating guidelines into practice: A systematic review of theoretic concepts, practical experience and research evidence in the adoption of clinical practice guidelines. *CMAJ* **157**: 408–16.

Davis D.A., Thomson M.A., Oxman A.D., and Haynes R.B. (1995) Changing physician performance: A systematic review of the effect of continuing medical education strategies. *The Journal of the American Medical Association* **274**: 700–705.

Davis D.A., Thomson M.A., Oxman A.D., and Haynes R.B. (1992) Evidence for the effectiveness of CME: A review of 50 randomized controlled trials. *The Journal of the American Medical Association* **268**: 1111–17.

Davis J. *Necessary Competencies for Physicians in Health Care Organizations.* Presentation at the American College of Surgeons course, October 24: Chicago.

Davis K., Anderson G.F., Rowland D., and Steinberg E.P. (1990) *Health Care Cost Containment.* Baltimore, MD: The Johns Hopkins University Press.

Dean P.J. (1992) Making codes of ethics real. *Journal of Business Ethics* **11**: 285–90.

Delbanco T.L. (1991) Enriching the doctor-patient relationship by inviting the patient's perspective. *Annals of Internal Medicine* **116**: 414–18.

Delbecq A.L. (2004) Inspired leadership. *Physician Executive* **30**(4): 22–5.

Delbecq A.L. (1980) Effective meeting leadership, 203–227. In: *The Physician In Management.* Tampa, FL: American Academy of Medical Directors.

Delbecq A.L. (1967) The management of decision making within the firm: Three strategies for three types of decision making. *Academy of Management Journal* **10**(4): 329–39.

Delbecq A.L. and Gill S. (1985) Justice as a prelude to teamwork in medical centers. *Health Care Management Review* **10**(1): 45–51.

Delbecq A.L. and Pierce J. (1977) Organization structure, individual attitudes and innovation. *Academy of Management Journal* **2**(1): 27–37.

Deluca J.M. and Enmark R. (2002) *The CEO's Guide to Health Care Information Systems.* San Francisco: Jossey-Bass Wiley & Sons, Inc.

Desmond J. and Copeland L.R. (2000) *Communicating with Today's Patient: essentials to save time, decrease risk, and increase patient compliance.* Washington, DC: Association of Reproductive Health Professionals.

Detmer D.E. and Noren J. (1981) An administrative medicine program for clinician-executives. *Journal of Medical Education* **56**: 640–45.

Dolan T. (2000) The myths of mentoring. *Healthcare Executive* **6**: 5.

Dolan T. (1993) Career development: A professional and personal responsibility. *Journal of Health Administration Education* **11**(2): 287–92.

Downs R.L. (1984) The role of physician managers in larger multi-specialty groups. *College Review* **1**(2): 83–95.

Drucker P. (1967) *The Effective Executive.* New York: Harper & Row.

Dubrin A.J. (2001) *Leadership: research findings, practice, and skills*. Boston: Houghton Mifflin Company.

Dugdale D.C., Epstein R., and Pantilat S.Z. (1999) Time and the patient-physician relationship. *Journal of General Internal Medicine* **14**(suppl 1): S34-S40.

Duncan W.J., Ginter P.M., and Swayne L.E. (2001) *Handbook of Health Care Management*. Malden, MA: Blackwell Publishers Inc.

Dunham N., Kindig D., and Schulz R. (1994) The value of the physician executive's role to organizational effectiveness and performance. *Health Care Management Review* **19**(4): 56–63.

Dye C.F. (1996) Cultivating physician talent: Five steps for developing successful physician leaders. *Healthcare Executive* **11**(3): 18–21.

Dye C.F. (2002) *Winning the Talent War: ensuring effective leadership in healthcare*. Chicago: Health Administration Press.

Edge R. and Groves J. (1999) *Ethics of Healthcare: a guide for clinical practice*. Albany, New York: Delmar Publishers.

Edgley G.J. (1992) Type and temperament. *Association Management* **44**(10): 83–92.

Ehman J.W., Ott B.B., Short T.H., Clampa R.C., and Hansen-Flaschen J. (1999) Do patients want physicians to inquire about their spiritual or religious beliefs if they become gravely ill? *Archives of Internal Medicine* **159**(15): 1803–6.

Eliason B. (2000) Personal values of family physicians, practice satisfaction, and service to the underserved. *Archives of Family Medicine* **9**(3): 228–32.

Ellis A. (2004) *Rational Emotive Behavior Therapy: it works for me – it can work for you*. New York: Prometheus Books.

Ellis A. and Harper R.A. (1997) *A Guide to Rational Living*. 3rd edn. Hollywood, CA: Melvin Powers Wilshire Book Company.

Ellis D. (2000) *Technology and the Future of Health Care: preparing for the next thirty years*. New York: John Wiley & Sons, Inc.

Elnicki D.M., Curry R.Y., Fagan M., Friedman E., Jacobson E., Loftus T., Ogden P., Pangaro L., Papadakis M., Szauter K., Wallach P., and Linger B. (2002) Medical students' perspectives on and responses to abuse during the internal medicine clerkship. *Teaching and Learning in Medicine* **14**(2): 92–7.

Epstein R.M. (1999) Mindful practice. *The Journal of the American Medical Association* **282**: 833–9.

Epstein R.M. and Hundert E.M. (2002) Defining and assessing professional competence. *The Journal of the American Medical Association* **287**(2): 226–35.

Estes M.L. (1997) Core competencies for physician practice success. *Physician Executive* **23**(1): 9–14.

Ettore B. (1996) When an M.D. just isn't enough. *Management Review* **85**(3): 9.

Eubanks P.A. (1990) The new hospital CEO: Many paths to the top. *Hospitals* **December 5, 64**: 26–31.

Ewart C.K., Taylor C.B., Kraemer H.C., and Agras W.S. (1991) High blood pressure and marital discord: Not being nasty matters more than being nice. *Health Psychology* **10**: 155–63.

Fairchild D.G., Benjamin E.M., Gifford D.R., and Huot S.J. (2004) Physician leadership: Enhancing the career development of academic physician administrators and leaders. *Academic Medicine* **79**(3): 214–18.

Fang D. and Meyer R.E. (2003) PhD faculty in clinical departments of U.S. medical schools, 1981–1999: Their widening presence and roles in research. *Academic Medicine* **78**: 167–76.

Farber N.J., Weiner J.L., Boyer E.G., Willard P.G., Robinson E.J., and Diamond M.P. (1986) Values and CPR decisions: A comparison of physicians and administrators in training. *Journal of Health Administration Education* **4**: 205–15.

Fargason C.A., Jr., Evans H.H., Ashworth C.S., and Capper S.A. (1997) The importance of preparing medical students to manage different types of uncertainty. *Academic Medicine* **72**: 688–92.

Farrell J.P. (1993) Leadership competencies for physicians. *Healthcare Forum* **36**(4): 39–42.

Ferlie E., Fitzgerald L., Wood M., and Hawkins C. (2001) *The diffusion of innovation in health care: The impact of professionals*. Paper presented at the Academy of Management Annual Congress. August.

Fernandez C.R. (1998) Make physician-administrator teams work. *MGM Journal* **45**(5): 12–14.

Ferrell O.C., Fraedrich J., and Ferrell L. (2002) *Business Ethics: Ethical decision making and cases*. Boston: Houghton Mifflin Company.

Fine A. (1990) New challenges for medical directors. *Physician Executive* **16**(2): 36–7.

Fine D.G. (2001) Experiential learning in healthcare administration. *Journal of Health Administration Education* **special issue**: 93–106.

Fine D.J. (2002) Establishing competencies for healthcare managers. *Healthcare Executive* **March/April**: 66–7.

Fiore N. (1989) *The Now Habit: a strategic program for overcoming procrastination and enjoying guilt-free play*. New York: Putnam Books.

Fisher R. and Ury W. (1991) *Getting to Yes: negotiating agreement without giving in*. New York: Penguin Books.

Flannery T. (ed.) (2002) *Executive Compensation: guidelines for healthcare leaders and trustees*. Chicago: Health Administration Press.

Forbes S., Bern-Klug M., and Gessert C. (2000) End-of-life decision making for nursing home residents with dementia. *Journal of Nursing Scholarship* **32**(3): 251–8.

Fottler M., Heaton C., and Ford R. (2002) *Achieving Service Excellence: strategies for healthcare*. Chicago: Health Administration Press.

Fox R.D. (2000) Theory and practice in continuing professional development. *Journal of Continuing Education in the Health Professions*, **20**: 238–46.

Fox W.L, O'Rourke P.T., Collins M., and Gooding K. (1998) Encouraging physician leadership: Catholic healthcare systems explore balanced relationships. *Health Progress* **79**(2): 40–47.

Frankford D.M. and Konrad T.R. (1998) Responsive medical professionalism: Integrating education, practice, and community in a market-driven era. *Academic Medicine* **73**: 138–45.

Freedman N. and Grand S. (1977) *Communicative Structures and Psychic Structures*. New York: Plenum.

Freidson E. (1994) *Professionalism Reborn: theory, prophecy and policy*. Chicago: The University of Chicago Press.

Freidson E. (1970) *Professional Dominance: the social structure of medical care*. New York: Aldine Publishing Company.

Freund C.M. (1988) Decision-making styles: Managerial application of the MBTI and type theory. *Journal of Nursing* **18**(12): 5–11.

Fried B.J. and Gaydos L. (2002) *World Health Systems: challenges and perspectives*. Chicago: Health Administration Press.

Fried B.J. and Johnson J.A. (eds) (2002) *Human Resources in Healthcare: managing for success*. Chicago: Health Administration Press.

Friedman E. (1986) Physicians as administrators. *Medical World News* **June 23**.

Frist W.H. (1989) *Transplant: a heart surgeon's account of the life-and-death dramas of the new medicine*. New York: The Atlantic Monthly Press.

Fritts H. (1997) *On Leading a Clinical Department*. Baltimore: Johns Hopkins University Press.

Gabel S. (2003) Making waves: Stages and process of organizational change. *MGMA Connexion* **3**(9): 31–2.

Gaillour F.R. (2004) Want to be CEO? Focus on finesse. *Physician Executive* **30**(4): 14–16.

Gaillour F.R. (2003) Zen and the Art of Dealing with Difficult Physicians: A 3-fold Path for Enlightened Leaders. *Physician Executive* **29**(5): 22–6.

Gaillour F.R. (2003) How do we get into ethically murky situations, anyway? *HealthLeaders News*. Posted 11/22/2003 at www.healthleaders.com.

Gaillour F.R. (2003) The perfect storm in healthcare: crisis or opportunity? *HealthLeaders News*. Posted 11/22/2003 at www.healthleaders.com.

Gardner J.W. (1990) *On Leadership*. New York: Collier MacMillan/The Free Press.

Gardner W.L. and Martinko M.J. (1996) Using the Myers-Briggs Type Indicator to study managers: A literature review and research agenda. *Journal of Management* **22**(1): 45–83.

Gauvreau E. (2002) On board: How a physician becomes an effective member of your medical group's board of directors. *MGMA Connexion* **February**, 38–9.

Gawande A. (2002) *Complications: a surgeon's note on an imperfect science*. New York: Picador, Henry Holt & Company.

Gehlbach S.H., Bobula J.A., and Dickinson J.C. (1980) Teaching residents to read the medical literature. *Journal of Medical Education* **55**: 362–5.

Gelmon S. and Mickevicius V. (1984) Do physicians manage? A perspective on physician-managers in teaching hospitals. *Health Management Forum* **5**(4): 55–65.

Gentry S. (1999) Defining core knowledge, helping teams meet ACMPE goals. *MGM Journal* **46**(2): 52–5.

Gevitz N. (1982) *The D.O.'s: osteopathic medicine in America*. Baltimore: The Johns Hopkins University Press.

Giacalone R.A., Jurkiewicz C.L., and Knouse S.B. (2003) A capstone project in business ethics: Building an ethics training program. *Journal of Management Education* **27**(5): 590–607.

Gill S. (1998) Managing the transition from clinician to manager and leader. In LeTourneau B. and Curry W. *In Search of Physician Leadership*. Chicago: Health Administration Press.

Ginter P.M., Swayne L.E., and Duncan W.J. (1998) *Strategic Management of Health Care Organizations*. Malden, MA: Blackwell Publishers Inc.

Glaser J.P. (2002) *The Strategic Application of Information Technology in Health Care Organizations*. New York: John Wiley & Sons, Inc.

Glasser W. (1989) *Reality Therapy: a new approach to psychiatry*. New York: Perennial Publishing.

Goldsmith J.C. (1985) The future corporate structure of the hospital and implications for education in management. *Journal of Health Administration Education* **Spring**, **3**: 93–102.

Goldstein D.E. (2000) *E-healthcare: Harness the power of Internet e-commerce and e-care*. Gaithersburg, MD: Aspen Publications, Inc.

Goldstein J. (1994) *The Unshackled Organization: facing the challenge of unpredictability through spontaneous reorganization*. Portland, OR: The Productivity Press.

Goleman D. (1998) *Working with Emotional Intelligence*. New York: Bantam Books.

Goleman D. (1995) *Emotional Intelligence*. NY: Bantam Books.

Goleman D., McKee and Boyatzis. (2002) *Primal Leadership: realizing the power of emotional intelligence*. Harvard Business School Press.

Gonzi A. (1993) *The Development of Competence-based Assessment Strategies for the Professions*. Canberra: Australian Government Publishing Service, National Office of Everseas Skills Recognition Research Paper # 8.

Goold S.D. (2000) Handling conflict in end-of-life care. *Journal of the American Medical Association* **283**(24): 3199–200.

Gossin M.E. (1962) Administration and the physician. *Journal of Public Health* **52**(2): 183–91.

Grad R., Macaulay A.C., and Warner M. (2001) Teaching evidence-based medical care: Description and evaluation. *Family Medicine* 33: 602–6.

Greene J. (1998) Coaching the entire team. *Healthcare Executive* 13(1): 16–19.

Greene J. (1997) Marcus Welby, MBA. *Hospitals & Health Networks* 7(15): 36–8.

Greene M.L. and Ellis P.J. (1997) Impact of an evidence-based medicine curriculum based on adult learning theory. *Journal of General Internal Medicine* 12: 742–50.

Greener I. (2004) Talking to health managers about change: Heroes, villains and simplification. *Journal of Health, Organisation and Managment* 18(5): 321–35.

Greenhalgh T. and Macfarlane F. (1997) Towards a competency grid for evidence-based practice. *Journal of the Evaluation of Clinical Practice* 3: 161–5.

Greenhaus J.H., Collins K.M., and Shaw J.D. (2003) The relation between work-family balance and quality of life. *Journal of Vocational Behavior* 63: 510–31.

Griest D.L. and Belles D.R. (1990) Health care executives: A personality profile. *Hospitals* 64(3): 74–5.

Griffith J.R. (1998) Can you teach the management technology of health administration? A view of the 21st century. *Journal of Health Administration Education* 16: 323–38.

Griffith J. and White K. (2002) *The Well Managed Healthcare Organization*. Chicago: Health Administration Press.

Grodin M. (1993) Religious advance directives: The convergence of law, religion, medicine, and public health. *Journal of Public Health*, 83: 899–903.

Groopman J. (2004) God at the bedside. *New England Journal of Medicine* 350(12): 1176–8.

Gruen R.L., Pearson S.D., and Brennan T.A. (2004) Physician-citizens: Public roles and professional obligations. *Journal of the American Medical Association* 291(1): 94–8.

Gruppen L.D., Frohna A.Z., Anderson R.M., and Lowe K.D. (2003) Faculty development for educational leadership and scholarship. *Academic Medicine* 78: 137–41.

Guthrie M.B. (1999) Challenges in developing physician leadership and management. *Frontiers of Health Services Management* 15(4): 3–26.

Hackman J.R. (2002) *Leading Teams: setting the stage for great performances*. Boston: Harvard Business School Press.

Hackman M.Z. and Johnson C.E. (2000) *Leadership: a communication perspective*. 3rd edn. Crossland Heights, IL: Waveland Press Inc.

Haddock C., McClean R., and Chapman R. (2002) *Careers in Healthcare Management: how to find your path and follow it*. Chicago: Health Administration Press.

Hagland M. (1991) Physician execs bring insight to non-clinical challenges. *Hospitals & Health Networks* September 20: 42–8.

Haisfield-Wolfe M.E. (1996) End-of-life care: Evolution of the nurse's role. *Oncology Nursing Forum* 23(6): 931–5.

Halpern R., Lee M.Y., Boulter P.R., and Phillips R.R. (2001) A synthesis of nine major reports on physicians' competencies for the emerging practice environment. *Academic Medicine* 76(6): 606–15.

Hamel R. and Lysaught M. (1994) Choosing palliative care: Do religious beliefs make a difference? *Journal of Palliative Care* 19: 61–6.

Hammer M. and Champy J. (2001) *Reengineering the Corporation: a manifesto for business revolution*. New York: HarperBusiness.

Handley P. (1989) *INSIGHT Inventory™ Technical Manual*. Kansas City, MO.

Haney J. (2002) *Making Culture Pay: solving the puzzle of organizational effectiveness*. Lee's Summit, MO: Visionomics, Inc.

Hardy C., Lawrence T.B., and Grant D. (2005) Discourse and collaboration: The role of conversations and collective identity. *Academy of Management Review* 30(1): 58–77.

Harris D.M. (1999) *Healthcare Law and Ethics: issues for the age of managed care*. Chicago: Health Administration Press.

Hartfield J. (1988) The costs, challenges and rewards of management. *Physician Executive* **14**(4): 3–5.

Harvey J.D. (1985) National leadership in health care: The role of the hospital CEO. *Hospital & Health Services Administration* **30**: 77–84.

Hatala R. and Guyatt G. (2002) Evaluating the teaching of evidence-based medicine. *The Journal of the American Medical Association*, **288**: 1110–1112.

Hateley B.J. and Schmidt W.H. (1997) *A Peacock in the Land of Penguins: a tale of diversity and discovery*. San Francisco: Berrett-Koehler Publishers.

Havens L. (1978) Explorations in the uses of language in psychotherapy: Simple empathic statements. *Psychiatry* **41**: 336–45.

Healy B. (2004) Keynote presentation at the Medical Group Management Association annual convention.

Heller R. (1999) *Learning to Lead*. New York: D K Publishing.

Helzberg B. (2003) *What I Learned Before I Sold to Warren Buffett: an entrepreneur's guide to developing a highly successful company*. Hoboken, NJ: John Wiley & Sons.

Henry R. (1988) *Roads to Medical Management: physician executives' career decisions*. Tampa: American College of Physician Executives Press.

Hershey N. (1990) Documenting roles and responsibilities. *Physician Executive* **16**(4): 7.

Herzlinger R. (1997) *Market-Driven Healthcare: who wins, who loses in the transformation of America's largest service industry*. Reading, MA: Perseus Books.

Heyland D.K., Tranmer J., and Feldman-Stewart D. (2000) End-of-life decision making in the seriously ill hospitalized patient: An organizing framework and results of a preliminary study. *Journal of Palliative Care* **October 16**, Supplement: S31–9.

Hinz C.A. (2000) *Communicating With Your Patients: skills for building rapport*. Chicago: American Medical Association.

Hirsch G. (2000) *Strategic Career Management for the 21st Century Physician*. Chicago: The American Medical Association.

Hirsch G. (1999) Physician career management: Organizational strategies for the 21st century. *Physician Executive* **25**(2): 30–35.

Hoff T.J. (1998) Physician executives in managed care: Characteristics and job involvement across two career stages. *Journal of Healthcare Management* **43**(6): 481–97.

Holman P. and Devane T. (eds) (1999) *The Change Handbook: group methods for shaping the future*. San Francisco: Berrett-Koehler Publishers, Inc.

Hosmer L.T. (2003) *The Ethics of Management*. New York: McGraw-Hill Irwin.

Howell J.M. and Shamir B. (2005) The role of followership in the charismatic leadership process: Relationships and their consequences. *Academy of Management Review* **30**(1): 96–112.

Hudak R.P., Brooke, Jr., and Finstuen K. (2000) Identifying management competencies for health care executives: Review of a series of Delphi studies. *Journal of Health Administration Education* **18**: 213–43.

Hudak R.P., Brooke P.P., Jr., Finsteun K., and Trounson J. (1997) Management competencies for medical practice executives: Skills, knowledge and abilities required for the future. *Journal of Health Administration Education* **15**(4): 219–39.

Hudson T. (1999) Leadership 99. *Hospitals & Health Networks* **November**: 36–44.

Hyland P., Davison G., and Sloan T. (2003) Linking team competences to organisational capacities in health care. *Journal of Health, Organisation and Management* **17**(3): 150–63.

Ibbotson T., Grimshaw J., and Grant A. (1998) Evaluation of a programme of workshops for promoting the teaching of critical appraisal skills. *Medical Education* **32**: 486–91.

Institute of Medicine (2003) Academic Health Centers: leading change in the 21st century. Washington D.C.: National Academies Press.

Jacobs M.O. and Mott P.D. (1987) Physician characteristics and training emphasis considered desirable by leaders of HMOs. *Academic Medicine* **62**: 725–31.

Jaklevic M.C. (1998) Focus on doc leadership. *Modern Healthcare* **28**(7): 40.

James J. (2001) Leadership skills for a new age. *Health Forum Journal*.

Jansen A.R., Siegler M., and Winslade W.J. (1982) *Clinical Ethics*. NY: MacMillan Publishing Company, Inc.

Jeffers S.J., Hightower D.P., Kelley G.R., McKenna M.K., Nelson M.E., and Schwartz A.M. (2005) Patients and spirituality. *The Leading Edge, American College of Physician Executives Online Journal for Medical Management* **2**(1): posted online 1/01/05 at www.acpe.org.

Jessee W.F. (2004) *From Competition to Partnership: A Clinical Case Study of Physician-Hospital Relations*. Presented for the L.R. Jordan Distinguished Lecture. Sandestin, FL, August 4.

Jillson J. (1986) *Fine Art of Flirting*. New York: Fireside Publishing.

Johnson J.A. (1998) Interview with Warren Bennis, Chairman, The Leadership Institute. *Journal of Healthcare Management* **43**(4): 293.

Johnson S. and Blanchard K.A. (1998) *Who Moved My Cheese? An amazing way to deal with change in your work and in your life*. New York: Putnam Publishing Group.

Johnson S.C. and Pfeifer M.P. (1998) Patient and physician roles in end-of-life decision making. End-of-life study group. *Journal of General Internal Medicine* **13**(1): 43–5.

Judge W.Q. and Ryman J.A. (2001) The shared leadership challenge in strategic alliances: Lessons from the U.S. healthcare industry. *Academy of Management Executive* **15**(2): 71–9.

Kagarise M.J. and Meyer A.A. (2004) Academic Medical Centers. In Keagy B.A. and Thomas M.S. *Essentials of Physician Practice Management*. San Francisco: Jossey-Bass Publishers.

Kamin C., O'Sullivan P., Deterding R. and Younger M. (2003) A comparison of critical thinking in groups of third-year medical students in text, video, and virtual PBL case modalities. *Academic Medicine* **78**: 204–11.

Kaplan S.H., Greenfield S., Gandek B., Rogers W.H., and Ware J.W. (1996) Characteristics of physicians with participatory decision-making styles. *Annals of Internal Medicine* **124**(5): 497–504.

Kaplan S.H., Greenfield S., and Ware J.E. Jr. (1989) Assessing the effects of physician-patient interactions on the outcomes of chronic disease. *Medical Care* **27**: S110–S127 with correction **27**: 679.

Katzenbach J.R. (1997) *Real Change Leaders: how you can create growth and high performance at your company*. New York: Random House, Inc.

Kaufman A. (1998) Leadership and governance. *Academic Medicine* **73** (9 Suppl.): 11S–15S.

Keagy B.A. and Thomas M.S. (2004) *Essentials of Physician Practice Management*. San Francisco: Jossey-Bass Publishers.

Keck K. (2001) Physician group practice turnaround. *MGM Journal* **March/April**: 24–8.

Kegan R. and Lahey L.L. (2001) *How the Way We Talk Can Change the Way We Work: seven languages for transformation*. San Francisco: Jossey-Bass Publishers.

Keirsey D. and Bates M. (1998) *Please Understand Me: character and temperament types*. Del Mar, CA: Prometheus Nemesis Book Company.

Kemper D.W. and Mettler M. (2002) *Information Therapy: prescribed information as a reimbursable medical expense*. Boise, ID: Healthwise, Inc.

Kielcolt-Glaser J., Malarkey W.B., Chee M.A., Newton T., Cacioppo J.T., Mao H., and Glaser R. (1993) Negative behavior during martial conflict is associated with immunological down-regulation. *Psychosomatic Medicine* **55**: 395–409.

Kindig D.A. (1997) Do physician executives make a difference? *Frontiers of Health Services Management* **13**(3): 38–42.

Kindig D.A. and Dunham N.D. (1991) How much administration is today's physician doing? *Physician Executive* **17**(1): 3–7.

Kindig D.A. and Lastiri S. (1986) Administrative medicine: A new medical specialty? *Health Affairs* **5**(4): 146–56.

Kindig D.A. and Lastiri-Quiros S. (1989) The changing managerial role of physician executives. *Journal of Health Administration Education* **7**(1): 36–46.

King D.E. and Bushwick B. (1994) Beliefs and attitudes of hospital inpatients about faith healing and prayer. *Journal of Family Practice*, **39**: 349–352.

King M., Speck P., and Thomas A. (1994) Spiritual and religious beliefs in acute illness: Is this a feasible area for study? *Social Science Medicine* **38**: 631–6.

Kirschman D. (1999) Leadership is the key to chief medical officer success. *Physician Executive* **25**(9): 34–6.

Kirschman D. (1996) Physician leadership: Physician executives share insights. *Physician Executive* **22**(9): 27–30.

Kirschman D. and Grebenschikoff J. (1990) *Physician Executive Guide: everything you need to know about creating and filling a physician executive position*. Tampa: Physician Executive Management Center.

Kitchens J.M. and Pfeifer M.P. (1989) Teaching residents to read the medical literature: A controlled trial of a curriculum in critical appraisal/clinical epidemiology. *Journal of General Internal Medicine* **4**: 384–7.

Klass D. (2000) Re-evaluation of clinical competency. *American Journal of Physical Medicine Rehabilitation* **79**: 481–6.

Kofoddimos J. (1993) *Balancing Act: how managers can integrate successful careers and fulfilling personal lives*. San Francisco: Jossey-Bass Publishers.

Kohn L.T. and Donaldson S.M. (eds) (2000) *To Err Is Human*. Washington, DC: National Academy Press.

Komisar R. (2001) *The Monk and the Riddle: The art of creating a life while making a living*. Boston: Harvard Business School Press.

Koska M.T. (1992) New approaches to developing physician leaders. *Hospitals* **66**(9): 76–8.

Koster J. (2001) Taking the lead: Fortune 500 offers tips for developing healthcare executives. *Modern Physician* **February 12**: 20–21.

Kotter J. (1996) *Leading Change*. Boston: Harvard Business School Press.

Kouzes J.M. and Posner B.Z. (2003) *Credibility: how leaders gain it and lose it, why people demand it*. San Francisco: Jossey-Bass.

Kouzes J.M. and Posner B.Z. (2002) *The Leadership Challenge: how to keep getting extraordinary things done in organizations*. San Francisco: Jossey-Bass.

Kruger J. and Dunning D. (1999) Unskilled and unaware of it: How difficulties in recognizing one's own incompetence lead to inflated self-assessments. *Journal of Personality and Social Psychology* **77**(6): 1121–34.

Kubler-Ross E. (1997) *The Wheel of Life: a memoir of living and dying*. New York: Station Hill Press, Inc.

Kuhl I. (1986) *The Executive Role in Health Service Delivery Organizations*. Association of University Programs in Health Administration Press.

Kuntz R., Fritsche L., and Neumayer H.H. (2001) Development of quality assurance criteria for continuing education in evidence-based medicine. *Z Arstl Fortbild Qualitattssich* **95**: 371–5.

Kurtz M.E. (1980) A behavioral profile of physicians in management roles. In: *The Physician in Management*. Tampa, FL: American Academy of Medical Directors.

Kusy M., Essex L.N., and Marr T.J. (1995) No longer a solo practice: How physician leaders lead. *Physician Executive* **21**(12): 11–15.

Laing A., Marnoch G., McKee L., Joshi R., and Reid J. (1997) Administration to innovation: The evolving management challenge in primary care. *Journal of Managing Medicine* **11**(2): 71–87.

Lane D.S. and Ross V. (1998) Defining competencies and performance indicators for physicians in medical management. *American Journal of Preventative Medicine* **14**(3): 229–36.

Lanser E.G. (2000) Reaping the benefits of mentorship. *Healthcare Executive* **15**(3): 18–23.

Larson D.B., Chandler M., and Forman H.P. (2003) MD/MBA programs in the United States: Evidence of a change in health care leadership *Academic Medicine* **78**(3): 335–41.

Larson D.B., Hohmann A.A., Kessler L.G., Meador K.G., Boyd J.H., and McSherry E. (1988) The couch and the cloth: The need for linkage. *Hospital Community Psychiatry* **29**: 1064–9.

Laschinger H.K.S., Finegan J., Shamian J., and Wilk P. (2003) Workplace empowerment as a predictor of nurse burnout in restructured healthcare settings. *Longwoods Review* **1**(3): 2–11.

Latham G.P. (2004) The motivational benefits of goal-setting. *Academy of Management Executive* **18**(4): 126–29.

Laubach C. (2002) *Mastering the Negotiation Process: a practical guide for the healthcare executive*. Chicago: Health Administration Press.

Lazarus A. (2004) The changing landscape of pharmaceutical medicine. *Physician Executive* **30**(7): 40–43.

Leach D.C. (2002) Competence is a habit. *The Journal of the American Medical Association* **287**(2): 243–4.

Lee R.J. and King S.N. (2001) *Discovering The Leader In You: a guide to realizing your personal leadership potential*. San Francisco: Jossey-Bass Inc.

Leebov W. and Scott G. (1990) *Health Care Managers in Transition: shifting roles and changing organizations*. San Francisco: Jossey-Bass Publishers.

Leibman M.S. (1990) Personality profile shows up and comers lead by example. *Modern Healthcare* **20**: June 18, 38.

Leider R.J. (1995) *Repacking Your Bags: lighten your load*. San Francisco: Berrett-Koehler Publishers.

Leider R.J. (1997) *The Power of Purpose: creating meaning in your life and work*. San Francisco: Berrett-Koehler Publishers, Inc.

Lencini P. (2002) *The Five Dysfunctions of a Team: a leadership fable*. San Francisco: Jossey-Bass Publishers.

Lencioni P. (2004) *Death By Meeting: a leadership fable about solving the most painful problem in business*. San Francisco: Jossey-Bass Publishers.

Lepinot A. (1987) Does your hospital need a full-time physician manager? *Training* **40**(2): 19–23.

LeTourneau B. (2004) What doctors want. *Journal of Health Care Management* **49**(4): 218–20.

LeTourneau B. and Curry W. (1998) *In Search of Physician Leadership*. Chicago: Health Administration Press.

LeTourneau B. and Curry W. (1998) The new management team. *Physician Executive* **24**(5): 24–7.

LeTourneau B. and Curry W. (1997) Physicians as executives: Boon or boondoggle? *Frontiers of Health Services Management* **13**(3): 3–25.

LeTourneau B. and Curry W. (1997) Do physician executives make a difference? Reply. *Frontiers of Health Services Management* **13**(3): 43–5.

Levey S., Hill J., and Green B. (2002) Leadership in healthcare and the leadership literature. *Journal of Ambulatory Care Management* **25**(2): 68–75.

Levin A. (2000) Medicine and MBAs. *Annals of Internal Medicine*, **132**: 1015.

Levin J.S. (1997) Religion and health: Is there an association: Is it valid, and is it causal? *Social Science Medicine* **38**: 1475–82.

Levin J.S., Larson D.B., and Puchalski C.M. (1997) Religion and spirituality in medicine: Research and education. *Journal of the American Medical Association* **278**: 792–3.

Levinson W. (1997) Physician-patient communication: The relationship with malpractice claims among primary care physicians and surgeons. *Journal of the American Medical Association* **277**(7): 553–9.

Lewis J.M. (1998) For better or worse: Interpersonal relationships and individual outcome. *American Journal of Psychiatry* **155**(5): 582–8.

Lewis J.M. (1986) Family structure and stress. *Family Process* **25**: 235–47.

Linney B. (1996) *Hope For The Future: a career development guide for physician executives*. Tampa: American College of Physician Executives Press.

Linney G.E., Jr. (1995) Communication skills: A prerequisite for leadership. *Physician Executive* **21**(7): 48–9.

Linney G.E., Jr., and Linney B.J. (2000) *Physician Executives: what, why, how*. Tampa: American College of Physician Executives Press.

Lipson R. (1997) Back to school. *Health Systems Review* **30**(6): 49–51.

Lister E.D. (2000) Effective health care leadership requires well-organized team. American College of Physician Executives, *Click Online Medical Management Magazine* **July**.

Lloyd P.A. (1994) Management competencies in health for all: New public health settings. *Journal of Health Administration Education*, 12(2): 187–207.

Loebs S.F. (2001) The continuing evolution of health management education. *Journal of Health Administration Education* **Special issue**: 33–50.

Loebs S.F. and Dalston J.W. (1993) Issues in management development for health services executives. *Journal of Health Administration Education* 11(1): 235–253.

Loewy E.H. (1997) *Moral Strangers, Moral Acquaintances and Moral Friends: connectedness and its conditions*. New York: State University of New York Press.

Loewy E.H. (1992) Healing and Killing, Harming and Not Harming: Physician Participation in Euthanasia and Capital Punishment. *Journal of Clinical Ethics* 3: 29–34.

Lombardo M.M. and Eichinger R.W. (1989) *Eighty-eight Assignments for Development in Place*. Greensboro, NC: Center for Creative Leadership.

Longest B.B., Jr. (1998) Managerial competence at senior levels of integrated delivery systems. *Journal of Healthcare Management* **43**: 115–35.

Longshore G.F. (1999) *Top Docs: managing the search for physician leaders*. 2nd edn. Longshore & Simmons.

Luborsky L. (1977) Measuring a pervasive psychic structure in psychotherapy: The core conflictual relationship theme. In: *Communicative Structures and Psychic Structures*. NY: Plenum.

Lundin S.C., Paul H., and Christensen J. (2000) *Fish! A remarkable way to boost morale and improve results*. NY: Hyperion.

Lussier and Achua. (2004) *Leadership: theory, application, skill development*. 2nd edn. Thomson South-Western.

Lynch D.C., Pugno P.A., Beebe D.K., Cullison S.W., and Linn J.J. (2003) Family practice graduate preparedness in the six ACGME competency areas: Prequel. *Family Medicine* **35**(5): 324–9.

Lyons M.F. (1999) Transitional leaders for transitional times. *Frontiers of Health Services Management* **15**(4): 36–41.

Lyons M.R., Ford D., and Singer G.R. (1996) Physician Leadership: how do physician executives view themselves? *Physician Executive* **22**(9): 23–6.

MacArthur J. (2004) *The Book on Leadership: the power of a godly influence*. Nashville, TN: Thomas Nelson Publishing.

Magnis E. (2003) *Information Technology: tools for the medical practice*. Englewood, CO: Medical Group Management Association.

Maguire P. (2001) Five strategies for physicians to overcome burnout. *ACP-ASIM Observer*, **March**. Online at www.acponline.org.

Mangham I.L. (1986) In search of competence. *Journal of General Management* 12(2): 6.

Marcinko D.E. (2000) *The Business of Medical Practice: profit maximizing skills for savvy doctors*. New York: Springer Publishing Company, Inc.

Margulies N. and Adams J. (1982) *Organizational Development in Health Care Organizations*. Reading, MA: Addison-Wesley Publishing.

Marston W.M. (2002) *Emotions of Normal People*. London: Routledge.

Martin C. (2004) *Healing America, a Biography: the life of Senate Majority Leader William H. Frist M.D. and the issues that shape our times*. Nashville: W Publishing Group.

Martin W.F. and Keogh T.J. (2004) Managing medical groups: 21st century challenges and the impact of physician leadership styles. *Journal of Medical Practice Management* 20(2): 102–106.

Marvel M.K., Doherty W.J., and Weiner E. (1998) Medical interviewing by exemplary family physicians. *Journal of Family Practice*, 47(5): 343–348.

Masaoka J. (2004) *The Best of the Board Café: hands-on solutions for non-profit boards*. St. Paul, MN: The Wilder Foundation and CompassPoint.

Masaoka J. (2000) *All Hands On Board: a handbook for boards of all-volunteer organizations*. St. Paul, MN: National Center for Nonprofit Boards.

Masaoka J. and Allison M. (2004) *Why Boards Don't Govern*. St. Paul, MN: National Center for Nonprofit Boards and CompassPoint.

Matey D.B. (1991) Significance of transactional and transformational leadership theory on the hospital manager. *Hospital & Health Services Administration* 34: Winter, 600–606.

Matheson G. and Gill S. (1988) Good management for good medicine, the role of the vice president of medical affairs. *Healthcare Executive* 3(5): 31–3.

Matthews D., McCullough M., Larson D., Koenig H., Sywers J., and Milano M. (1998) Religious commitment and health status: A review of the research and implications for family medicine. *Archives of Internal Medicine* 7: 118–24.

Matthews D. (1998) Religion and spirituality in the care of patients with chronic renal failure. *Dialysis Transplant* 27: 136.

Matzo M.L., Sherman D.W., Nelson-Marten P., Rhome A., and Grant M. (2004) Ethical and legal issues in end-of-life care: Content of the end-of-life nursing education consortium curriculum and teaching strategies. *Journal of Nurses Staff Development* 20(2): 59–66.

Maxwell J.C. (2001) *The Right To Lead: a study in character and courage*. Tennessee: Thomas Nelson Publishing.

Maxwell J.C. (1993) *Developing the Leader Within You*. Nashville, TN: Injoy, Inc.

Mazmanian P.E. (2002) Continuing medical education and the physician as a learner. *The Journal of the American Medical Association* 288(9): 1057–60.

McBride J.L., Arthur G., Brooks R., and Pilkington L. (1998) The relationship between a patient's spirituality and health experiences. *Family Medicine* 30: 122–6.

McCall M. (1990) Why physician managers fail – part I. *Physician Executive* 16(3): 8–11.

McCaulley M.H. (1983) *Application of the Myers-Briggs Type Indicator to Medicine and Other Health Professions*. Gainesville, FL: Center for Applications of Psychological Type.

McCaulley M.H. (1981) *The Myers-Briggs Type Indicator in Medical Career Planning*. Gainesville, FL: Center for Applications of Psychological Type.

McCaulley M.H. (1978) *Application of the Myers-Briggs Type Indicator to medicine and other health professions (monograph I)*. Gainesville, FL: Center for Applications of Psychological Type.

McColl A., Smith H., White P., and Field J. (1998) General practitioners' perceptions of the route to evidence-based medicine: A questionnaire survey. *British Medical Journal* 316: 361–5.

McCue J.D., Magrinat G., Hansen C.J., and Bailey R.S. 1986) Residents' leadership styles and effectiveness as perceived by nurses. *Academic Medicine* 61: 53–8.

McDaniel R.R., Jr. (1985) Management and medicine, never the twain shall meet. *Journal of the National Medical Association* 77(2): 107–12.

McDaniel R.R. and Driebe D.J. (2001) Complexity science and health care management.

Advances in Health Care Management **2**: 11–36.

McGaghie W.C. and Frey J.J. (eds) *Handbook for the Academic Physician*. New York: Springer-Verlag.

McGinn P. (2004) *Leading Others, Managing Yourself*. Chicago: Health Administration Press.

McGinn T., Seltz M., and Korenstein D. (2002) A method for real-time, evidence-based general medical attending rounds. *Academic Medicine* **77**: 1150–2.

McKay M., Davis M., and Fanning P. (1995) *Messages: the communications skills book*. 2nd edn. New Harbinger Publications, Inc.

McKenna M.K. (2003) *High Tech Medicine: building your practice with computers and the Internet*. Kansas City: Rockhurst University Press.

McKenna M.K., Gartland M.P., and Pugno P.A. (2004a) Development of physician leadership competencies: Perceptions of physician leaders, physician educators and medical students. *The Journal of Healthcare Administration Education* **21**(3): 343–54.

McKenna M.K., Gartland M.P., and Pugno P.A. (2004b) Defining and developing physician leadership competencies. American College of Physician Executives, *Click Online Medical Management Magazine* **February/March**.

McKenna M.K. and Pugno P.A. (2002) Strengthen physician relations by helping residents develop ACGME-mandated competencies. *The Society for Healthcare Strategy and Market Development Spectrum* **November/December**.

McKenna M.K., Shelton C.D., and Darling J. (2002) Leading in an age of paradox: Optimizing behavioral style, job fit and cultural cohesion. *The Journal of Leadership and Organization Development* **23**(6).

McKenna M.K., Shelton C.D., and Darling J. (2002) The impact of behavioral style assessment on organizational effectiveness: A call for action. *The Journal of Leadership and Organization Development* **23**(6).

Medical Leadership Forum (1999) *Medical Leadership Trends in Hospitals and Health Systems across North America*. Lacombe, LA: The Medical Leadership Forum.

Menzies B. (2004) Physician leaders. *Physician Executive* **July–August, 30**(7): 38–9.

Merrill D.W. and Reid R. (1981) *Personal Styles and Effective Performance*. Radnor, PA: Chilton.

Merrill M.J. and Moosbruker J. (1982) Building an organizational development effort in a teaching hospital, pp. 75–104. In: *Organizational Development in Health Care Organizations*. Reading, MA: Addison-Wesley Publishing.

Merry M. (1996) Physician Leadership: The time is now. *Physician Executive* **22**(9): 4–9.

Meyer G., Lewin D., and Eisenberg J. (2001) To err is preventable. *American Journal of Medicine* **110**: 597–603.

Mick S.S. and Wyttenbach M.E. (eds) (2004) *Advances in Health Care Organization Theory*. San Francisco: Jossey-Bass Publishers.

Millenson M.L. (1999) *Demanding Medical excellence: doctors and accountability in the Information Age*. Chicago: The University of Chicago Press.

Miller G.E. (1990) The assessment of clinical skills/competence/performance. *Academic Medicine* **65**(suppl): S63–S67.

Mitchill S.L. (2003) *Letter from Dr. Samuel L. Mitchill of New York to Samuel M. Burnside*. Temecula, CA: Reprint Services Corp.

Mitlyng J. and Wenzel F. (1999) It takes more than money: Keys to success in leading and managing physician groups. *MGM Journal* **46**(2): 30–2, 34–8.

Mohlenbrock B. (2000) Physician-led quality improvement. *Medical Leadership Forum* **Winter**.

Moise H. (1999) *Physician-patient Relations: a guide to improving satisfaction*. Chicago: American Medical Association.

Montgomery K. (2001) Physician executives: The evolution and impact of a hybrid profession. *Advances in Health Care Management* **2**: 215–41.

Moore G.A. (1995) *Inside the Tornado: marketing strategies from Silicon Valley's cutting edge.* HarperCollins Publishers.

Moore T. and Wood D. (1979) Power and the hospital executive. *Hospital & Health Services Administration* 30–41.

Morahan P.S., Kasperbauer D., McDade S.A., Aschenbrener C.A., Triolo P.K., Monteleone P.K., Counte M., and Meyer M.J. (1998) Training future leaders of academic medicine: Internal programs at three academic health centers. *Academic Medicine* **73**: 1159–68.

Morrison I. (2000) *Health Care in the New Millennium: vision, values, and leadership.* San Francisco: Jossey-Bass Publishers.

Mosher S.A., and Colton D. (2001) Quality improvement in the curriculum: A survey of AUPHA programs. *The Journal of Healthcare Administration Education* **19**(2): 203.

Mullan F. (2002) *Big Doctoring in America: profiles in primary care.* Berkley, CA: University of California Press.

Myers I.B. and Davis J.A. (1976) *Relation of Medical Students' Psychological Type to their Specialties Twelve Years Later.* Gainesville, FL: Center for Applications of Psychological Type.

Myers I.B. (1962) *Manual: the Myers-Briggs type indicator.* Palo Alto, CA: Consulting.

Nash D.B., Markson L.E., Howell S., and Hildreth E.A. (1993) Evaluating the competence of physicians in practice: From peer review to performance assessment. *Academic Medicine* **68** (2 Suppl.): 19S-22S.

National Academy Press (ed.) (2001) *Crossing the Quality Chasm.* Washington, DC: National Academy Press.

Neufeld V.R. and Norman G.R. (eds) (1985) *Assessing Clinical Competence.* NY: Springer.

Neuhauser D. (1983) *Coming of Age: a 50-year history of the American College of Hospital Administrators and the profession it serves, 1933–1983.* Chicago: Pluribus Press.

Newton L.H. and Schmidt D.P. (2004) *Wake-up Calls: classic cases in business ethics.* Mason, OH: Thomson Southwestern.

Nolan T. (1998) Understanding medical systems. *Annals of Internal Medicine* **128**(4): 293–8.

Norman G.R. (1985) Defining competence: A methodological review, pp.15–35. In: Neufeld V.R. and Norman G.R. (eds) *Assessing Clinical Competence.* NY: Springer.

Norman G.R. and Shannon S.I. (1998) Effectiveness of instruction in critical appraisal (evidence-based medicine) skills: A critical appraisal. *CMAJ*, **158**: 177–81.

Northouse P.G. (2004) *Leadership: theory and practice.* 3rd edn. California: Sage Publications.

Novak D.H., Epstein R.M., and Paulsen R.H. (1999) Toward creating physician-healers: Fostering medical students' self-awareness, personal growth, and well-being. *Academic Medicine* **74**: 516–20.

Novak D.H., Suchman A.L., Clark W., Epstein R.M., Najberg E., and Kaplan C. (1997) Calibrating the physician: Personal awareness and effective patient care. *The Journal of the American Medical Association* **278**: 502–9.

Nuland S.B. (1988) *Doctors: the biography of medicine.* New York: Random House.

O'Brien M.A., Freemantle N., and Oxman A.D. (2002) *Continuing education meetings and workshops: Effects on professional practice and health care outcomes* (Cochrane Review). Oxford, England: Cochrane Library, Update Software: 2002 Issue 1.

O'Connor S.J., Shewchuk R.M., and Raab D.J. (1992) Patterns of psychological type among health care executives. *Hospital & Health Services Administration* 37(4): 431–47.

O'Connor S.J. and Shewchuk R.M. (1993) Enhancing administrator-clinician relationships: The role of psychological type. *Health Care Management Review* 18(2): 57–65.

Ogrinc G., Splaine M.E., Foster T., Regan-Smith M., and Batalden P. (2003) Exploring and embracing complexity in a distance-learning curriculum for physicians. *Academic Medicine* **78**: 280–5.

Olive K.E. (1995) Physician religious beliefs and the physician-patient relationship: A study of devout physicians. *South Medicine Journal* **88**: 1249–55.

Olson E.E. and Eoyang G.H. (2001) *Facilitating Organization Change: lessons from complexity science*. San Francisco: Jossey-Bass Publishers.

Paauw D.S. (1999) Did we learn evidence-based medicine in medical school? Some common medical mythology. *Journal of the American Board of Family Practice* **12**: 143–9.

Page L. (1987) From lab coat to suit. *American Medical News* **April 10**: 34–43.

Paller M.S., Becker T., Cantor B., and Freeman S.L. (2000) Introducing residents to a career in management: The physician management pathway. *Academic Medicine* **75**(7): 761–3.

Papa F.J. and Harasym P.H. (1999) Medical curriculum reform in North America, 1765 to the present: A cognitive science perspective. *Academic Medicine* **74**(2): 154–64.

Parkes J., Hyde C., Deeks J., and Milne R. (2001) *Teaching critical appraisal skills in health care settings*. Cochrane Database Systemic Review, 3: CD001270.

Parrott L. (1996) *High Maintenance Relationships: how to handle impossible people*. Tyndale Publishing.

Parry S.B. (1998) Just what is a competency? *Training* **35**(6): 58–64.

Parson M.J. (1989) *An Executive's Coaching Handbook*. NY: Facts on File Publications.

Paulson T. (1996) *Paulson On Change*. Glendale, CA: Griffin Publishing Inc.

Pellegrino E. and Thomasma D.C. (1988) *For the Patient's Good: the restoration of beneficence in health care*. New York: Oxford University Press.

Pennington and Bockmon. (1995) *On My Honor, I Will: leading with integrity in changing times*. New York: Treasure House.

Percy B.J. (1984) The role of the physician manager. *Health Management Forum* **5**(3): 48–55.

Percy I. (1997) *Going Deep: exploring spirituality in life and leadership*. Scottsdale, AZ: Inspired Productions Press.

Perrone J. (2003) Creating a mentoring culture. *Healthcare Executive* **18**(3): 84–5.

Perry F. (2002) *The Tracks We Leave: ethics in healthcare management*. Chicago: Foundation of the American College of Healthcare Executives.

Peters T. (1991) *Thriving On Chaos: handbook for a management revolution*. New York: HarperCollins.

Peters T. and Waterman. (1989) *A Passion For Excellence: lessons from America's best run companies*. New York: Warner Books.

Petzinger T., Jr. (1999) *The New Pioneers: the men and women who are transforming the workplace and marketplace*. New York: Simon & Schuster.

Pointer D.D. and Orlikoff J.E. (2002) *Getting to Great: principles of health care organization governance*. San Francisco: Jossey-Bass Publishers.

Pointer D.D. and Williams S.J. (2004) *The Health Care Industry: a primer for board members*. San Francisco: Jossey-Bass Publishers.

Pollard J.W. (1995) *The Physician Manager in Group Practice*. Englewood, CO: The Center for Research in Ambulatory Health Care Administration.

Porter R.D. and Schick I.C. (2003) Revisiting Bloom's taxonomy for ethics and other educational domains. *Journal of Health Administration Education* **20**(3): 167–88.

Post S.G., Puchalski C.M., and Larson D.B. (2000) Physicians and patient spirituality: Professional boundaries, competency and ethics. *Annals of Internal Medicine* **132**(7): 578–83.

Powell K. (2001) Communicating with your staff: Skills for increasing cohesion and teamwork. Chicago: American Medical Association.

Pritchett P. (1993) *Culture Shift: the employee handbook for changing corporate culture*. Plano, TX: Pritchett Rummler-Brache.

Propp D.A. and Uehara D.T. (2001) Creating a model physician executive. American College of Physician Executives, *Click Online Medical Management Magazine* **February**.

Prybil L.D. (2001). Building bridges between health management education and practice. *Journal of Health Administration Education* **19**(2): 253–61.

Prybil L.D. and Warden G.L. (eds) (1993) Postgraduate management development. *Journal of Health Administration Education* **11**(2): 157–342.

Puchalski C.M. and Larson D.B. (1998) Developing curriculum in spirituality and medicine. *Academic Medicine* **73**: 970–4.

Pugno P.A., Burnett W., Gilanders W.R., and Mitling J.E. (2001) What every chief medical officer (CMO) needs to know. American College of Physician Executives, *Click Online Medical Management Magazine* **February**.

Pugno P.A. (2004) Advance directives in the primary care setting. *Wien Klin Wochenschr* **116**(13): 417–9.

Pugno P.A. (1981) Psychologic stresses encountered by resident physicians. *Family Medicine* **13**(1): 9–12.

Putnam R. (1995) *Bowling Alone: the collapse and revival of American community*. New York: Touchstone Publishing.

Rakich J.S., Longest B.B., and Darr K. (1993) *Managing Health Services Organizations*. Baltimore: Health Professions Press.

Ramsey P.G., Wenrich M., Carline J.D., Inul T.S., Larson E.B., and LoGerfo J.P. (1993) Use of peer ratings to evaluate physician performance. *The Journal of the American Medical Association*, **269**: 1655–60.

Reardon C. (2003) Listening to Obatala. *Ford Foundation Report* **Winter**: 32–7.

Reinertsen J.L. (2003) Zen and the art of physician autonomy maintenance. *Annals of Internal Medicine* **138**: 992–5.

Reinertsen J.L. (1998) Physicians as leaders in the improvement of health care systems. *Annals of Internal Medicine* **128**: 833–8.

Reinertsen J.L. (1995) Transformation: The new knowledge needed for health care administrators. *Journal of Health Administration Education* **13**(1): 39–51.

Richie N., Tagliareni J., and Schmitt J. (1979) Identifying health administration competencies via a delphi survey. *Association of University Programs in Health Administration Program Notes* **82**: 8–18.

Rideout C.A. and Richardson S.A. (1989) A teambuilding model: Appreciating differences using the Myers-Briggs Type Indicator with developmental theory. *Journal of Counseling and Development* **67**: 529–33.

Risser D.T., Smon R., Rice M.M., and Salisbury M.L. (1999) A structured teamwork system to reduce clinical errors, 235–277. In: *Error Reduction in Health Care: a systems approach to improving patient safety*. NY: John Wiley & Sons.

Ritchey T. and Axelrod A. (2002) *I'm Stuck, You're Stuck: break through to better work relationships and results by discovering your DISC behavioural style*. San Francisco: Berrett-Koehler Publishers.

Robbins C.A., Bradley E.H., and Spicer M. (2001) Developing leadership in healthcare administration: A competency assessment tool. *Journal of Healthcare Management* **46**(3): 188–202.

Roberts N. and Melnick G. (1989) The evolving role of the medical director. *Physician Executive* **15**(3): 18–21.

Robinson J.C. (1999) *The Corporate Practice of Medicine: competition and innovation in health care*. Berkley: The University of California Press.

Roche W.P., Scheetz A.P., Dane F.C., Parish D.C., and O'Shea J.T. (2003) Medical students' attitudes in a PBL curriculum: Trust, altruism, and cynicism. *Academic Medicine* **78**: 398–402.

Rohrer J.E. (1989) The secret of medical management. *Health Care Management Review* **14**(3): 7–13.

Romeo S.J.W. (1988) The challenges of medical management. *MGM Journal* **35**(6): 14–18.

Rooney M.C. (2004) Recovering from a career setback: A mistake doesn't have to derail your career plans. *Healthcare Executive* **19**(2): 57–58.

Rosef A.B. and Felch W.C. (1992) *Continuing Medical Education: a primer.* 2nd edn. Westport, CT: Praeger Publishers.

Rosell T.D. (2002) *Physician/clergy Dialogue: For patients' sake.* EthicsDaily.com, an imprint of the Baptist Center for Ethics, November 11.

Ross A., Wenzel F.J. and Mitlyng J.W. (2001) *Leadership for the Future: core competencies in health care.* Washington, DC: Health Administration Press.

Ross A., Wenzel F.J., and Mitlyng J.W. (2002) *Leadership for the Future: core competencies in healthcare.* Chicago: The Foundation of the American College of Healthcare Executives.

Ross R. and Verdieck A. (2003) Introducing an evidence-based medicine curriculum into a family practice residency: Is it effective? *Academic Medicine* **78**: 412–17.

Rossiter A.M., Greene B.R., and Kralewski J.E. (2000) The American College of Medical Practice Executives' competency study. *Journal of Ambulatory Care Management* **23**(4): 1–8.

Rothman E.L. (1999) *White Coat: becoming a doctor at Harvard Medical School.* New York: Harper Collins Publishers Inc.

Royer T. (1995) Physician executives of the future moving from management to leadership. *MGM Journal* **10**: 12.

Royer T.C. (2003) Good doctor/good leader: It's not an oxymoron. *MGMA Connexion* **3**(8): 26–7.

Rucker L. and Shapiro J. (2003) Becoming a physician: Students' creative projects in a third-year IM clerkship. *Academic Medicine* **78**: 391–97.

Ruelas E. and Leatt P. (1985) The roles of physician-executives in hospitals: A framework for management education. *Journal of Health Administration Education* **3**(2): 151–69.

Ruiz M.A. (2001) *The Four Agreements.* Carlsbad, CA: Hay House, Inc.

Rumsey J. (1987) Group practices need medical director as go-between. *American Medical News* **30**(35): 32.

Saccardi T.A. and Banai M. (1996) The effects of hospital executives' personality traits on their perceptions and trust. *Hospital & Health Services Administration* **41**(2): 197.

Sackett D.L. (1997) *Evidence-based Medicine: how to practice and teach EBM.* NY: Churchill Livingstone.

Sackett D.L., Straus S.E., Richardson W.S., Rosenberg W., and Haynes R.B. (2000) *Evidence-based Medicine: how to practice and teach EBM.* Edinburgh: Churchill Livingstone.

Sackett D.L. and Straus S.E. (1998) Finding and applying evidence during clinical rounds: The 'evidence cart'. *The Journal of the American Medical Association* **280**: 1336–8.

Sackett D.L., Rosenberg W.M.C., Gray J.A.M., Haynes R.B., and Richardson W.S. (1996) Evidence based medicine: What it is and what it isn't. *British Medical Journal* **312**: 71–2.

Safran D.G., Montgomery J.E., Chang H., Murphy J., and Rogers W.H. (2001) Switching doctors: Predictors of voluntary dis-enrollment from a primary physician's practice. *Journal of Family Practice* **50**: 130–6.

Safran D.G., Taira D.A., Rogers W.H., Kosinski M., Ware J.E., and Tarlov A.R. (1998) Linking primary care performance to outcomes of care. *Journal of Family Practice* **47**: 213–20.

Sanborn M. (2002) *The Fred Factor: how passion in your work and life can turn the ordinary into the extraordinary.* Colorado Springs: Waterbrook Press.

Saultz J.W. (1995) Effective leadership in a reformed health care system: New skills for family physicians. *Family Medicine* **27**(6): 393–6.

Sayles L.R. (1993) *The Working Leader.* New York: The Free Press.

Schenke R. (ed.) (1980) *The Physician in Management.* Washington, DC: American Academy of Medical Directors.

Schick I.C., Porter R., and Chaiken M. (2002) Core competencies in ethics. *Journal of Health Administration Education* **Special Issues**: 149–58.

Schneck L.H. (2002) Follow the Torch: Identifying and developing physician leaders. *MGMA Connexion* **August**: 33–5.

Schneerson M.M. (2001) *The Unbreakable Soul: a chasidic discourse by Lubavitcher Rebbe Rabbi Menacham M. Schneerson of Chabad-Lubavitch*. New York: Kehot Publication Society.

Schneller E. (1991) The leadership and executive potential of physicians in an era of managed care systems. *Hospital & Health Services Administration* **36**(1): 43–55.

Schneller E., Greenwald H. Richardson M., and Orr J. (1997) The physician executive: Role in the adaptation of American medicine. *Health Care Management Review* **22**(2): 90–6.

Schneller E. (1997) Accountability for health care: A white paper on leadership and management for the U.S. health care system. *Health Care Management Review* **22**(1): 38–48.

Schon D.A. (1983) *The Reflective Practitioner*. NY: Basic Books.

Schreiber K. (1991) Religion in the physician-patient relationship. *Journal of the American Medical Association*, **266**: 3062–6.

Schultz F.C. (2004) Who should lead a healthcare organization: MDs or MBAs? *Journal of Healthcare Management* **49**(2): 103–17.

Schuster J. (2003) *Answering Your Call: a guide for living your deepest purpose*. San Francisco: Berrett-Kohler Publishing.

Schwartz R.W., Pogge C.R., Gillis S.A., and Holsinger J.W. (2000) Programs for the development of physician leaders: A curricular process in its infancy. *Academic Medicine* **75**: 133–40.

Schwartz R. (1998) Physician leadership: A new imperative for surgical educators. *American Journal of Surgery* **176**(1): 38–40.

Scott S. (2002) *Fierce Conversations: achieving success at work and life one conversation at a time*. New York: Viking Press.

Scott H.M., Tangalos E.G., Blomberg R.A., and Bender C.E. (1997) Survey of physician leadership and management education. *Mayo Clinic Proceedings* **72**(7): 659–62.

Senge P. (1990) *The Fifth Discipline: the art and practice of the learning organization*. New York: Doubleday.

Sentell J. and Finstuen K. (1998) Executive skills 21: A forecast of leadership skills and associated competencies required by naval hospital administrators into the 21st century. *Military Medicine* **163**(1): 3–8.

Shalowitz J., Nutter D., and Snarr J. (1996) Medicine and management: A combined educational program. *Journal of Health Administration Education* **14**(3): 305–14.

Shamir B., House R.J., and Arthur M.B. (1993) The motivational effects of charismatic leadership: A self-concept based theory. *Organization Science* **4**: 577–94.

Sheldon A. (1986) *Managing doctors*. Homewood, IL: Dow Jones-Irwin.

Shell G. and Klasko S. (1996) Negotiating: Biases physicians bring to the table. *Physician Executive* **22**: 4–7.

Shelton C. (1999) *Quantum Leaps: seven skills for workplace recreation*. Boston: Butterworth-Heineman.

Shelton C.D., McKenna M.K., and Darling J. (2004) Learning from complex systems: Quantum skills for quantum organizations. *The Central Business Review/University of Central Oklahoma* **23**(1): 6–12.

Shelton C.D., McKenna M.K., and Darling J. (2003) Leading in the age of paradox: Optimizing behavioral style, job fit and cultural cohesion. *The Leadership and Organizational Development Journal* **23**(7): 372–9.

Shelton C.D. and McKenna M.K. (2002) *Quantum Organizations: Creating Networks of Passion and Purpose*. Managing the Complex Conference Proceedings.

Sherman F. (2004) Wanted in academic medicine: Doctors with management training. *The American College of Physician Executive's The Leading Edge* 1(3). Accessed online at www.acpe.org/leadingedge/Oct_2004_Vol1_No3/academic.htm.

Sherrill W.W. (2004) MD/MBA programs growing, students explain why: Perspectives on the future generation of medical leaders. *The American College of Physician Executive's The Leading Edge* 1(2). Accessed online at www.acpe.org/leadingedge/Jan_2004_Vol1_No2/academic.htm.

Sherrill WW. (2004) MD/MBA students: An analysis of medical student career choice. *Medical Education Online* 9(14). Retrieved from www.med-ed-online.org 01/14/04.

Sherrill J.W. (2001) Tolerance of ambiguity among MD/MBA students: Implications for management potential. *The Journal of Continuing Education in the Health Professions* 21: 117–22.

Sherriton J. and Stern J.L. (1997) *Corporate Culture, Team Culture: removing the hidden barriers to team success.* New York: American Management Association.

Shields M.C. (1994) The physician-administrator team revisited. *MGM Journal* 41(5): 100–110.

Shortell S.M. and Kaluzny A.D. (1997) *Essentials of Healthcare Management.* Albany, NY: Delmar Publishers.

Shortell S. and Kaluzny A. (eds) (1994) *Healthcare Management: organization design and behavior.* New York: Delmar Publishers.

Shortell S.M. (1996) The role of research and scholarship in health administration programs. *Journal of Health Administration Education,* 14: 25–34.

Shriberg A., Shriberg D., and Lloyd C. (2002) *Practicing Leadership: principles and applications.* New York: John Wiley & Sons, Inc.

Shumway J.M. (2001) Thinking outside the box: Reflections on teaching. *Medical Teacher* 23(3): 229–30.

Shumway J.M. and Harden R.M. (2003) AMEE Guide No. 25: The assessment of learning outcomes for the competent and reflective physician. *Medical Teacher* 25(6): 569–84.

Silversin J. and Kornacki M.J. (1990) The HMO physician as team player. *HMO Practice* 4: 226–30.

Silversin J. and Kornacki M.J. (2000) *Leading Physicians Through Change: how to achieve and sustain results.* Florida: American College of Physician Executives.

Simoni P.S. and Paterson J.J. (1997) Hardiness, coping and burnout in the nursing workplace. *Journal of Professional Nursing* 13(3): 178–85.

Sloan R.P., Gabiella E., and Powell T. (1999) Religion, spirituality, and medicine. *Lancet* 353: 664–7.

Slomka J. (1992) The negotiation of death: Clinical decision making at the end of life. *Social Science Medicine* 35(3): 251–9.

Smith C.A., Ganschow P.S., Reilly B.M., Evans A.T., McNutt R.A., and Osei A. (2002) Teaching residents evidence-based medicine skills: A controlled trial of effectiveness and assessment of durability. *Journal of General Internal Medicine* 15: 710–15.

Smith H.L., Yourstone S., Lorber D., and Mann B. (2001) Managed care and medical practice guidelines: The thorny problem of attaining physician compliance. *Advances in Health Care Management* 2: 93–118.

Smith J.E. (1997) Managing physician group practices. *Healthcare Executive* 12(5): 46–7.

Smith R.P. and Edwards M.J. (1999) *The Internet for Physicians.* New York: Springer-Verlag.

Spallina J.M. (2002) Organizing clinical programs: Requirements for contemporary leaders and successful organizations. *Spectrum* 8–9.

Spath P.L. (ed.) (1999) *Error Reduction in Health Care: a systems approach to improving patient safety.* NY: John Wiley & Sons.

Spencer L.M. (1993) *Competence at Work.* New York: John Wiley & Sons.

Spreitzer G. (1995) Psychological empowerment in the workplace: Dimensions, measurement and validation. *Academy of Management Journal* **38**(5): 1442–62.

Stack L. (2004) *Leave the Office Earlier: the productivity pro shows you how to do more in less time … and feel great about it*. NY: Broadway Books.

Stahl M. and Dean P.J. (1999) *The Physician's Essential MBA: what every physician leader needs to know*. Gaithersburg, MD: Aspen Publishers, Inc.

Starfield B., Wray C., Hess K., Gross R., Birk P.S., and D'Lugoff B.C. (1981) The influence of patient-practitioner agreement on outcome of care. *American Journal of Public Health* **71**: 127–31.

Starfield B. (1998) *Primary Care: balancing health needs, services and technology*. New York: Oxford University Press.

Starr P. (1984) *The Social Transformation of American Medicine*. New York: Basic Books.

Steinert Y., Nasmith L., McLeod P.J., and Conochie L. (2003) A teaching scholars program to develop leaders in medical education. *Academic Medicine* **78**: 142–9.

Sterns T.H. (1999) How physician/administrator teams work in small groups: Six steps to make it happen. *MGM Journal* **46**(3): 44–50.

Stevens D. and Lewis G. (2001) *Jesus M.D.: a doctor examines the great physician*. Grand Rapids, MI: Zondervan Publishing House.

Stevens D.P. (2002) Finding safety in medical education. *Quality and Safety in Health Care* **11**: 109–11.

Stevens R. (1989) *In Sickness and in Wealth: American hospitals in the twentieth century*. Baltimore: The Johns Hopkins University Press.

Stewart M. (1995) Effective physician-patient communication and health outcomes: A review. *CMAJ* **152**: 1423–33.

Stewart M., Brown J.B., and Donner A. (2000) The impact of patient-centered care on outcomes. *Journal of Family Practice* **49**: 796–804.

Stewart M., Brown J.B., Boon H., Galajda J., Meredith L., and Sangster M. (1999) Evidence on patient-doctor communication. *Cancer Prevention Control* **3**: 25–30.

Strack G. and Fottler M.D. (2002) Spirituality and effective leadership in healthcare: Is there a connection? *Frontiers of Health Services Management* **18**(4): 3–18.

Straus S.E., Green M.L., Bell D.S., Badgett R., Davis D., Gerrity M., Ortiz E., Shaneyfelt T.M., Whelan C., and Rajesh M. (2004) Evaluating the teaching of evidence based medicine: Conceptual framework. *British Medical Journal* **329**: 1029–32.

Straus S.E. and McAlister F.A. (2000) Evidence-based medicine: A commentary on common criticisms. *CMAJ*, **163**: 837–41.

Strosberg M.A. and Teres D. (1997) *Gate-keeping in the Intensive Care Unit*. Chicago: Health Administration Press.

Suchman A.L., Botelho R.J., and Hinton-Walker P. (1998) *Partnerships in Healthcare: transforming relationship process*. Rochester, NY: University of Rochester Press.

Sullivan M.D. (2002) The illusion of patient choice in end-of-life decisions. *American Journal of Geriatric Psychiatry* **10**(4): 365–72.

Swartz H.M. and Gottheil D.L. (1991) The need to educate physician-scholars for leadership in the health care system (editorial) *Annals of Internal Medicine* **114**(4): 333–4.

Sweeney D. (1988) Why every group needs a managing doctor. *Medical Economics* **65**(19): 60–7.

Swenson R.A. (2002) *Margin: the overload syndrome*. Colorado Springs: NavPress.

Swenson R.A. (1999) *Restoring Margin to Overloaded Lives*. Colorado Springs: NavPress.

Tabenkin H. (1987) *Task and managerial characteristics of physician managers in primary and ambulatory care organizations*. Master's thesis, Case Western Reserve University.

Tabenkin H., Zyzanski S.J., and Alemagno S.A. (1989) Physician managers: Personal characteristics versus institutional demands. *Health Care Management Review* **14**(2): 7–12.

Tangalos E.G., Blomberg R.A., Hicks S.S., and Bender C.E. (1998) Mayo leadership programs for physicians. *Mayo Clinic Proceedings* **73**(3): 279–84.

Taylor A.D. (2000) *How to Choose a Medical Specialty*. 3rd edn. Philadelphia: W.B. Saunders Company.

Taylor C. (1994) Ministering to persons who face death: Practical guidance for care givers of persons making end-of-life treatment decisions. *Health Progress* **75**(4): 58–62.

Taylor R., Reeves B., Ewings P., Binns S., Keast J., and Mears R. (2000) A systematic review of the effectiveness of critical appraisal skills training for clinicians. *Medical Education* **34**: 120–5.

Taylor R.B. (2003) Leadership is a learned skill. *Family Practice Management* **10**(9): 43–8.

Tett R.P., Jackson D.N., and Rothstein M. (1991) Personality measures as predictors of job performance: A meta-analytic review. *Personnel Psychology* **Winter**: 703–42.

Thiel M.M. and Robinson M.R. (1997) Physicians' collaboration with chaplains: Difficulties and benefits. *Journal of Clinical Ethics* **8**: 94–103.

Thompson L.L. (2004) *Making the Team: a guide for managers*. 2nd edn. Florida: Harcourt, Inc.

Thrall T.H. (2001) Leadership survey: An evaluation of health care executives' challenges. *MGM Journal* **May/June**: 38–42.

Tichy N.M. and Cardwell N. (2002) *The Cycle of Leadership: how great leaders teach their companies to win*. New York: HarperCollins Publishers, Inc.

Tobis F. (2004) Lost docs: Physicians need special training to handle today's stressful and chaotic business environment. *ACPE Click* **February/March**, **5**(1): accessed online from www.acpe.org/click/volume%204/issue4volume4/Tobis/Page1.html.

Treister N.W. (1995) Development of a local physician executive leadership program. *Physician Executive* **21**(4): 22–4.

Trent W.C. (1986) Some unique aspects of health care management. *Hospital & Health Services Administration* **31**(1): 122–32.

Tresolini C.P. and the Pew-Fetzer Task Force (1994) *Health Professional Education and Relationship-centered Care*. San Francisco: Pew Health Professions Commission and the Fetzer Institute.

Tuttas C.A. (2002) The facts of end-of-life care. *Journal of Nursing Care Quality* **16**(2): 10–16.

Ulrich D., Senger J., and Smallwood N. (1999) *Results-based Leadership: how leaders build the business and improve the bottom line*. Boston: Harvard Business School Publishing.

Van Eynde D.F. and Tucker S.L. (1996) Personality patterns of health care and industry CEOs: Similarities and differences. *Health Care Management Review* **21**(2): 87–95.

Versel N. (2003) Hand in hand: VHA's physician leadership builds a bridge between suits and coats. *Modern Physician* **May**: 16–18.

Viggiano T.R., Shub C., and Giere R.W. (2000) The Mayo Clinic's clinician-educator award: A program to encourage educational innovation and scholarship. *Academic Medicine* **75**: 940–3.

Vinson C. (1994) Administrative knowledge and skills needed by physician executives. *Physician Executive* **20**(6): 37.

Volpp. K.G.M. and Grande D. (2003) Residents' suggestions for reducing errors in teaching hospitals. *New England Journal of Medicine* **348**: 851–5.

Wade D. and Recard R. (2001) *Corporate Performance Management: how to build a better organization through measurement-driven strategic alignment*. Boston: Butterworth-Heineman.

Waldhausen J. (2001) Leadership in medicine. *Bulletin of the American College of Surgeons* **86**(3): 13–19.

Waldman D.A. (2003) Does working with an executive coach enhance the value of multi-source performance feedback? *Academy of Management Executive* **17**(3): 146–8.

Walker E., Darling J., and McKenna M.K. (2002) Keys to organizational excellence: Leadership values and strategies. *The Journal of Business and Society* **Fall**, **15**(1).

Wallace L. (1987) Physician executives. *Modern Healthcare* **May 6**: 48.

Wallick W.G. (2001) *CEO's Perceptions of Trainer Roles in Selected Multi-hospital Healthcare Systems*. Ann Arbor, MI: University Microfilms.

Wallick W.G. (2002) Healthcare managers' roles, competencies, and outputs in organizational performance improvement. *Journal of Healthcare Management* 47(6): 390–401.

Walsh A.M. and Borkowski S.C. (1999) Mentoring in health administration: The critical link in executive development. *Journal of Healthcare Management* 44(4): 269–81.

Wan T.T.H. (2000) Evolving health services administration education: Keeping pace with change. *Journal of Health Administration Education* 18(1): 11–36.

Warden G.L. (2000) The interface between health administration education and practice in the new millennium. *Journal of Health Administration Education* 18(3): 303–20.

Warden G.L. and Griffith J.R. (2001) Ensuring management excellence in the healthcare system. *Journal of Healthcare Management* 46(4), 228–37.

Was M., Combs A., and Combs J.N. (1999) *Finding Your Strong Suit*. Los Angeles: Renaissance Books.

Watson L. (1992) *The Dreams of Dragons: an exploration and celebration of the mysteries of nature*. Rochester, VT: Destiny Books.

Watson M. and Wooten K. (2000) An accidental team: Physician executives tackle teamwork. American College of Physician Executives, *Click Online Medical Management Magazine* **September**.

Weil P. and Herman A. (1996) Forecast: Physician, hospital relationships. *Healthcare Executive* 6(4): 26–8.

Weil T. (1997) Physician executives: Additional factors impinging on their future success. *Frontiers of Health Services Management* 13(3): 33–7.

Weinberg A.D., Ullian L., Richards W.D., and Cooper P. (1981) Informal advice and information-seeking between physicians. *Academic Medicine* 56: 174–80.

Weisbord M. (1976) Why organization development hasn't worked (so far) in medical centers. *Health Care Management Review* 3(1): 17–38.

Weiss J.W. (2003) *Business Ethics: a stakeholder and issues management approach*. Mason, OH: Thomson Southwestern.

Wenzel F., Grady R., and Freedman T. (1995) Competencies for health management practice: A practitioner's perspective. *Journal of Health Administration Education* 13: 612–29.

Wheatley M. (1999) *Leadership and the New Science: discovering order in a chaotic world*. San Francisco: Berrett-Kohler Publishing.

Whitcomb M.E. (ed.) (2003) The information technology age is dawning for medical education. *Academic Medicine* 78: 247–8.

Whitcomb M.E. (ed.) (2003) More on improving the education of doctors. *Academic Medicine* 78: 349–50.

White B. (2004) Making evidence-based medicine doable in everyday practice: Finding the evidence you need is getting easier than you ever thought possible. *Family Practice Management* **February**. Accessed online at www.aafp.org/fpm.

Williams E.S., Konrad T.R., Linzer M., McMurray J., Pathman D.E., Gerrity M., Schwartz M.D., Scheckler W.E., Van Kirk J., Rhodes E., and Douglas J. (1999) Refining the measurement of physician job satisfaction: Results from the Physician Worklife Survey. *Medical Care* 37(11): 1140–54.

Williams S.J. (2001) Training needs for physician leaders. *Journal of Health Administration Education* 19(2): 195–202.

Wilson B. and Laschinger H.K.S. (1994) Staff nurse perception of job empowerment and organizational commitment: A test of Kanter's theory of structural power in organizations. *Journal of Nursing Administration* 24(4): 39–45.

Wilson-Evered E., Hartel C.E J., and Neale M. (2001) A longitudinal study of work group innovation: The importance of transformational leadership and morale. *Advances in Health Care Management*, 2: 315–40.

Winters D. and Latham G.P. (1996) The effect of learning versus outcome goals on a simple versus a complex task. *Group and Organization Management* **21**: 236–50.

Wipf J.E., Pinsky L.E., and Burke W. (1995) Turning interns into senior residents: Preparing residents for their teaching and leadership roles. *Academic Medicine* **70**: 591–6.

Woods M.S. (2000) *Applying Personal Leadership Principles to Healthcare: the DEPO principle*. The Woods Development Institute.

Yamazaki Y. and Kayes D.C. (2004) An experiential approach to cross-cultural learning: A review and integration of competencies for successful expatriate adaptation. *Academy of Management Learning and Education* **3**(4): 362–79.

Zaccaro S.J. and Klimoski R.J. (2001) *The Nature of Organizational Leadership: understanding the performance imperatives confronting today's leaders*. San Francisco: Jossey-Bass Publishers.

Zenger J.H., Musselwhite E., Hurson K., and Perrin C. (1994) *Leading Teams: mastering the new role*. New York: Zenger-Miller Inc.

Zuckerman C. and Wollner D. (1999) End of life care and decision making: How far we have come, how far we have to go. *Hospital Journal* **14**(3–4): 85–107.

Next Steps

If you have stories, poems, or essays to share
about your own experiences as a physician leader,
please let us know.

To discover more resources for physician leadership development,
or to become involved in supporting
the development of other emerging physician leaders
please contact us at:

Healthcare Leadership Group
12203 Wyandotte Court
Kansas City, MO 64145
(816) 309–9925
www.PhysiciansAsLeaders.com

Dr. McKenna not only teaches Health Care Leadership to physicians, nurse
executives, medical students and residents at Rockhurst University, she is also
a professional speaker, and frequently delivers general session keynote
presentations at medical conferences and full day Continuing Medical
Education training seminars for organizations across the country.
Both Dr. McKenna and Dr. Pugno would like to hear from you, if you share
their interest in equipping physicians to become more effective, fulfilled
leaders.

Biographical Summaries of the Physician Leaders Who Contributed Insights for This Book

"To create a legacy is to plant a tree under which you will never sit. It is to look past your interests, your hopes and your lifetime ... to put into motion changes that will be an indelible inspiration to those who follow."

Christopher J. Hegarty
in *Cavett Robert: Leaving a Lasting Legacy*
by Cavett Robert and Lee E. Robert

We wish to express our *heartfelt gratitude* to these physician leaders, and to those who've gone before them. They are truly creating legacies, and enabling others to do the same.

Monte L. Anderson, MD
Gastroenterologist
Consultant in Gastroenterology, Hepatology and Transplantation
Mayo Clinic Scottsdale
Scottsdale, Arizona 85259

Dr. Anderson maintains an active consulting practice in gastroenterology and hepatology and transplantation medicine, while participating as an investigator in clinical research projects, teaching residents and fellows, publishing, and participating in various academic conferences.

Dr. Anderson completed his fellowship in Gastroenterology at Brooke Army Medical Center in San Antonio; residency in Internal Medicine at Creighton University School of Medicine in Omaha; and his medical school education at the University of Nebraska, College of Medicine in Omaha. He completed specialty training with the Mayo Clinic Rochester and the Armed Forces Institute of Pathology in Washington, D.C. He was honorably discharged from the United States Army Medical Corps where he served as a Commissioned Captain in the U.S. Army Infantry.

Dr. Anderson is a fellow of the American College of Physicians and a Diplomate of the American Board of Internal Medicine, with subspecialties in Gastroenterology and Internal Medicine. He is a Board Director for the Mayo Clinic Alumni Association; Regional Coordinator, Mexico and Central America, for the Mayo Clinic Foundation; and Director of International Affairs for the Mayo Clinic Scottsdale.

He was Chairman, Department of Gastroenterology, Director of Endoscopy Services, and Physician Coordinator of International Activities, for the Mayo Clinic Scottsdale; a member of the Physician Advisory Committee to Arizona Rep. J.D. Hayworth; and a Board Director of the Arizona Chapter of the American Liver Foundation.

Dr. Anderson has been listed each year since 1996 in *The Best Doctors in America: Pacific Region;* and is an Honorary Member of medical societies in Ecuador and Columbia. He received the Best Speaker Award from the Mayo Clinic Cancer Reviews; the Merck Award for Outstanding Achievement in Medical Education; and the Ernest B. Manning Public Health Scholarship, University of Nebraska College of Medicine.

He has held Academic Appointments as an Assistant Professor in Mayo Medical School, overseeing staff physicians' formal didactic teaching of fellows, residents, and medical students; teaching practicing physicians the subspecialty of Gastroenterology, Hepatology, and Liver Transplantation; and holding Invited Professorships in Argentina, Colombia, Ecuador, Guatemala, and Mexico.

Dr. Anderson has authored and co-authored many published articles, case reports, posters, abstracts, book chapters, and studies. He has served as an Invited Reviewer for several medical journals; and as a member of the Medical Advisory Board for eHealthCoach.com and the Editorial Board for Scottsdale Memorial Hospital System's *Scope Magazine*.

Dr. Anderson and his wife, Patricia, have three children: Elizabeth, Mark, and Chris.

Bruce Bagley, MD
Family Physician
Medical Director for Quality Improvement
The American Academy of Family Physicians
Leawood, Kansas 66211

Dr. Bagley is currently the Medical Director for Quality Improvement for the American Academy of Family Physicians (AAFP), and organization that represents more than 94,000 family physicians, family practice residents, and medical students nationwide.

Throughout his clinical career, Dr. Bagley has provided the full range of family medicine services in a single specialty group practice in Albany, New York. Under his leadership, the 10-partner group has been a pioneer in the community in adapting to the challenges of managed care, quality improvement, and informatics.

In his active leadership role with the AAFP, Dr. Bagley was elected president-elect in 1998, served as president in 1999–2000 and as Chair of the Board in 2000–2001. Dr. Bagley chaired AAFP Task Forces on Hospitalist Physicians, Obstetrics in Family Medicine, Quality Enhancement, and Quality in Family Medicine. He also chaired the Ad Hoc committee on electronic medical records for the AAFP.

Dr. Bagley has spoken extensively on the topics of quality improvement, office redesign, electronic medical records, and leadership.

Nancy J. Baker, MD
Family Physician
University of Minnesota
Minneapolis, Minnesota 55455

Dr. Baker is a second generation Family Physician. After graduating from St. Olaf College, she attended the University of Missouri, Columbia for medical school She completed her Family Medicine residency at St. Paul Ramsey Medical Center in St. Paul, Minnesota. For three years she has served as faculty in the Family Medicine residency at Lutheran General Hospital in Park Ridge, Illinois. She spent 15 years as faculty at St. Paul Ramsey Medical Center.

Dr. Baker is a Clinical Associate Professor. She teaches at Smiley's Clinic at the University of Minnesota. Dr. Baker has held multiple leadership positions within the Minnesota Academy of Family Physicians and the American Academy of Family Physicians. She is currently enrolled in the Physician Leadership College at the University of St. Thomas.

Mark H. Belfer, DO, FAAFP
Family Physician
Residency Director
Akron General Medical Center/NEOUCOM
Akron, Ohio 44307

Mark H. Belfer, DO, FAAFP assumed the directorship of the Akron General Medical Center's Family Practice Residency Program in May 2002 after his arrival from Kansas City, Missouri, where he also served as a program director for several years. He has practiced in the private sector and has held several positions in both university and community hospital teaching programs.

Dr. Belfer attended Michigan State University (Bachelor of Science degree) and the College of Osteopathic Medicine and Surgery in Des Moines, Iowa (Doctor of Osteopathy degree). He completed his internship at Grand Rapids (Michigan) Osteopathic Hospital and his residency training at Martin Army Community Hospital in Ft. Benning, Georgia. He is a Fellow of the American Academy of Family Physicians and is certified by the American Board of Family Practice.

Besides currently serving as Professor of Clinical Family Medicine on the faculty of NEOUCOM, Dr. Belfer has held several leadership positions, including president of the Ohio Academy of Family Physicians. He is active within the American Academy of Family Physicians, currently serving on the board of directors of the AAFP Foundation and the AAFP Commission on Education. His teaching interests include procedural skills, practice management, and curriculum development.

Richard B. Birrer, MD, MPH, MMM, CPE
Family, Emergency, Sports and Geriatric Medicine Physician
Locust Whey, New York 11560

Dr. Richard Birrer is board certified in Family Medicine, Emergency Medicine, Sports Medicine and Geriatric Medicine. He is a fellow of the American College of Physician Executives. Formerly the Chief Executive Officer of St. Joseph's University Medical Center in New Jersey, Dr. Birrer devotes his full-time professional activities to helping healthcare organizations in need of management guidance for performance turnaround situations.

Dr. Birrer is an advocate of lifelong learning. His work has been published in *Health Progress* and other prestigious journals. Dr. Birrer served on the Medical Advisory Board of eHealthCoach.com, an organization that operated from 2000 through 2003 in order to help physicians and medical managers learn how to select and use computer systems to improve the quality and cost-effectiveness of care.

Edward T. Bope, MD
Family Physician
Program Director
Riverside Family Practice Residency Program
697 Thomas Lane
Columbus, Ohio 43214

Edward T. Bope, MD graduated twice from the Ohio State University and then completed a family practice residency at Riverside Methodist Hospital in Columbus, Ohio. After residency he joined the faculty at Riverside and became the director in 1985. He served on the American Board of Family Practice Board of Directors from 1990–1995 and was President of the Board in 1995. He was president of the Association of Family Practice Residency Directors (AFPRD) in 1998. He served on the RRC for Family Practice from 1991 to 2001 and was Chair of the RRC in the final two years.

Dr. Bope currently serves on the board of directors of the ACGME. He is the co-author/editor of *Conn's Current Therapy*, *The Saunders Review of Family Practice* and the *Family Practice Desk Reference*. Dr. Bope is most proud of leading the Riverside Residency to local and national prominence and helping other program directors pursue excellence through the National Institute of Program Director Development. Two passions for Dr. Bope are student teaching and the Physicians Free Clinic where he serves as volunteer medical director.

John R. Bucholtz, DO
Family Physician
Director of Medical Education
Program Director, Family Practice Residency Program
1900 10th Avenue, Suite 100
Columbus, Georgia 31902

John R. Bucholtz, DO is currently Director of Medical Education and Program Director for the Family Practice Residency Program at The Medical Center in Columbus, Georgia.

Dr. Bucholtz is a 1982 graduate of the Philadelphia College of Osteopathic Medicine and completed residency training in Family Practice at Martin Army Community Hospital, Fort Benning, Georgia. He spent a total of 20 years on active duty and reserve time. While in the Army he completed a faculty development fellowship at the University of North Carolina, Chapel Hill.

Dr. Bucholtz has served the Georgia AFP chapter and the American Academy of Family Physicians on numerous committees and commissions. He is a past president of the Association of Family Medicine Residency Directors. He was a member of the Project Leadership Committee for the Future of Family Medicine Project for which he served as chair of the residency education task force.

Daniel S. Durrie, MD
Ophthalmologist
President, Durrie Vision Center
Overland Park, Kansas 66211

Dr. Durrie is an expert, standard bearer, pioneer; making medical advances in vision correction via his research, clinical care, and mentoring.

He is an advocate for excellence, which requires focus, and sometimes involves risk and sacrifice (to eliminate everything else). He believes in the importance of mentoring, which requires trust-based relationships.

Dr. Durrie is a past board member of the International Society for Refractive Surgery, and a frequent expert advisor to the FDA.

David G. Fairchild, MD, MPH
Internist
Chief of General Medicine
Tufts – New England Medical Center
Boston, Massachusetts 02115

Dr. Fairchild is the Chief of General Medicine at Tufts, New England Medical Center in Boston and an Assistant Professor of Medicine at Harvard Medical School. He previously served as Director of Primary Care at Brigham & Women's Hospital, where he led the transition from a flat salary system to a variable physician compensation model, and guided the group as it moved its administrative infrastructure and billing operation from the hospital in to the Brigham & Women's physician organization.

Dr. Fairchild's work has appeared in over 20 publications in peer-reviewed journals, including his article "Physician Leadership: Enhancing the Career Development of Academic Physician Administrators and Leaders" published in *Academic Medicine.*

In addition to his accomplishments as a clinical leader and health services researcher, Dr. Fairchild also makes contributions to the advancement of healthcare through his involvement in the Society of General Internal Medicine (SGIM), the national society for academic general internists, physician administrators, and leaders.

Kevin S. Ferentz, MD
Family Physician
Past President, Maryland Academy of Family Physicians
Residency Director, Department of Family Medicine and Associate Professor, University of Maryland School of Medicine
Baltimore, Maryland 21201

Dr. Ferentz received his MD from SUNY at Buffalo School of Medicine. He completed his Family Practice residency, as well as a fellowship in Faculty

Development, at the University of Maryland, where he has been a faculty member since 1987 and Residency Director since 1993. He is an Associate Professor and has authored more than two dozen articles and book chapters.

Dr. Ferentz has received numerous teaching awards, including the Exemplary Teaching Award from the AAFP and the Outstanding Program Director Award from the Association of Family Practice Residency Directors. He was named one of the Best Family Physicians by Baltimore Magazine in 1997, 2000, and 2002. The Ladies Home Journal also named him one of the best Family Physicians in America in 2002. He was listed in Who's Who in America in 2004.

Dr. Ferentz is the designer of an award winning smoking cessation program, "1, 2, 3 . . . Tobacco Free," which has been implemented in Baltimore area high schools. Dr. Ferentz is recognized as a national thought leader regarding the care of mental illness in primary care.

Dr. Ferentz is a past-President of the Maryland Academy of Family Physicians and has served on several committees and commissions for the AAFP.

Michael O. Fleming, MD
Family Physician
President, American Academy of Family Physicians
Shreveport, Louisiana 71103

Michael O. Fleming, MD, a family physician in Shreveport, Louisiana, is the 2004 president of the American Academy of Family Physicians. He is managing senior partner for The Family Doctors, a group practice of 10 family physicians. He is also assistant clinical professor in the Department of Family Medicine at Louisiana State University Health Science Center and in the Department of Family and Community Medicine at Tulane University Medical School.

Dr. Fleming is a past president of the Louisiana Academy of Family Physicians, and past chair of the Board of Directors for the Academy Foundation. He was Louisiana Family Doctor of the Year in 1996. Dr. Fleming attended Louisiana State University in Baton Rouge, and received his medical degree from Louisiana State University in Shreveport in 1975. He completed a family medicine residency at Louisiana State University Affiliated Hospitals in Shreveport, and is certified by the American Board of Family Practice and an AAFP Fellow.

In addition to his active practice, Fleming participates in international activities promoting medical education and primary care worldwide. He works with numerous local community organizations, and has served as medical director for facilities providing care to mentally retarded individuals and patients with behavioral disorders.

Senator William H. Frist, MD
Thoracic Surgeon
Senate Majority Leader, U.S. Congress
Washington, D.C. 20008

William H. Frist, MD graduated in 1974 from Princeton University, where he specialized in healthcare policy at the Woodrow Wilson School of Public and International Affairs, and in 1978 from Harvard Medical School, spending the next seven years in surgical training at Massachusetts General Hospital; Southampton General Hospital, Southampton, England; and Stanford University Medical Center. He is board certified in both general surgery and heart surgery.

In 1985, Dr. Frist joined the faculty at Vanderbilt University Medical Center where he founded and directed the multi-disciplinary Vanderbilt Transplant Center, which under his leadership became a nationally renowned center of multi-organ transplantation. He has performed over 150 heart and lung transplant procedures, including the first successful combined heart-lung transplant in the Southeast. Dr. Frist has written five books and more than 100 articles, chapters, and abstracts on medical research.

First elected to the U.S. Senate on November 8, 1994, and re-elected on November 7, 2000, Dr. Frist was the first practicing physician elected to the Senate since 1928. In 2000, Dr. Frist was unanimously elected chairman of the National Republican Senatorial Committee (NRSC) for the 107th Congress and in 2002 was unanimously elected Majority Leader of the U.S. Senate. Dr. Frist is particularly passionate about confronting the global AIDS pandemic. He frequently takes medical mission trips to Africa to perform surgery and care for those in need. As Senate Majority Leader, he continues to raise awareness about the HIV/AIDS crisis throughout the world.

Senator Frist and his wife, Karyn, have three sons: Harrison, Jonathan, and Bryan. He enjoys flying, writing, running marathons, and medical mission trips to Africa.

Francine R. Gaillour, MD, MBA, FACPE
Internist
Founder & Director of Creative Strategies in Physician Leadership
President & CEO, The Gaillour Group
Bellevue, Washington 98008

A certified Executive Coach, leadership consultant, and professional speaker, Dr. Gaillour has long worked with physicians who want to improve their effectiveness as leaders and business professionals. Out of that experience, Dr. Gaillour founded and directs Creative Strategies in Physician Leadership™, an organization that serves as a forum for the provision of executive coaching and strategic consulting resources for healthcare leaders in a variety of professional endeavors. Dr. Gaillour also serves as a strategic advisor for healthcare industry executives, and is a nationally recognized speaker in the areas of healthcare leadership, technology, innovation, cultural change, customer-focused strategy, marketing, and the future of medical practice.

Dr. Gaillour's professional experience spans over 18 years in healthcare delivery and healthcare technology business management. Before launching her consulting and coaching firm, she previously held the position of Medical Director and Senior Vice President of Research and Development with HBS International, overseeing new product development, healthcare outcomes research, and clinical effectiveness programs. Prior to that, she served as Medical Director for PHAMIS/IDX, responsible for electronic medical record development and market strategy for the integrated delivery system market. Her transition into the business world came after years of practicing clinical medicine where she witnessed first hand the tremendous capacity of her patients to tap into their potential and transform their lives, families, work and community.

Dr. Gaillour is board certified in Internal Medicine and spent over 10 years in clinical practice. She completed her residency training at the University of Washington. Her undergraduate work was in biomedical engineering at the University of New Mexico; her medical training was also at the University Of New Mexico School Of Medicine, where she was elected to the Alpha Omega Alpha Medical Honor Society. In 1998 Dr. Gaillour received a Masters in Business Administration from the University of Tennessee. Her executive coach training has been through the Academy for Coach Training and the Graduate School of Corporate Coaching.

Dr. Gaillour is a Fellow and Board Member of the American College of Physician Executives, the leading organization of health system medical officers and leaders. She speaks and writes for organizations across the United States, striving to lay a foundation for adaptive change in order to usher in the new era of professional accountability in healthcare.

J. Peter Geerlofs, MD
Family Physician
Chief Medical Officer
Allscripts Healthcare Solutions Inc.
Libertyville, Illinois 60048

Dr. Geerlofs is a board certified family physician. He is the former Health Officer for Jefferson County, and founder of Port Townsend Family Physicians, Inc. He practiced medicine for many years before transitioning into his current work as an activist for significant change in healthcare – particularly through leveraging the powerful potential of information systems technology in the delivery of care.

While practicing medicine in the state of Washington during the early 1980s, Dr. Geerlofs began using information systems technology to enhance the quality, timeliness, and accessibility of educational information for patients. Since then, he has lectured and written widely on the use of computers in clinical medicine. His passion has always been the creation of systems that are affordable, and can help introduce clinical computing to typical practicing physicians.

Dr. Geerlofs founded Medifor, a medical software company and developer of Patient Education®, with that vision in mind. He also helped lead the design of the original Clinical Health Care System (CHCS) order entry system for the Department of Defense.

When Medifor was acquired by Allscripts Healthcare Solutions in 2000, Dr. Geerlofs became that company's Chief Medical Officer, where he continues to champion practical, affordable technology solutions for use by practicing physicians.

Dr. Geerlofs currently serves on the Steering Committee of the "Connecting for Healthcare" project sponsored by the Markle Foundation, and on the Steering Committee of the "ePrescribing" task force led by the eHealth Initiative.

Roland A. Goertz, MD, MBA
Family Physician
President, McClennan County Medical Education and Research Foundation
Waco, Texas 76707

Roland A. Goertz, MD, MBA is Chief Executive Officer of three foundations that oversee all operations of the Waco Family Practice Center, which includes a family practice residency training program, a Federally Qualified Health Center, the Family Medicine Faculty Development Center of Texas, and the Brazos Area Health Education Center. He holds an appointment as Associate Clinical Professor at the University of Texas Southwestern Medical School in Dallas, Texas.

Dr. Goertz graduated medical school from the University of Texas Health Science Center at San Antonio in 1981 and then completed Family Practice residency training in Fort Worth, Texas at John Peter Smith Hospital. He also completed a clinical teaching fellowship in family medicine. In 2003, Dr. Goertz received an MBA from Baylor University.

In Dr. Goertz's career, he has been a physician in a rural private practice, a family practice residency program director at two highly regarded residencies, and chair of the Department of Family and Community Medicine at the University of Texas Medical School at Houston. Dr. Goertz and his spouse, Rose, have been married 23 years and they have three adult daughters.

Larry A. Green, MD
Family Physician
Director, The Robert Graham Center for Policy Studies in Family Practice and Primary Care
Washington, D.C. 20101

Larry A. Green, MD is the founding director of The Robert Graham Center for Policy Studies in Family Medicine and Primary Care, which opened in 1999 in Washington, D.C. He completed his residency in family medicine at the University of Rochester and Highland Hospital and entered practice in Arkansas in the National Health Services Corps, after which he joined the faculty at the University of Colorado.

Dr. Green was the Woodward-Chisholm Chairman of the Department of Family Medicine at the University of Colorado for 14 years, and continues to serve on the faculty as Professor of Family Medicine and Director of the National Program Office for Prescription for Health. Much of his career has been focused on developing practice-based, primary care research networks.

Dr. Green practices as a certified Diplomat of the American Board of Family Practice. He is a member of the American Academy of Family Physicians, the Society of Teachers of Family Medicine, the World Organization of Family Doctors, and the North America Primary Care Research Group.

Dr. Green received his BA from the University of Oklahoma and his MD from Baylor College of Medicine, Houston, Texas. He is a member of the Institute of Medicine.

Reverend Pamela S. Harris, MD
Physical Medicine and Rehabilitation Physician
Clinic Chief, Kansas City Veteran's Administration Hospital
Minister of Health, United Methodist Church of the Resurrection
Roeland Park, Kansas 66205

Dr. Harris is a native Kansan. She attended the University of Kansas for undergraduate, medical school, and residency programs. Dr. Harris was in private
practice in inner city Kansas City, Kansas for many years prior to taking the
position of Clinic Chief of Physical Medicine and Rehabilitation at the Kansas
City VA Medical Center in 2000.

More recently, she has completed Basic Theological Studies at Saint Paul School
of Theology in Kansas City, Missouri. Dr. Harris is a probationary deacon within
the Kansas East Conference of the United Methodist Church, seeking ordination
in 2007. She serves as Minister of Health for the United Methodist Church of the
Resurrection, providing health education to the congregation and larger community and providing pastoral care to those experiencing healthcare crises.

Dr. Harris and her husband, Tom, have two daughters, Emily and Bethany.

Douglas E. Henley, MD, FAAFP
Family Physician
Executive Vice President
American Academy of Family Physicians
Leawood, Kansas 66211

Douglas E. Henley, MD is Executive Vice President (EVP) of the American
Academy of Family Physicians, representing more than 93,700 physicians and
medical students nationwide. As EVP, Dr. Henley serves the Academy as chief
executive officer. He also provides representation for the AAFP to other organizations, including medical, public, and private sectors, and he serves on the
board of directors of the AAFP Foundation, the charitable arm of the Academy.

Dr. Henley has been an AAFP physician member and volunteer since 1973.
He was on the AAFP Board of Directors from 1991 to 1997, serving as chair
from 1993 to 1994 and 1996 to 1997, and as president from 1995 to 1996.

Prior to assuming the position of EVP, Dr. Henley was in private practice for
20 years in his hometown of Hope Mills, North Carolina. He is the first practicing family physician to be named EVP and the first AAFP past-president and
board chair to serve in that position.

Dr. Henley is a graduate of the University of North Carolina, School of Medicine,
Chapel Hill, and the university's family medicine residency program. He is board
certified by the American Board of Family Practice and is an AAFP Fellow.

Steven G. Hull, MD, FCCP, FAASM
Director of Sleep Disorders, Pain Management and Vaccine Research
Vince and Associates Clinical Research
Medical Director, somniTech, Inc.
Overland Park, Kansas 66211

Dr. Hull is a clinical expert in the emerging field of sleep disorders. He champions the improvement of clinical outcomes by raising awareness among both
physicians and patients.

Dr. Hull is one of only 2,300 board certified sleep medicine diplomats in the world. Active in clinical studies, frequent speaker on sleep disorders.

Charles Jaffe, MD, PhD
Vice President Life Sciences
SAIC
West Chester, Pennsylvania 19382

Dr. Jaffe is involved with academia and industry, helping standardize clinical informatics. He is active in many HCIT standards groups such as HL-7.

William F. Jessee, MD, FACMPE
Pediatrician, Emergency Medicine and Preventive Medicine Physician
President, Medical Group Management Association
Englewood, Colorado 80112

William F. Jessee, MD, FACMPE, brings a wide range of experience to his job as President of the Medical Group Management Association, which represents the interests of 185,000 physicians in more than 7,100 medical groups and other organizations.

Before joining MGMA last year, Dr. Jessee served for three years as Vice President for quality and managed care standards at the American Medical Association, where he led the development and implementation of the American Medical Accreditation Program. Dr. Jessee's clinical background includes stints as a practicing pediatrician and emergency physician. A founding board member of the International Society for Quality in Health Care, Dr. Jessee was its president from 1989 to 1991.

Dr. Jessee is an adjunct professor of health policy and administration at the University of North Carolina's School of Public Health, where he taught full-time from 1980 to 1986. Dr. Jessee is a 1972 graduate of the University of California, San Diego Medical School. He served in the U.S. Public Health Service from 1973 to 1976.

Norman B. Kahn, Jr., MD
Family Physician
Vice President, Science and Education
American Academy of Family Physicians
Leawood, Kansas 66211

Dr. Norman Kahn serves as Vice President for Science and Education of the American Academy of Family Physicians. He is responsible for the educational, scientific, public health and research activities of the AAFP, and represents the Academy on those issues to a number of national organizations.

Dr. Kahn received his medical degree from the University of Kansas. He completed his internship and residency in family practice at San Francisco General Hospital, affiliated with the University of California, San Francisco. After completing this highly regarded, urban-oriented family practice residency program, Dr. Kahn established a rural practice in Hughson, California, population 2,940.

Dr. Kahn has been the director of both a community and a university-based family practice residency program. In addition, he directed a network of university-affiliated residency programs. He also served as assistant dean for the statewide Area Health Education Center (AHEC) in California. After five years in the Department of Family Medicine at the University of California, Davis, Dr. Kahn joined the national staff of the American Academy of Family Physicians as Director of the Division of Education, a position he held until April 1999 when he assumed the responsibilities of Vice President for Science and Education.

Kieren P. Knapp, DO, FACOFP
Family Physician
Past President, American College of Osteopathic Family Physicians
Jacobus, Pennsylvania 17407

Dr. Knapp is a private practice Family Physician and a Past President of the American College of Osteopathic Family Physicians. Graduating from Iowa State University with a BS in Zoology and a BS in Bacteriology, Dr. Knapp received his Doctor of Osteopathic Medicine degree from the College of Osteopathic Medicine and Surgery in Des Moines, Iowa.

After completing his training in Family Medicine at Memorial Osteopathic Hospital in York, Pennsylvania, he began a rural practice in Jacobus, Pennsylvania, where he still practices. Dr. Knapp served as chairman of the Department of Family Practice and as President of the staff at Memorial Hospital, and is Assistant Director of the Family Practice Residency Program there.

While on the ACOFP Board of Governors, Dr. Knapp served as the editor of *Osteopathic Family Practice News*, Treasurer, and finally President of ACOFP. Recently, Dr. Knapp has been appointed to the Medicare Coverage Advisory Committee of CMS.

Dr. Knapp and his wife, Jane, have been married since 1976, and reside on a small farm in southern Pennsylvania. They have two children, Jason and Kiera.

Melanie Susan Kraft, MD, MRO, AMEt
Faculty Physician, Baptist-Lutheran Family Medicine Residency Program
Kansas City, Missouri 64131

Dr. Susan Kraft has worked as a full-time faculty physician with Baptist Lutheran Medical Center since September 2003, but her association with the residency program began years earlier. After growing up in Tulsa, Oklahoma and attending medical school at the University of Texas Medical School in Houston, Dr. Kraft completed her medical residency at the Trinity Lutheran Family Practice Residency Program in 1996. She has been involved with the program as part-time faculty over the years, while practicing medicine in rural Kansas and Missouri, and consulting with physicians about the selection, implementation, and utilization of electronic medical records.

Dr. Kraft's professional interests include Sports Medicine, Occupational Medicine, Aviation Medicine, Medical Review of Drug Testing, Medical Informatics (Technology and Medicine), and Physician Leadership.

Dr. Kraft has co-authored numerous articles and monographs on use of computer systems in medicine, such as the 1999 and 2003 monographs entitled

"How to Select a Computer System for a Family Physician's Office" and the 2001 article entitled "Electronic Medical Records: The FPM vendor survey," which reported on 23 conventional patient record systems and five Internet-based systems.

Jeffrey B. Kramer, MD
Cardothoracic Surgeon
Kansas University Medical Center
3901 Rainbow Boulevard
Kansas City, Kansas 66160

Jeffrey B. Kramer, MD earned a Bachelor of Arts degree from Haverford College in 1976. He completed his Medical Education at Washington University School of Medicine in 1980. Dr. Kramer then went to Barnes Hospital where he completed his General Surgery Residency in 1988 and his Cardiothoracic Fellowship in 1990.

Dr. Kramer is currently pursuing a Masters degree in Business Administration (MBA) from the Health Care Leadership PMBA Program at Rockhurst University, while maintaining his full-time cardiothoracic surgery practice at the Kansas University Medical Center.

Dr. Kramer is a member of the Cardiothoracic Surgery Network and the Society of Thoracic Surgeons. He enjoys spending time with his wife and their two children.

Alma B. Littles, MD
Family Physician
Associate Dean of Academic Affairs
Florida State University
Tallahassee, Florida 32352

As Associate Dean for Academic Affairs, Dr. Littles is the chief academic officer of the FSU College of Medicine, with overall responsibility for overseeing the design, development, implementation, and evaluation of the four-year comprehensive curriculum leading to the MD degree.

A statewide and national leader in organized medicine, Dr. Littles came to FSU from Tallahassee Memorial Hospital, where she directed the Family Practice Residency Program. She has been involved in medical education since 1989, when she began precepting medical students and residents in her solo family practice in Quincy, Florida.

Dr. Littles joined the faculty of the Family Practice Residency Program at Tallahassee Memorial Healthcare in 1996, and became director in 1999. Former president of the Florida Academy of Family Physicians and 1993 Florida Family Physician of the Year, Dr. Littles is a longtime patient advocate.

Erich H. Loewy, MD
Internist and Bioethicist
Professor of Medicine (emeritus)
Founding Alumni Association Chair of Bioethics
Associate, Department of Philosophy
University of California, Davis 95817

Dr. Loewy is a recognized international expert in medical bioethics. He is author of the 1997 book *Moral Strangers, Moral Acquaintances and Moral Friends: connectedness and its conditions* and of the 1992 article "Healing and killing, harming and not harming: Physician participation in euthanasia and capital punishment," published in the *Journal of Clinical Ethics*.

Donald R. Lurye, MD, MMM
Family Physician
Chief Medical Officer
Welborn Clinic
Evansville, Indiana 47713

Donald R. Lurye, MD is the Chief Medical Officer for the Welborn Clinic – a large multi-specialty physician group, with nine locations and over 100 healthcare providers in 30 medical and surgical specialties and numerous ancillary services. He is currently involved in multiple quality improvement activities and in the implementation of an electronic medical record. He was previously Medical Director at Meridian Medical Group in Atlanta, Georgia and has practiced family medicine in several different settings.

Dr. Lurye completed his medical education at Tufts University School of Medicine in 1980, and completed his residency at the University of Maryland Hospital in Baltimore. He is board certified in Family Medicine. Dr. Lurye recently completed a Master of Medical Management degree at Carnegie Mellon University.

Bridgett M. McCandless, MD
Internist
Medical Director
Jackson County Free Health Clinic
Independence, Missouri 64050

Bridget McCandless, MD is board certified in Internal Medicine. In addition to maintaining an active practice in her role as Medical Director of the Jackson County Free Health Clinic, she has extensive experience in volunteer work, leading initiatives and advocating programs to address the unmet healthcare needs of those in her community.

Dr. McCandless was appointed in 2003 to serve on the Board of Directors of the Health Care Foundation of Greater Kansas City, Missouri. She co-chairs, along with Al Van Iten, a coalition launched in 2003 to reduce diabetes and other chronic diseases in her community. The coalition identifies ways local citizens can improve their health through nutritious eating, increased physical activity, and reduced tobacco consumption.

McCandless co-authored "A prospective, randomized, multi-centered controlled trial to compare the annual outcomes of patients with diabetes mellitus monitored with weekly fructosamine testing versus usual care: A 3-month interim analysis," which appeared in the October 2002 issue of *Diabetes Technology & Therapeutics* (Vol. 4, No.5, pages 637–642).

Deborah S. McPherson, MD, FAAFP
Family Physician
Associate Director, Family Medicine Residency Program
Kansas University Medical Center
Kansas City, Kansas 66160

Deborah S. McPherson, MD recently joined the KU Medical Center staff as Associate Director of the Family Medicine Residency Program. Previously, Dr. McPherson was the Assistant Director of Medical Education for the American Academy of Family Physicians (AAFP), while maintaining a part-time clinical practice in family medicine.

Dr. McPherson also served as a faculty member of the AAFP Chief Resident Leadership Development Program and held a faculty appointment at the University of Kansas School of Medicine. She has published numerous articles in medical education research, and has been a contributing author for several textbooks on family medicine.

Dr. McPherson completed her family practice residency at the University of Nebraska Medical Center in Omaha, Nebraska, where she also received her medical degree. As a resident, she served as a delegate to the AAFP Congress of Delegates and was the Resident Member of the AAFP Board of Directors.

Dr. McPherson is extensively involved in resident and student leadership development and frequently conducts workshops and presentations for medical schools and professional medical organizations across the county and internationally.

Gary B. Morsch, MD, MPH
Family and Emergency Medicine Physician
U.S. Army Military Reserves
Founder, Heart to Heart International, Physicians Who Care, and Priority Physician Placement
Bucyrus, Kansas 66013

Dr. Morsch was student body President in college and a Rhodes Scholar national finalist before the University of Oklahoma Medical School named him a MAP International/Reader's Digest Fellow to Africa. He earned a Master's Degree in Public Health at Loma Linda University and completed his Family Practice residency in 1984 at Florida Hospital in Orlando. He co-founded a family practice group, but left in 1993 to devote more time to an organization he founded that mobilizes volunteers and resources to address critical needs in the United States and around the world. That organization, Heart to Heart International, has personally delivered thousands of tons of medicine and supplies, valued at more than $360 million, to hospitals and clinics for the poor in over 100 countries. To support his humanitarian work, Dr. Morsch founded Docs Who Care, through which physicians provide family practice, emergency room and *locum tenens* staffing for rural hospitals in seven states.

He has been involved in many refugee feeding programs, healthcare training programs, and disaster response programs around the world. He has served on numerous corporate, community, and university boards, including the Johnson County Health Partnership non-profit clinic, the Lamb's Center, and Goodwill Global, Inc.

Dr. Morsch has received the Mead Johnson Award, the President's Volunteer Action Award, the Points of Light Community Leadership Award, the International Relations Council Community Service Award, the Salvation Army's Others Award, the American Academy of Family Physicians Humanitarian Award, the Washington Times Foundation's National Service Award, the Medical Missions Foundation Humanitarian Award, and the Cincinnatus Award.

His latest book, *Heart and Soul: awakening your passion to serve*, celebrates the awesome power of each individual to make a positive difference for humanity.

Gary and his wife Vickie reside in Kansas with their youngest son and enjoy frequent visits from their three daughters and sons-in-law.

Tim A. Munzing, MD
Family Physician
Director, Medical Education
Kaiser Permanente – Orange County
Santa Ana, California 92705

Dr. Munzing has been a family physician with Kaiser Permanente in Orange County, California for the past 19 years and currently is a past-President of the Orange County Academy of Family Physicians. For the last 15 years he has been the program director of the Kaiser Permanente Orange County Family Medicine Residency Program. He spent five years on the National Board of Directors of the Association of Family Medicine Residency Directors and chaired the Medical Student Resident Advisory Committee for the California Academy of Family Physicians.

Dr. Munzing maintains a busy clinical practice and for a decade was the medical director for primary services at Kaiser's 30-physician Tustin-Santa Ana Medical Office. He holds the appointment of Associate Clinical Professor at the University of California, Irvine College of Medicine.

Dr. Munzing has been an invited speaker at numerous venues, including the American Academy of Family Physicians Annual Scientific Assemblies, at an international conference on Family Medicine held in Cairo, Egypt, as the guest of the Egyptian Minister of Health, and in Tuscany, Italy.

His outside activities include travel, sports, information technology, and his son's sports and scouting activities.

John R. Musich, MD, MBA
Obstetrician and Gynecologist
Chair, Council for Resident Education in Obstetrics and Gynecology
Troy, Michigan 48098

John R. Musich, MD, MBA is a graduate of the University of Minnesota Medical School and the obstetrics and gynecology residency program at the University of Michigan, and obtained his MBA from Michigan State University.

He currently serves as the Corporate Director of Medical Education for the William Beaumont Hospital system, a two-hospital, 1,350-bed independent academic medical center in Royal Oak/Tory, Michigan. A recent 21–year Department of Obstetrics and Gynecology Chair and Residency Program Director at Beaumont, Dr. Musich has been involved in medical education and its administration at the undergraduate, graduate, and continuing medical education levels his entire professional career.

A former examiner for the American Board of Ob/Gyn and Chair of the Council for Resident Education in OB/Gyn, Dr. Musich is currently a member of the ACGME's Institutional Review Committee and ACOG's Executive Board.

His clinical practice is in the area of reproductive endocrinology and infertility, in which he has subspecialty certification.

Randall Oates, MD
Family Physician
President and CEO, Docs, Inc.
Springdale, Arkansas 72764

Randall Oates, MD has been a practicing Family Physician for more than 20 years. He started implementing information technologies in his practice in 1982. This project evolved into a software company that now delivers an electronic health record system to thousands of doctors.

Over the years, Dr. Oates has been involved with many initiatives to educate his peers and others who are involved in efforts to improve healthcare.

Elissa J. Palmer, MD, FAAFP
Family Physician
Director, Altoona Family Physicians Residency, Pregnancy Care Center and Women's Health and Wellness of Altoona Regional Health System
Altoona, Pensylvania 16601

Elissa J. Palmer, MD, FAAFP is the Director of the Altoona Family Physicians Residency, Pregnancy Care Center, and Women's Health and Wellness of Altoona Hospital in Pennsylvania. She serves on various Continuous Process Improvement Leadership Teams.

Dr. Palmer has been the Chair of the Pennsylvania Program Director's Association and a member of the Society of Teachers of Family Medicine Public Policy and Legislative Commission, in addition to being a Member-at-Large on the national board for the Association of Family Medicine Residency Directors, faculty on the Academic Council of the National Institute for Program Director Development, and advisory board member for several national genetics initiatives. She has lectured at state, national, and international meetings on primary care, genetics, leadership, and obstetrical care.

Dr. Palmer's practice experience includes private, hospital, and academic settings. She earned her MD from the Johns Hopkins University School of Medicine, followed by residency at the University of Wisconsin. Dr. Palmer completed the National Institute of Program Director Development Fellowship, and is board certified in Family Medicine.

John M. Pascoe, MD, MPH
Pediatrician
Professor of Pediatrics and Chief, General and Community Pediatrics
Wright State University School of Medicine (WSUSOM)
Dayton, Ohio 45404

John M. Pascoe, MD, MPH is Professor of Pediatrics and Chief, General and Community Pediatrics at Wright State University School of Medicine (WSUSOM), Dayton, Ohio.

Dr. Pascoe received his medical degree from the University of Michigan and a Master in Public Health (Maternal and Child Health) from the University of North Carolina at Chapel Hill, where he was a Robert Wood Johnson Clinical Scholar. Dr. Pascoe has been appointed to the pediatric faculty at Michigan State University and the University of Wisconsin-Madison before joining the faculty at WSUSOM in 2000.

Dr. Pascoe's research has focused on the impact of mothers' social support and depressive symptoms on their children's health.

He was a member of the national Executive Committee for the HRSA-funded national medical education project, Undergraduate Medical Education for the 21st Century (UME-21).

Ronald N. Riner, MD
Cardiologist
President, The Riner Group
St. Louis, Missouri 63117

Dr. Riner is President of his own consulting firm which he began in 1980. The firm serves as advisors and consultants to medical practices, hospitals, academic medical centers, health systems, and professional medical associations throughout the United States. The company focuses on strategy and business development, as well as performance improvement, with particular expertise in the interface of the business community with those providing healthcare services, or developing new methods of delivery health services.

Dr. Riner has served as a member of the executive management team of one of the largest healthcare systems in the United States, and is the editor for the Practice Management and Economics Section of the *Journal of Invasive Cardiology*, which has a domestic and international readership.

A graduate of Princeton University, Dr. Riner attended Cornell University Medical College, and performed his internship and residency training at the New York Hospital/Memorial Sloan-Kettering Cancer Center. He undertook his specialty training in cardiovascular diseases at the Mayo Clinic in Rochester, Minnesota. Dr. Riner has received formal business education at the Olin School of Business at Washington University, Kellogg School of Business in Chicago, Babson University in Boston, and Harvard University in Boston.

Dr. Riner is a Fellow of the Institute for Advanced Study on International Business Development at Washington University. He is a former Program Director and Chairman of a Department of Medicine, and had over 15 years of private medical practice experience before devoting himself entirely to the business of medicine.

Burton N. Routman, DO, FACOFP
Family Physician
Professor of Family Medicine
Western University of Health Sciences College of Osteopathic Medicine of the Pacific
RCH Cucamonga, California 91730

Burt Routman, DO, FACOFP is currently Professor of Family Medicine at the College of Osteopathic Medicine of the Pacific at Western University of Health Sciences. He received his BA degree from The Johns Hopkins University, and his DO degree from Des Moines University, College of Osteopathic Medicine.

Dr. Routman has been in academic medicine for 25 years, and has been on the faculty of Des Moines University, College of Osteopathic Medicine and Ben Gurion University of the Negev in Beer Sheva, Israel.

Dr. Routman represents the American College of Osteopathic Family Physicians on the Primary Care Organizations' Consortium.

Daniel Z. Sands, MD, MPH
General Internist
Beth Israel Deaconess Medical Center
Assistant Professor of Medicine, Harvard Medical School
Chief Medical Officer and Vice President, Clinical Strategies, Zix Corporation
Boston, Massachusetts 02215

Dr. Sands is a Fellow of the American College of Medical Informatics. During the 1990s, Dr. Sands led the development and dissemination of the first widely-adopted guidelines for electronic physician–patient communications.

Dr. Sands received the President's Award from the American Medical Informatics Association in 1998, and is a recipient of the Information Technology Innovator Award from *Healthcare Informatics Magazine*. He currently serves on the Board of Directors of the American Medical Informatics Association.

Dr. Sands recently joined Zix Corporation as Chief Medical Officer and Vice President of Clinical Strategies, while continuing his faculty appointment as an Assistant Professor of Medicine for Harvard Medical School.

Dr. Sands provides clinical care for patients through his General Internal Medicine practice at Beth Israel Deaconess Medical Center.

Andrew M. Schwartz, MS, MD
Cardiothoracic Surgeon and Vice President, Medical Staff Services
Shawnee Mission Medical Center
Shawnee Mission, Kansas 66204

Andrew M. Schwartz, MS, MD is a native of Long Island, New York. Dr. Schwartz received his undergraduate education in The City University of New York. He earned his Masters of Science degree in Physiology and his Doctor of Medicine degree from Georgetown University.

After seven years of surgical training, Dr. Schwartz fulfilled his dream by entering into the practice of cardiothoracic surgery. Kansas is now his home. During his journey, Dr. Schwartz met a wonderful woman, Janet, whom he married. He believes that his wife and their two children are truly the most precious gifts given to him by God.

Dr. Schwartz says his time is well spent with family, friends, sports, his Judaic faith, and in his roles as a physician and a member of his organization's medical staff leadership.

Michael J. Scotti, Jr., MD
Family Physician
Retired Vice President for Medical Education and Senior Vice President for Professional Issues, American Medical Association
2540 North Randolph Street
Arlington, Virginia 22207

Michael J. Scotti, Jr., MD was born in New York City and educated in the public schools, Fordham College, and Georgetown University School of Medicine, where he graduated cum laude.

Dr. Scotti joined the U.S. Army during medical school. During the next three years, he rotated as an intern, ran an emergency room and served in Viet Nam as a Battalion Surgeon and Medical Company Commander. Dr. Scotti completed his residency in Internal Medicine and was grandfathered into Family Medicine. Over the next 30 years, Dr. Scotti's assignments with the U.S. Army included leadership of a Family Practice Residency Program, and the Army's graduate medical education program, Chief of Quality Assurance, Hospital Commander, Chief of the Medical Corps, and Commander of Army medicine in Europe during the first Gulf War. He retired from the Army as a major general.

Dr. Scotti was subsequently employed by the American Medical Association as Vice President for Medical Education and Senior Vice President for Professional Issues. He retired from the AMA in 2004.

Kevin J. Soden, MD, MPH, MPA
Emergency Medicine Physician
Medical Correspondent, NBC News
Soden Consulting Services
2510 Danbury Street
Charlotte, North Carolina 28211

Kevin J. Soden, MD, MPH, MPA is a national Medical Correspondent for NBC and is seen regularly on NBC's *Today Show.* He received the National Award for

Excellence in Medical Reporting from the National Association of Medical Communicators and was a Finalist for the prestigious International Freddie Award in 2001. He wrote *The Art of Medicine: what every doctor and patient should know* – the critically acclaimed text on doctor–patient communications, and was the primary author of *Special Treatment: how to get the special care your doctor gets.* He is the worldwide Medical Director for Texas Instruments and the Celanese Corporation.

Dr. Soden served 23 years in emergency medicine and is the founder of the oldest, largest physician-owned managed care organization in the Carolinas. He has spoken to organizations and companies all over the country, and his clients include numerous Fortune 500 companies.

Dr. Soden graduated from the University of Florida, College of Medicine, and received a Masters in Public Health from the Medical College of Wisconsin and a Masters in Personnel Administration from Florida State University.

His biggest successes are his five children. He is married to Dr. Meg Humphrey and they live happily and relatively stress-free in Charlotte, North Carolina.

Jeannette E. South-Paul, MD
Family Physician
Chair, Department of Family Medicine
University of Pittsburgh School of Medicine
Pittsburgh, Pennsylvania 15213

Jeanette E. South-Paul, MD became Professor and Chair of the Department of Family Medicine at the University of Pittsburgh, School of Medicine in July 2001, upon retiring from the U.S. Army after 22 years of active service.

During her 15 years at the Uniformed Services University of the Health Sciences in Bethesda, Maryland, Dr. South-Paul served as Vice President for Minority Affairs for five years and as Chair of Family Medicine for six years. She also serves as Medical Director of the Division of Community Health Services of the UPMC.

Dr. South-Paul maintains an active clinical practice, including maternity care. She is involved in clinical teaching and does research in culture competence. She currently serves on the WONCA Scientific Programs Committee of the Public Health of the American Academy of Family Physicians (AAFP) and is Senior Advisor for the AAFP Quality Care for Diverse Populations project that recently launched a new cultural competence video teaching module. She is Chair of the Association of American Medical Colleges (AAMC) Advisory Committee for Development of a Cultural Competence Curriculum.

Dr. South-Paul was recently installed as President of the Society of Teachers of Family Medicine, the academic organization of more than 5,000 medicine educators across the nation.

Penny Tenzer, MD
Family Physician
Vice Chair, Department of Family Medicine and Community Health
Director, Family Medicine Residency Program
University of Miami School of Medicine
Miami, Florida 33101

Penny Tenzer, MD is Associate Professor, Vice Chair, Director of the Residency Program, and Director of Continuing Medical Education for the Department of Family Medicine and Community Health at the University of Miami School of Medicine in Miami, Florida. She is an Attending Physician in the Department of Family Medicine at Jackson Memorial Hospital.

Dr. Tenzer was named the American Academy of Family Physicians 2003 Full Time Exemplary Teacher of the Year and received the 2003 Exemplary Educator Award from the Florida Academy of Family Physicians. She received the Golden Apple Teaching Award twice and is a recipient of the Illinois Academy of Family Physicians "President's Award." Florida Monthly Magazine June 2004 named Dr. Tenzer one of Florida's Best Doctors. In 2001, Miami Metro Magazine recognized her as one of "Miami Dade's Most Influential Females." Dr. Tenzer has served as an author and editor for a variety of journals and book publications such as *Clinics of North America*.

She has served as a member of the board of directors of the Association of Family Medicine Residency. In June 2004 Dr. Tenzer was elected to the position of President Elect of the AFMRD and assumes the Presidency in June 2005.

Nikitas J. Zervanos, MD
Family Physician
Semi-Retired Director Emeritus, Family Practice Residency Program
Lancaster General Hospital
Lancaster, Pennsylvania 17603

Nikitas J. Zervanos, MD is the semi-retired Director Emeritus of the Family Practice Residency Program at Lancaster General Hospital in Lancaster, Pennsylvania. He served as its Founder and Director from 1969 to 2002. Dr. Zervanos is a 1962 graduate of the University of Pennsylvania, School of Medicine, where each year a medical student with promise as a leader in family practice is selected for the Annual Family Practice Award named in his honor.

Dr. Zervanos has been recognized for his leadership in family practice with the Certificate of Excellence from the Society of Teachers of Family Medicine. He has also been recognized by the Pennsylvania Academy of Family Physicians, for which the annual Student Interest Award is named in his honor, and by the American Academy of Family Physicians with both the Thomas Johnson Award and the John Walsh Award. Dr. Zervanos was the first recipient of the Outstanding Program Director Award given by the Association of Family Practice Residency Directors, which is now named in his honor. He was among the first recipients of the Accreditation Council on Graduate Medical Education's Parker Palmer Courage to Teach Award.

On a part-time basis, Dr. Zervanos continues to care for patients through his small Greek-immigrant practice. He teaches physical diagnosis to third year medical students and precepts his residents, and serves as Director of the TU/LGH Semi-annual Family Practice Review.

Index